Gordon W. Russell

The
Social Psychology
of Sport

With 20 Figures

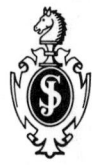

Springer-Verlag

New York Berlin Heidelberg London Paris
Tokyo Hong Kong Barcelona Budapest

Gordon W. Russell
Department of Psychology
University of Lethbridge
Lethbridge, Alberta
Canada T1K 3M4

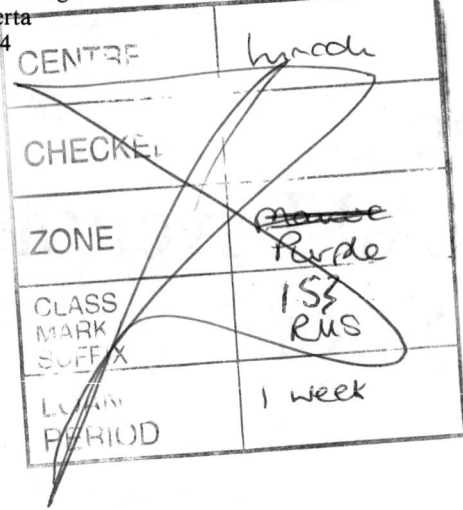

Library of Congress Cataloging-in-Publication Data
Russell, Gordon W., 1931–
    The social psychology of sport/Gordon W. Russell.
    p. cm.
    Includes bibliographical references (p.) and indexes.
    ISBN 0-387-97792-9. – ISBN 3-540-97792-9
    1. Sports – Psychological aspects. 2. Social psychology.
    I. Title.
    GV706.4.R87   1993
    796'.01 – dc20   92-34893

Printed on acid-free paper.

Production managed by Francine McNeill; manufacturing supervised by Gail Simon.
Camera-ready copy prepared using WriteNow.
Printed and bound by Edwards Brothers, Inc., Ann Arbor, MI.
Printed in the United States of America.

9 8 7 6 5 4 3 2 (Second corrected printing)

ISBN 0-387-97792-9 Springer-Verlag New York Berlin Heidelberg
ISBN 3-540-97792-9 Springer-Verlag Berlin Heidelberg New York

£36·50 ·

704800 ·

796·01

The Social Psychology of Sport

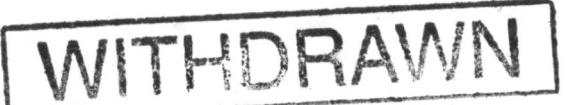

To Audrey and to the Memory of my Parents

Preface

This book is written from the perspective of a social psychologist. As a consequence, the topics covered in the upcoming chapters were chosen from among those traditionally of interest to the discipline of social psychology. A criterion for inclusion was the topic's usefulness in providing insights and/or understanding of the social processes at work in sports settings. To this end, I have drawn extensively from mainstream journals in social psychology (e.g., *Journal of Personality and Social Psychology*), and grounded the discussion of topics and issues on the methodologically sound studies/experiments they generally provide. There is also an equally strong interdisciplinary emphasis that features research from physical education, sociology, management science, and education. I have made a further attempt, not as successful as I would have liked, to incorporate a substantial amount of the fine sports research that has been conducted overseas, particularly in Europe and Australia. I am hopeful that in bringing together the works of international scholars from a variety of disciplines a clearer and balanced outline of this field will take shape.

And now a word about the audience for this text and how to get the most from its pages. I would suggest that the reader have taken a course in social psychology following an introductory-level course. An introductory course in research methodology would also be helpful. As regards statistics, I have provided a brief review of the correlational method that underlies many of the findings reported on the pages to follow. You may wish to leap ahead to the section in Chapter 7 entitled "A Crash Course on Correlation" (pp. 163–164). In short, the more background the students have along the lines of these courses, the more they can expect to derive from the book and the references they are encouraged to pursue. Of course, senior undergraduates and graduate students in the social sciences, the best prepared of all, stand to benefit the most and, indeed, were my focus in writing this text.

Next, a few words about the overall organization of this book. The first six chapters deal with topics that have a direct or indirect bearing on athletic performance. Thereafter, questions related to interpersonal and collective aggression begin to receive more attention. The basic data and theory of social psychology are woven throughout the development of these themes. The opening chapter begins with a review of several of the leading theories of motivation that provide some understanding of the bases for our initial choice and persistence in a sport. A number of the major theories or models having implication specifically for athletic performance are described against the background of sports research in Chapters 2 and 3. Chapters 4 to 6 examine our behaviors in groups and the influence that leaders and those who serve as exemplars have on our activities. The themes of performance and aggression are bridged by Chapter 7, on personality. The remaining chapters deal with one of the more troubling aspects of sport, interpersonal aggression. Chapter 8 provides an overview of the topic of aggression in considering its measurement, theoretical views, and basic findings derived from sports settings. The popular belief in catharsis (i.e., that sports serve as a "safety valve" for pent-up aggressive urges) is reviewed in Chapter 9, both with respect to its historical origins and the evidence that bears on the validity of the concept. In the concluding chapter, sports crowds are examined in regard to their composition and behavior at sports events, in particular, their behavior on those occasions when collective actions (e.g., panics, riots) have tragic consequences.

While I am reluctant to burden you with matters of definition, my overly generous use of the term *sports* should be acknowledged at the outset. Although several theorists have undertaken the formidable task of providing a formal definition of sports (e.g., Loy, McPherson, & Kenyon, 1978), I have chosen instead to throw a wider-than-usual net in my selection of studies, one that encompasses the likes of professional wrestling, aerobatic flying, cheerleading, nail hammering, chess, and horse racing. Admittedly, some of these would be better described as entertainment, games, or leisure activities rather than as sport.

The organization of this book includes three special features, the first of which is intended to offer an occasional diversion. Most chapters contain one or more boxes entitled "Speaking Tangentially." These showcase intriguing research findings that are an offshoot of the topic being discussed on nearby pages. It is my hope that they will challenge a number of your assumptions and/or sufficiently pique your interest to pursue the issues they raise.

The second feature is an index of sports mentioned throughout the text. The listing is restricted to those sports that researchers used in a substantive way as the setting for their studies. While it is always interesting to see the ways in which our favorite sport(s) has (have) contributed to research, it is additionally interesting to note how certain sports, because of their structure or the sorts of people they attract, have provided ideal opportunities for testing sports-related theory.

The third feature is a selection of suggested readings that appears at the end of each chapter. Entries have been carefully chosen to represent state-of-the-art reviews of a topic or to introduce several thought-provoking works and to provide examples of the best in investigative techniques.

Writing a text is anything but a solo undertaking. Others offer suggestions, give criticism, and bring obscure references to an author's attention. All of this help plays a major part in shaping the final form of a manuscript. My greatest debt is to the legions of colleagues in the social sciences whose fine work I have been privileged to cite. Their work has formed the foundation for this book and has allowed me to provide the reader with more facts and fewer speculations than might otherwise have been the case. Also important is the ongoing feedback I have received from students over a period of several years. Their detailed knowledge of contemporary sports has kept me in constant touch with the real world of sports. Incidentally, let me say that I am a good listener. I would welcome and be pleased to reply to any comments, suggestions, or criticisms that you would care to bring to my attention.

I wish also to single out a number of friends and colleagues for special thanks for their willingness to review individual chapters of the manuscript. In this regard, I am grateful to Robert Barney, Ivan Kelly, Chris Knapper, Professor Whimsy, and Neil Widmeyer. Others undertook even more extensive critiques that covered major portions of the book. I am deeply indebted to Susan Butt, Peter Mudrack, Raymond Novaco, and Garry Smith for the Herculean efforts on my behalf.

The final tip of my cap is to my wife, Audrey, and our children, Shelley and Cameron, for their continuing support and encouragement. Their patience with my Type A behaviors exceeded what I had any right to expect.

Lethbridge, Alberta, Canada   Gordon W. Russell

Contents

1

Motivation: The Why of Behavior

It seems only logical to open the topic of sports psychology with an overview of several theoretical views that have addressed that most fundamental and intriguing question: What causes us to behave as we do? Literally volumes have been written on *motivation*, a term that applies to a wide range of problems and that has been of central interest to a variety of disciplines, for example, comparative psychology, learning theory, industrial organizational psychology, and psychiatry. However, our coverage of motivation will necessarily be highly selective and restricted to those theoretical perspectives that have direct relevance and application to sporting activities. As with all of the upcoming chapters, motivational models and the predictions they provide will be illustrated and evaluated, wherever possible, in the context of studies conducted in sports.

But first the reader should bear in mind that our attempts to identify motives, either informally as observers or more formally as researchers, must rely ultimately on the inferences we draw. For example, why has Arthur chosen to dedicate himself to high jumping when he has shown equal if not greater promise in a number of other sports? Several pieces of information might guide us in reaching a conclusion about his choice of sport. Arthur is known to have a fondness for wildlife, especially birds, and dreams of pursuing a career in ornithology. He also comes from a family with limited financial means. Most of us would be drawn to the conclusion that his choice of sport was motivated by the prospect of a track and field scholarship. Arthur himself may describe his reason for concentrating on the high jump in much the same way. Again, both we as outside observers of his circumstances and Arthur's own self-report involve inferences regarding his motivation.

However, we could both be wrong. It is always possible that other motives, operating consciously or unconsciously, may be directing Arthur's efforts. He may simply derive more personal satisfaction from high jumping than from the other sports in which he has participated. Or Arthur may be secretly hoping to win the heart of a girl who he knows is a fan of the event.

Even though the motives of others may seem terribly obvious to everyone concerned, the interpretations of outside observers may still miss the mark. The most convincing illustration of this point is seen in a study of the motivations that underlay the heroic acts of Christians in rescuing Jews from the Nazis in World War II. Many men and women risked, and indeed many lost, their lives in hiding Jews during the German occupation of their homelands. Could any of us doubt for a moment that these deeds were an expression of strong altruistic and/or patriotic motives? Postwar interviews with these people suggest something quite different (London, 1970). Surprisingly, the principal motive for their involvement proved to be a zest for the excitement and danger associated with their rescue efforts.

Before we proceed too far with a discussion of motivation, let us be clear as to its meaning. There are two distinct processes that need to be recognized and addressed by a theory of motivation. First, the emergence of needs, innate in origin or arising through individuals interacting with their environment, serves an *energizing* function. Second, motivational theory must account for the particular *directions* individuals pursue in attempts to satisfy their needs. It is not enough simply to describe the processes by which the person is prompted to take action. Rather, the motivated state must additionally be described in terms of the individual being energized with respect to a specific purpose or directed toward some goal (Deci & Ryan, 1985). Let's assume for the sake of argument that our original inference about the reason for Arthur's dedication to high jumping was correct. Not only is he expending great effort in following a demanding training regimen, but he undertakes it with a particular goal in mind, that of earning a college scholarship. These underlying directional and energizing components of motivation are brought together in a definition of *motivation* proposed by Baron (1983): "a set of processes concerned with the force that energizes behavior and directs it toward attaining some goal" (p. 123).

An understanding of the dynamics of motivation can bring us closer to answers to a variety of questions surrounding sports activities. What, for example, prompts some people to take up a sports activity in the first instance, whereas others painstakingly avoid any such involvement? Why do some persist at an activity, whereas others fall by the wayside? What prompts the choice of one particular sport from among all those that are available to us?

The answers to these questions can have important and far-reaching social implications. For example, public health authorities periodically launch various fitness programs as a preventive health measure. An understanding of motivational processes should enable them to maximize the impact of their promotional campaigns by reaching and involving many of those who might otherwise be reluctant to participate. Questions such as these will be touched on in the course of this chapter.

The upcoming discussion of selected motivational models will follow a rough chronological order, starting with Abraham Maslow's need hierarchy. Near the end of the chapter, this pattern will be broken and we will turn to consider several views that attempt to account for the special attraction that high-risk sports hold for some people. But now let us consider the first of the major theoretical viewpoints that have addressed the question of human motivation.

The Need Hierarchy Theory

The starting point for our discussion of motivational theory begins with Maslow's (1968) need hierarchy. Maslow's model is important for both historical and heuristic reasons, as well as for its wide intuitive appeal. His theory proposes that people seek the satisfaction of a set of needs. However, these needs are arranged in a hierarchy such that the gratification of lower needs must be attained before one can move upward and strive to meet higher placed needs. The lower and more basic *deficiency* needs include physiological requirements such as air, food, water, and sex. Moving upward in the hierarchy, the individual next seeks the satisfaction of "safety" needs, that is, a work or play environment that is safe and free from physical or psychological threats. The most highly placed of the deficiency needs are "social" in character. This category includes the need for friendships and a sense of belonging to a social group.

The second, more highly placed, category includes two basic *growth* needs, namely, "esteem" needs and "self-actualization" needs. Esteem needs are met as the individual draws respect from others and is able to gain a measure of pride from his or her efforts. The highest level in Maslow's hierarchical ordering of needs is self-actualization. Attempts to satisfy this need involve individuals in efforts to make maximum use of whatever native talents they might possess. Self-actualization is realized as people develop a sense of who they are and their place in the grand scheme of things.

As mentioned earlier, Maslow saw individuals striving to fulfill needs on only one level at a time. Only when lower needs have been satisfied do needs at the next highest level come into play. For example, a miner threatened with the possibility of the roof of the shaft collapsing can scarcely afford the luxury of striving to fulfill belongingness needs. His immediate and overriding concern is for a safe working environment. More lofty needs must await the satisfaction of basic considerations. It also follows from the model that only a small fraction of the world's population can address growth needs. By and large, it is the affluent and privileged few who have the option of pursuing the satisfaction of esteem or self-actualization needs; others are engaged in a day-to-day struggle to fulfill deficiency needs.

Any good theory of human behavior produces testable predictions. It is, of course, the results of those empirical tests that either provide support for or detract from the adequacy of a theory. A review of the research conducted on the need hierarchy theory reveals very little support for its major tenets (Wahba & Birdwell, 1976). There is neither evidence of the five basic and discrete categories of need proposed by Maslow nor support for the upward sequential progression of individuals in their quest to fulfill activated needs. Fortunately, a more tenable compromise theory is at hand.

ERG Theory

Particular note should be taken of Alderfer's (1972) ERG theory inasmuch as it represents a refinement and simplification of Maslow's views. Alderfer recognizes three basic categories of needs: existence, relatedness and growth needs (hence, ERG). Each category has its counterpart in Maslow's need hierarchy theory, but there are three rather than five basic needs. For instance, physiological and safety needs are combined under existence needs. This reformulation of Maslow's theory offers us a simplified version of the structure of human needs, one more consistent with research findings.

Other features of the ERG model also recommend themselves. There is no restriction that the individual can seek to satisfy only one need at a time. For example, a person may pursue the fulfillment of friendship needs (relatedness) simultaneously with efforts to more fully develop his or her potential (growth needs). It follows, therefore, that Alderfer (1972) does not impose a requirement that needs at one level be satisfied before one activates needs at the next level in the hierarchy.

Measures have additionally been developed (Alderfer, 1972) to assess both the satisfactions that people are currently deriving from their day-to-day activities and their desire for particular satisfactions in the future. One's satisfaction with one's present circumstances is indicated by the extent of one's agreement or disagreement with an item such as "The major satisfaction in my life comes from my work." What Alderfer describes as relatively stable, *chronic* desires are measured by the priority that respondents assign, for example, to "opportunities to learn new things." *Episodic* desires are those that fluctuate with changing events and are rated in regard to their importance to the subject and his or her desire, for example, for "having a sense of security." All in all, Alderfer's ERG theory and means of assessing satisfactions represents an extension of Maslow's work that is both simpler and more compatible with the results of studies on the topic.

Although Maslow and Alderfer acknowledge the importance of sex needs in their motivational models, sexual motivation has been largely overlooked as an instructional and research topic by physical educators and those involved in recreational research. Susan Butt (1990) highlights the relevance of the subject and the implications for health and fitness in Speaking Tangentially 1.1.

Need for Achievement ("*n*" Ach.)

The theory of achievement motivation is rooted in an extensive research program dating at least as far back as the early 1950s (e.g., Atkinson, 1958; Atkinson & Feather, 1966; McClelland, 1953, 1987; McClelland, Atkinson, Clark, & Lowell, 1953). Building on earlier work on needs theory (Murray, 1938), David McClelland, John Atkinson, and others have developed a comprehensive motivational model that has explanatory value for understanding the strivings of some athletes. I stress *some* athletes to emphasize the fact that people participate or persist in sports for a variety of reasons. Need for achievement ("*n*" Ach.) is only one of a number of motivational systems that have been developed to account for the activities or directions that people pursue. Other motives may also be operating. For example, Winter (1973) has shown that students who lettered in varsity sports were higher in "*n*" Power than their classmates. Others, then, may participate in sporting activities on the basis of entirely different motives, for example, need for affiliation ("*n*" Aff.) or sensation seeking.

A clearer understanding of achievement-motivated individuals hopefully will emerge from a sketch of the situations that favor their activities, as well as some of the characteristics of high achievers themselves. It is to those situations and characteristics that we now turn.

****

Speaking Tangentially 1.1: Sex as Exercise
Based on an authoritative review of animal and physiological findings, Butt advances the reasonable proposition that the sexual response can be viewed as a form of exercise. She draws a compelling parallel between the associations of well-being and longevity with exercise and similar benefits to be realized from regular sexual activity. Sports practitioners specializing in fitness, physiology of exercise, and physical education are urged to incorporate the study of sexual behavior in their sphere of interest. As Butt concludes, sexual activity in long-term, mature relationships can represent "forms of competence expression, sport, enjoyment, and fun" (p. 341). Furthermore, contrary to locker-room lore, sexual activity in moderation prior to a competition is unlikely to have any adverse effects; in some instances, athletic performance may instead be enhanced.

****

Profile of the High "n" Ach. Individual

Among the situational characteristics that are preferred by those high in "n" Ach. is the availability of feedback on the success of their efforts. This preference for regular evaluative information on how well one is doing limits the number of situations that are attractive for the expression of achievement motives. For example, counselors of various sorts may labor long and hard in the interests of their clients yet receive little or no tangible feedback on the success of their efforts. Such feedback as they do receive may not materialize for months, perhaps years. Many of those in counseling and similar occupations where feedback is uncertain also strive for excellence in their profession but do so largely on the basis of other motivational systems. On the other hand, the world of commerce/business provides the entrepreneur or salesperson with yearly, monthly, weekly, or perhaps daily tallies of how well he or she has done (e.g., profit and loss statements, sales figures, etc.). Performance measures are similarly available at regular intervals to athletes, both when they enter into competitions and during practice or training sessions. Sports, then, by this standard at least, provide a sphere of activity that may hold a strong appeal for those motivated by a need for achievement.

A second situational characteristic important to high achievers is the degree of risk of failure in the task. High "n" Ach. individuals prefer to take on reasonable challenges where the likelihood of success is intermediate. As a 10-handicap golfer, they would not relish a match with a duffer, nor would they care to play against the club professional. Either way, there is little challenge when the outcome is a virtual certainty.

This preference for moderately risky activities on the part of those high in "n" Ach. is seen in two early experiments (McClelland, 1958; Roberts, 1974). In the first of these, children were invited to play a ring-toss game and to stand at a distance of their own choosing. Those low in "n" Ach. tended to adopt one of two strategies. They chose either to stand at a considerable distance from the peg where they had little hope of success or to stand alongside the peg where complete success was all but assured. In marked contrast, those children high in achievement motivation set themselves an interesting challenge by taking up a position midway between the extremes, a position that guaranteed neither success nor failure.

Glyn Roberts (1974) examined this risk-taking hypothesis using an improved experimental design that, among other things, took individual differences in subjects' skill level into account. Risk-taking research typically considers the tendency to avoid failure (e.g., French, 1958) in addition to the need to achieve success. Using a modified shuffleboard game, Roberts found that those high in achievement motivation displayed a greater preference for intermediate distances than subjects highly motivated to avoid failure. Subjects tending to avoid failure preferred the high-risk distances. From their perspective, there is no disgrace in failing at a nearly impossible task; there is also little likelihood of failure at the closer distances.

Perhaps more to the point, challenges that contain a moderate chance of failure tell us a great deal about our abilities. Little is to be learned from a task at which nearly everyone succeeds; nor is there much to be learned from a task at which almost everyone fails. The individual is provided with the greatest amount of information about his or her abilities in attempting tasks of moderate difficulty. It appears that this *diagnostic* feature of moderately difficult tasks holds a special attraction for the achievement-oriented person (Trope, 1980).

Foremost among other characteristics of individuals with high "*n*" Ach. is that their satisfactions are derived from successfully completing the challenge they undertook and have less to do with any external rewards that may follow. Although success in most fields of endeavor brings its share of rewards (e.g., recognition, promotion, trophies), these are secondary in importance. It is success against an internal standard that provides satisfaction for those high in achievement motivation. Their concern is less with demonstrating their superiority over others than with attaining their own standards of performance. It is success in competing against some internal standard of excellence that provides satisfaction. In this regard, the increased professionalism of many sports has likely made them less and less attractive as settings for the expression of achievement motivation. The acclaim, the medals, and the prizes that are showered on those athletes who do well may work against their improving their performance or even remaining in the sport. For achievement-motivated individuals, the imposition of external rewards and standards against which their performance is judged may erode the very motivational basis that originally brought them to their present level of skill.

Turning to the question of success in competition, it appears that high "*n*" Ach. goes hand in hand with better performances (e.g., Ostrow, 1976). When a neutral task is made competitive, subjects high in achievement motivation show greater improvement following the change than do their low "*n*" Ach. counterparts (Ryan & Lakie, 1965). At the same time, subjects who exhibit a *combination* of high "*n*" Ach. and low anxiety show greater improvement following a change from neutral to competitive task instructions than do low "*n*" Ach./high-anxiety subjects. (High anxiety is presumed to represent a motive to avoid failure.) Achievement motivation in combination with anxiety, then, provides an even stronger prediction of competitive success.

Other characteristics of the high "*n*" Ach. person include a preference for working with a competent "stranger" rather than a friend. This preference applies only in the situation where the stranger possesses skills that can be applied to the successful completion of a task (French, 1956). Finally, high "*n*" Ach. people are better able to delay gratification (Mischel, 1961). Schoolchildren high in achievement motivation generally declined to accept a small chocolate bar given assurance that Mischel would return in a week with a much larger bar. Low "*n*" Ach. children took what was immediately available.

How Is "*n*" Ach. Measured?

Achievement motivation has traditionally been assessed by a projective measure, the Thematic Apperception Test (TAT). Originally developed by Murray (1938), the test calls for the subject to provide a story in response to vague, unstructured scenes depicted on a series of cards. Only a subset of the TAT cards is used to assess need for achievement. The stories or protocols are then scored for achievement imagery by judges specifically trained for the task. The scoring procedures are somewhat complex (McClelland, 1953), and extensive training is required on the part of those using the test. Generally, when the trainee can consistently demonstrate a very high degree of agreement with a qualified tester (i.e., high interscorer reliability), the trainee is judged to have sufficient skills to score the measure.

The means to assess need for achievement have since been extended to researchers lacking expertise with projective measures through the development of several inventories (e.g., Helmreich & Spence, 1978; Mehrabian, 1968). A sample item from Mehrabian's scale is "I think I love winning more than I hate losing." (Agreement is scored as high achievement.) To this point, nearly all investigations of achievement motivation in sports have used objective paper-and-pencil tests.

The Origins of Achievement Motivation

An important question for any motivational model concerns the conditions and social influences that foster the development of the "motivated" individual. In the present case, our focus is on the individual high in "*n*" Ach. Although there is a host of influences impinging on the developing youngster in the process of becoming socialized, several factors in particular stand out as major contributors to the development of achievement motivation. Among the influences shaping high need for achievement is early independence training. Mothers of high "*n*" Ach. children think it important that early on their youngsters "go it alone" in many of their activities. These mothers want their children to "stick up for their rights," "to know their own way around the community," and "to do well in competition" (Winterbottom, 1958).

Another likely influence on need for achievement is to be found in the response of mothers to the successful accomplishments of their children. While mothers of both high- and low-achieving sons use positive sanctions to reward accomplishments and negative sanctions in the case of setbacks, there is a subtle but crucial difference in their manner of expressing their approval. The same moms that stress early independence characteristically greet their sons' successes with a warm embrace and kisses. Moms of low-achieving sons are physically less effusive (Rosen & D'Andrade, 1959; Winterbottom, 1958).

Rosen and D'Andrade (1959) additionally observed the behaviors of parents while their sons built a tower of blocks blindfolded and with only one hand. Told that the average child can build an eight-block tower, parents of high "n" Ach. boys predicted that their sons would build higher towers than did parents of boys known to be low in "n" Ach. In other words, they expressed higher levels of aspiration for their sons.

Parents of high- and low-achieving sons differed in yet another way while observing the efforts of their youngster. The fathers of low-scoring boys essentially took charge of the situation. They made decisions, gave directions, and expressed their irritation when things went badly. The suggestion is clear: Dictatorial or controlling fathers are likely raising sons to be low in achievement motivation.

And Females?

Throughout the preceding section, I have made repeated and exclusive references to achievement motivation in males. Females have not been mentioned. The fact is that the early research literature on "n" Ach. focused almost exclusively on males with a view to predicting success in male-dominated domains (e.g., business, academia). It would, however, be misleading for me to leave you with the impression that the traditional projective measure is equally valid for women or that research with female subjects has produced similar findings. Serious doubts have been raised on both points.

Virginia O'Leary (1974) has reviewed the achievement literature in the context of identifying a number of attitudinal barriers facing women who aspire to higher occupational positions (e.g., fear of failure, role conflict, and sex-role stereotyping). With regard specifically to the assessment of achievement motivation, she observes that it involves "a projective technique subject to the vagaries of a scoring system developed on male data collected in response to male competitive cues" (pp. 819–820). She further notes that one can strive for excellence other than in the context of the masculine competitive model. For example, O'Leary suggests that many women seek to attain purely social goals, a context in which interpersonal skills are effective and facilitate success. For these women, then, affiliative needs ("n" Aff.)—assessed by alternative measurement procedures—may instead be a reflection of achievement motivation. This is not to say that females are not motivated to achieve excellence in their endeavors but that many do so on the basis of a motivational system(s) other than achievement motivation.

O'Leary (1974) also has critically evaluated the theoretical model used to quantify one's motivation to achieve. Two major components underlie the calculations: the tendency to achieve success (T_s) and the motivation to avoid failure (T_f). Each of these factors, T_s and T_f, is in turn a multiplicative function of three terms: (1) the motivation to achieve success or *avoid failure,* (2) the probability of success or *failure,* and (3) the incentive value of success or *failure.* The overall calculation that provides a prediction of one's achievement motivation simply combines in an additive fashion the strength of the tendencies to achieve success and to fear failure. Details of the model and examples of calculations are illustrated in several sources (e.g., Gill, 1986, pp. 60–64; LeUnes & Nation, 1989, pp. 135–136). However, despite the general popularity of the model, it may at the same time be seriously limited in its applications. As O'Leary observes in her authoritative review, "this model yields accurate predictions of the direction, magnitude, and persistence of achievement behaviors only for males. The expectancies for and incentive values of achievement-related success differ for males and females" (p. 821). Assuming her conclusions are sound, consistently clear findings are unlikely to emerge from investigations using females. On the other hand, if subjects are drawn from sports settings in which female athletes have bought into the masculine competitive mode, then the model may, in those circumstances, be effective in explaining the achievement motivation of females.

To this point we have looked at motivational models that deemphasize the immediate social context in which motivation occurs. Most of our behavior does not take place in a social vacuum. It seems appropriate, therefore, that we now turn our attention to a motivational theory that takes social factors into account in its attempt to explain our behavior. Equity theory is one such perspective.

Equity Theory

A fair day's wages for a fair day's work, it is as
just a demand as governed men ever made of governing.
It is the everlasting right of men.

Thomas Carlyle, *Past and Present*

I would imagine that all of us have at one time or another felt that we were being treated unfairly. That unfair situation may have arisen at school, at work, in a romantic relationship, or in sports. In any one of these situations, the sense of injustice we experienced cut deeply. Is it likely that we respond in some fashion out of our sense of being treated inequitably? The answer is yes; we do respond to the inequity we see in our own circumstances. The question of just how people act to restore fairness in inequitable situations, however, will be deferred for the moment.

Before moving to a consideration of how we restore justice in our lives, we might first consider the basis for judgments of unfair treatment. We are given "too little" recognition, pay, or playing time—but "too little" compared to what or to whom? Actually, our comparisons are to others in similar circumstances whose outcomes and contributions to institutional or group goals are known to us. This process of comparing what we've received for what we've given of ourselves with the like investments and returns realized by others involves *social comparison* (Suls & Wills, 1991). We know generally what other people receive for their efforts by way of compensation (e.g., fringe benefits, recognition) and also how much they have invested in time, training, and energy in pursuit of those rewards. The *outcomes* and *inputs* that we ourselves receive or expend for work in similar task situations are, of course, known to us. It is just this comparison with others, that is, our own outcomes/inputs ratio *versus* the outcomes/inputs ratio of co-workers that can form the basis of a judgment that we are being treated fairly or unfairly (Adams, 1965).

Consider the example of the professional basketball player who puts in the same grueling hours of practice and has the same shooting averages as a teammate yet is paid substantially less than that teammate. From the player's perspective, the situation is clearly inequitable. Note, however, that his highly paid teammate may also recognize the inequity insofar as he is overpaid by the standard of what his teammate earns. Generally speaking, then, an individual's judgment of (in)equitable treatment is based on a comparison of his own outcome/input *ratio* with that of one or more co-performers. If those ratios compare favorably or are in balance, all is well. Otherwise, the individual will feel he is being unfairly treated. Typically, one does not accept inequity. Rather, "if inequity (unequal ratios) exists, it produces tension that motivates an individual to alter inputs, outcomes, or social referents so as to restore equity, or to withdraw from an exchange in either psychological or actual terms" (Lord & Hohenfeld, 1979, p. 19).

Two additional considerations are also used as bases for people's judgments of fairness. Fairness may be seen to prevail when outcomes are distributed according to people's *needs*. By this standard, those most in need should be compensated the most for their efforts; those with fewer needs should receive correspondingly less.

Finally, an *equality* principle sometimes serves as the basis for the distribution of outcomes. Irrespective of the contributions made by individuals to the common goal, all share equally in the payoffs. Fairness, then, stems from everyone's being equally rewarded. This rule for judging fairness has special relevance for certain athletic team performances. In particular, consider those events in which success comes from a smooth coordination of the athletes' skills, where they are required to perform almost as one. The pairs competitions in synchronized swimming and ice skating place a premium on smooth, harmonious relations between the couple for the successful execution of their programs. Any inequality in the outcomes experienced by either party has the potential to create friction with obviously negative consequences for their overall performance. In events where the development of an intimate and compatible relationship is requisite for success, the equality rule may be the best means of distributing rewards.

How Can Fairness Be Restored?

People have at their disposal a number of ways in which they can act to restore equity. For those who feel undercompensated, the most obvious means is simply to reduce their inputs or contributions to the enterprise, that is, to perform at a lower level, thereby bringing their outcome/input ratio more in line with that of their co-performers. Of course, those who feel overcompensated have the corresponding option of increasing their inputs, that is, making a greater effort.

A second means of achieving a more just situation involves actively attempting to change one's outcomes. The athlete who feels financially unappreciated may seek a more lucrative contract. In the rarer case, the overpaid athlete may, however reluctantly, quietly settle for a cut in salary following a poor season.

Yet another response to an inequitable situation is simply to withdraw. If the situation is intolerable and not likely to be resolved, the athlete may ask to be traded, move and play beyond the jurisdiction of the league, or perhaps retire. Such cases are reported with some regularity on our sports pages.

The Implications of Inequity

What, then, are the implications for a player's satisfaction with his role on the team, and what effects might his satisfaction have on his performance? An investigation by Pritchard, Dunnette, and Jorgenson (1972) provides some of the clearest answers to these and related questions. Male subjects in this large-scale experiment were assigned to working conditions in which they were either overpaid, equitably compensated, or underpaid for their efforts. The performance was highest among the overpaid workers, lower among those paid an equitable wage, and lower yet again in the underpaid condition. So far, no surprises! However, *satisfaction* with the job was highest among those in the equitable pay condition; both being overpaid and underpaid led to lower levels of satisfaction with the task. Dissatisfaction on the part of inequitably compensated team members obviously sows the seed of later dissension and conflict within the group. Where individual members feel their treatment to be unjust, it would seem unlikely that team unity will remain strong for very long.

As interesting and impressive as the Pritchard et al. (1972) findings might be, the skeptics among us might still ask if individuals in the real world beyond the laboratory would react to inequities in the same way. Would dedicated professional athletes with reason to feel they are being treated unfairly be motivated to restore equity by adjusting their inputs, that is, the caliber of their play? A unique event in major league baseball history, the striking down of the "reserve clause," provided Lord and Hohenfeld (1979) with the opportunity to test a major prediction of equity theory.

Since 1897, team owners had had the rights to the services of their players indefinitely. However, in December of 1975 a judicial ruling—upheld in later appeals—allowed that the rights of owners to a player's services held for no more than one year. Thereafter, a player was free to negotiate with any team. A number of players chose to play under their old contracts for the renewal year, after which they planned to accept the best offer as free agents. Others signed with their teams. Those playing out their contracts took pay cuts of up to 20% under the new regulations. Two free agents (Catfish Hunter and Andy Messersmith) had earlier negotiated multiyear, multimillion-dollar contracts. Thus, by the standards of both their own previous salaries and the extravagant settlements reached with two of the game's superstars, the nonsigners should have experienced a profound sense of inequity. What did Lord and Hohenfeld's test of the effects of inequity on performance reveal?

These researchers used a time-series analysis whereby four measures of performance were tracked for three years prior to the renewal year (1976) and one year following. The effects of inequity on "runs batted in" can be seen in Figure 1.1. During the first part of 1976, substantial drops in performance can be seen in the playing records of signers and nonsigners alike. However, upon reaching a contract settlement with their teams, the signers regained their former levels of batting skill. The nonsigners who played out their contracts continued to exhibit inferior performances at the plate, returning to their pre-renewal-year levels only after they had signed with a new team in 1977. With equity reestablished by means of lucrative new contracts, the earlier motivation for unsigned players to restore equity by restricting their inputs (i.e., performing less well) was removed. Of course, the signers who came to terms with their teams during the renewal year returned to form immediately thereafter, that is, in the second half of 1976. Generally similar results were found for three other performance measures: batting average, home runs, and to a lesser extent runs scored.

A more recent study (Harder, 1991) suggests that the decline in performance predicted for free agents by equity theory may not occur in those performance categories that bear a strong relationship to outcome expectations (e.g., home run ratios *and* future salaries). Thus, while Harder found that home runs by free agents remained constant, batting averages showed the predicted decline. Batting averages are only weakly linked to future rewards, whereas power hitting has much stronger ties to future salary settlements.

It is tempting to leave the reader with the Lord and Hohenfeld (1979) findings as the last word on equity effects in baseball. Their findings are clear and provide strong support for equity theory predictions. However, at the risk of complicating an otherwise straightforward set of results, I am obliged to draw attention to a systematic replication by Duchon and Jago (1981). These investigators expanded the earlier design to include, among other things, the free agents from the 1977 and 1978 seasons. While they fully confirmed the findings of Lord and Hohenfeld for the 1976 season, players in the combined 1977 and 1978 seasons exhibited just the opposite patterns of performance, that is, overall *increases* in performance during the option year and *poorer* performances in their first year with their new teams.

In retrospect, it would seem that 1976 was in many respects an unusual year. As Duchon and Jago (1981) point out, not only was it the first year of free agency,

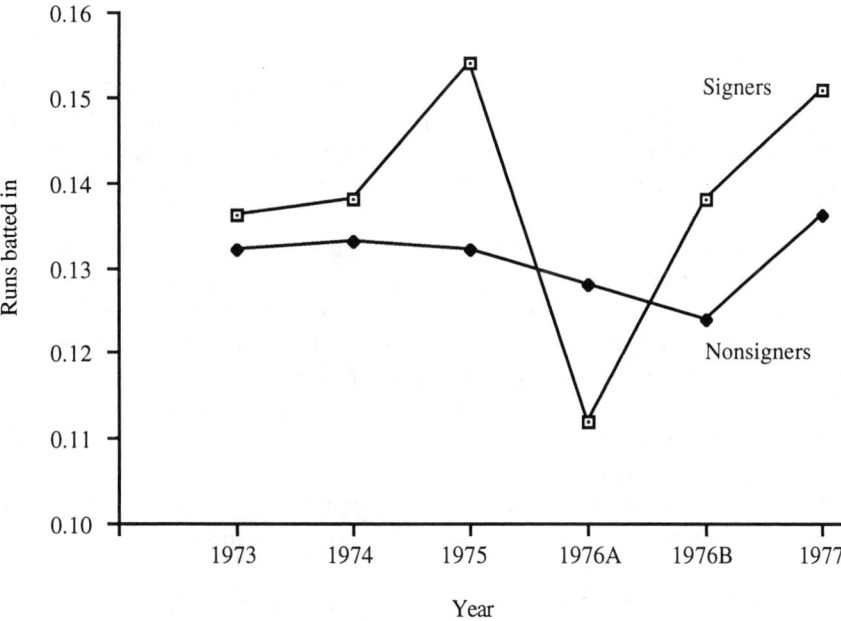

FIGURE 1.1 Batting performance 1973–1977 (adapted from Lord & Hohenfeld, 1979).

but players also took substantial pay cuts, a less common practice over the following two seasons. The players' sense of inequity may therefore have been especially acute in 1976. Moreover, free agents in 1977 and 1978 had a further advantage in knowing of the generous contract settlements of their predecessors in 1976. Perhaps it should not be surprising that their response to inequity took a different form. Inasmuch as equity theory allows that the individual can restore a sense of fairness through the *anticipation* of outcomes being favorably adjusted in the near future, the free agents of 1977 and 1978 were not motivated to adjust their performance inputs.

I might add as a postscript that people are generally less troubled by inequitable situations that favor them (i.e., overpayments) than by those situations in which they feel they are being shortchanged. It seems somewhat easier to come to terms with situations that provide us with an unfair advantage than those that are disadvantageous. Moreover, when inequities that leave us at a disadvantage result from our dealings with management, they are felt more acutely than similar dealings with co-performers. An inequitable situation occurring among team members will be seen as less unjust than the *same* inequity vis-à-vis an impersonal organization. Conversely, when the individual secures an unfair advantage over the organization he finds the situation easier to live with than the same inequity resulting from interactions with teammates (Greenberg, 1986).

Cognitive Evaluation Theory

Another theory that has considerable import and explanatory value for understanding motivation in sports is cognitive evaluation theory. Edward Deci and Richard Ryan (1985) have extended and refined earlier views (Deci, 1975) of the role played by intrinsic motivation in influencing human performance. From their perspective, intrinsic motivation performs a positive function, whereas extrinsic motivational factors serve generally to erode intrinsic motivation and produce deleterious effects on performance. Consider first their definition of intrinsic motivation. It "is the *innate* [italics added], natural propensity to engage one's interests and exercise one's capacities, and in so doing, to seek and conquer optimal challenges" (Deci & Ryan, 1985, p. 43). Intrinsic motivation, then, arises spontaneously from within the individual and is itself a motivational force sufficient to foster learning, intellectual growth, and the acquisition of skills over the course of human development.

The famous detective Sherlock Holmes revealed a strong intrinsic motivation following his brilliant solution of a notorious murder. Inspector Lestrade's offer to share authorship of the official report of the case led to this exchange:

> Lestrade: And you don't want your name to appear?
> Holmes: Not at all. *The work is its own reward* [italics added]. Perhaps I shall get the credit also at some distant day when I permit my zealous historian to lay out his foolscap once more—eh Watson? Well, now, let us see where this rat has been lurking.
> Sir Arthur Conan Doyle, *The Adventure of the Norwood Builder*

For Holmes and others, intrinsic motivation is all too easily weakened by ever present extrinsic factors (e.g., acclaim, awards, money).

Some representative research findings will be presented below to illustrate and hopefully clarify the major features of cognitive evaluation theory. First, however, I will describe the way in which intrinsic motivation is generally assessed.

Intrinsic motivation for an activity is measured typically by calculating the amount of time individuals freely choose to spend in working on a task they were engaged in on a previous occasion. The experimenter is "unexpectedly" called away from the lab, leaving the subject alone with the option of several activities. One of the available activities is the experimental task from the previous session. A hidden observer records the amount of time spent on the experimental task as opposed to other activities that are made available to the subject.

In order to illustrate how various factors influence intrinsic motivation, it might be helpful to describe a typical experiment, in particular, one testing the effects of monetary rewards on intrinsic motivation. Pritchard, Campbell, and Campbell (1977) presented their subjects with a series of chess problems in their study of the impact of money (i.e., an extrinsic incentive) on motivation. Basically, subjects were assigned randomly to either of two groups: one in which they could earn money for their efforts and one in which no mention was made of compensation for work on the problems. One week later these same subjects returned to the lab and were individually tested for intrinsic motivation by the free-choice measure. Subjects who had earlier been offered financial incentives for working on the problems were found to be less intrinsically motivated than subjects in the control group, who had not been offered extrinsic incentives. That is, those who had been paid chose to spend less time on the chess problems.

I would draw your attention to the fact that subjects in the Pritchard et al. (1977) experiment found the task to be extremely interesting. Of course, many tasks in the real world can also be interesting, but then again many can be incredibly boring. An investigation by Calder and Staw (1975) that took into account how interesting the task was revealed an important limitation to the general finding that financial incentives reduce intrinsic motivation.

Half of Calder and Staw's (1975) subjects assembled simple jigsaw puzzles with pieces that were blank. The other half worked on puzzle pieces of the same shape that when assembled depicted a variety of interesting pictures. The scenes ranged from sporting events to presidential photos to *Playboy* centerfolds. All subjects were either paid or unpaid for their efforts. We see again that money reduces intrinsic motivation for interesting tasks. Unpaid subjects found working on the picture puzzles to be more enjoyable than did those who were paid and in addition volunteered to spend more of their time in future sessions working on similar tasks. In the case of the uninteresting assignment (i.e., fitting blank jigsaw pieces), pay produced the opposite pattern of results. Now paid subjects found the task more enjoyable than did their unpaid peers and in addition tended to volunteer more of their time in the future to continue with similar tasks. In sum, although a financial incentive reduces intrinsic motivation, it does so only for interesting activities.

The question that follows, then, is why paying people money for their efforts might reduce their motivation to perform interesting tasks. The explanation for the tendency of monetary incentives to undermine intrinsic motivation is to be found in a change in subjects' perceived locus of causality. The direction of that change is from an internal to an external locus of causality. Intrinsic motivation arises from an individual's basic need to be *self-determining,* and when external rewards or constraints are introduced to an activity, it becomes difficult to maintain self-determination. The reward and/or other extrinsic incentives become ends in themselves. For many, an activity previously pursued for the interest and challenge of mastery it provided now is engaged in on the basis of a different motivational process.

The pressures are especially acute in the case of amateurs who turn professional and others who rise to the top of their sport, where the fruits of success await them. Doubts begin to creep in, raising the possibility that what was previously done for personal enjoyment is now being done for external rewards. It is at this point that we sometimes see the operation of what has come to be called the *over-justification effect.* When people are given numerous good reasons for their activity, they find it increasingly difficult to continue crediting internal factors for their participation. In effect, sports that were formerly undertaken on the basis of intrinsic motivation are now taken on for extrinsic reasons. Activity that was once done because it offered an interesting challenge is instead done for a financial or other external payoff.

The implications of these findings for sports and recreational organizations are important and far reaching. While the national work force and those in the employ of professional and semiprofessional organizations expect to be paid for the labors, legions of other workers do not. The reference here is to the hundreds of thousands of unpaid volunteers who are the lifeblood of community sports and recreational programs. Their motives for contributing their time, energies, and skills are obviously not monetary. The urge to find funds or other means to compensate volunteers for their dedicated efforts should probably be resisted. Suddenly being paid for work they took on for its inherent interest or challenge could bring about a fundamental reassessment of their reasons for serving as a volunteer in the first place. In effect, intrinsic motivation could suffer.

There are, of course, a variety of extrinsic factors that can decrease intrinsic motivation. Among these factors is an array of awards, ribbons, trophies, prizes, and publicity, all of which can serve to erode intrinsic motivation. A second class of factors operates with equal effectiveness to reduce self-determination and produce a shift in the perceived locus of causality for one's activities. For example, people engaged in an optimally challenging activity may see the presence of onlookers or the knowledge that their performance is being evaluated as controlling of their actions. For some, a perception of external causality may follow. In addition to reducing intrinsic motivation, an awareness that one is being critically evaluated may also lead to a less creative performance (Amabile, 1979). Thus, where artistic expression defines success in a sport, the implications are clear.

In a similar fashion, environmental controls in the form of deadlines for the completion of an interesting activity or the imposition of goals can further undermine intrinsic motivation. This is not to say that the setting of goals has no influence on performance. It does. Rather, while performance is improved by the imposition of difficult goals, the performer's intrinsic motivation for the activity and her subsequent satisfaction may, at the same time, decrease (Mossholder, 1980).

What are the effects on intrinsic motivation of *rivalry*, an attitude that regrettably pervades the play of many athletes? Note that in speaking of rivalry, we are more precisely referring to the participant's focus on defeating, hurting, or in some way beating his opponent (e.g., Katz & Schanck, 1938). A study by Edward Deci and his colleagues is particularly instructive in this regard (Deci, Betley, Kahle, Abrams, & Porac, 1981). College students worked on an interesting task alongside a confederate of the experimenter. Half of the subjects were told to try to *beat* the accomplice; the remaining subjects were not given competitive instructions. Subjects were allowed to win in both experimental conditions. During the subsequent free-choice period, those who had earlier performed under the competitive instructions exhibited decreased intrinsic motivation. Interestingly, the effect of rivalry in reducing intrinsic motivation was especially pronounced for females. Once again, as with money, prizes, evaluation, and so on, the activity itself becomes instrumental to the attainment of some end, in this case, beating another competitor. Reasons for participating in the activity that might otherwise apply are subverted in favor of extrinsic considerations. What was previously done for its inherent interest or the satisfactions it provided is now done merely as a means to achieve other ends.

Competence and Intrinsic Motivation

Cognitive evaluation theory recognizes that perceived competence is closely related to self-determination and that both are fundamental aspects of intrinsic motivation. For athletes, a growing sense of competence would seem necessary for their continuing development and for remaining in the sport. Evidence of one's competence is often provided through evaluative feedback. When feedback regarding the quality of a performance is positive, competence is implied. In such cases, intrinsic motivation for that activity will be enhanced. Not surprisingly, negative feedback and the incompetence implied by such information frequently results in decreased levels of intrinsic motivation. However, Deci and Ryan (1985, pp. 58–59) identify two conditions that must be present for intrinsic motivation to be affected by perceived competence in these ways. Not only must the task at hand represent an optimal challenge, but individual performers must also feel that their efforts can affect outcomes. Alternatively stated, the activity has to present a worthy challenge, and progress in that activity must be seen by the individual to result from, or be responsive to, her or his own efforts.

A study by Vallerand and Reid (1984) illustrates the differing effects of positive and negative feedback on intrinsic motivation. College students predictably experienced an increased sense of competence following positive feedback and a decreased perception of competence after receiving negative feedback. Furthermore, positive feedback increased intrinsic motivation, whereas negative feedback reduced intrinsic motivation. For a coach or trainer interested in increasing intrinsic motivation, the application of these findings is fairly straightforward.

But a question might still remain: How *much* positive feedback should one use? The more the better? Vallerand (1983) provides an answer. Varying amounts of positive verbal feedback were provided to teenage hockey players across 24 trials in a hockey simulation decision-making task. All subjects except those assigned to a *no*-feedback condition experienced increases in perceived competence and intrinsic motivation. However, subjects receiving the various amounts of positive feedback did not differ from one another. In short, once even a small amount of positive feedback is provided, additional praise contributes nothing further.

However, from the standpoint of an athlete learning a new skill, a coach may want to reinforce "correct" behaviors at various points in the learning process. While additional reinforcement may not appreciably increase intrinsic motivation, it will aid the learner in mastering the skill. Those additional reinforcements, however, will be more effective if they are offered intermittently rather than continuously (Hall, 1971). Learning that is acquired under conditions of occasional and irregular reinforcement is superior in the sense that it is more resistant to extinction or forgetting.

A Caveat

Until recently, conventional wisdom on the benefits of positive feedback on performance has never been seriously challenged. Indeed, when success is followed by feedback in the form of praise, the performer is likely to experience increases in intrinsic motivation (Deci & Ryan, 1985) and self-efficacy (Bandura, 1977). This, in turn, is apt to result in increased effort and persistence that can lead to improved performances. However, there is now reason to believe that the beneficial effects of praise may be limited to performances where the factors of effort and persistence are the major determinants of quality (Baumeister, Hutton, & Cairns, 1990). Where the quality of a performance is largely determined by *skill* (e.g., the pole vault versus the 100-meter dash), offering praise may actually impair performance. Early work on this question has led Baumeister et al. to favor a self-attention explanation. Praise may cause individuals to become self-conscious and to focus on the components of their performance. The already automatic and coordinated features of a skilled performance are thereby disrupted. Otherwise, if effort and persistence are the requisites for success, then praise remains a valuable instructional tool for coaches.

What are abundantly clear from the foregoing discussion of feedback are the implications for those who assume responsibility for teaching youngsters the skills of a sport. Coaches should be aware of the potentially harmful effects of negative feedback on perceptions of competence and, thereby, intrinsic motivation. In the interest of preserving a good learning environment, criticism should be framed in constructive terms and offered with considerable tact. If, as some writers have asserted (e.g., Curtis, Smith, & Smoll, 1979), some coaches of Little League and other sports are frequently deprecating in their remarks to youngsters, it does not bode well for the future development of either the children or the particular sport.

To recap, sports, hobbies, volunteer work, and numerous other activities are undertaken by people quite naturally and spontaneously for the intrinsic interest and satisfactions they provide. Such activities frequently involve a considerable investment of time and energy on the part of participants who strive to attain personal standards of excellence. Contemporary social commentary frequently notes the absence of satisfactions in the workplace. Some have suggested (e.g., Deci & Ryan, 1985, pp. 313–314) that sports and recreational pursuits offer one avenue of escape from the repetitive, sterile, and sometimes meaningless tasks that many of us perform from 9:00 to 5:00. As a consequence, it would seem ill-advised to continue following a course of increasing the professionalization of sports, with its emphasis on extrinsic factors. The inevitable erosion of intrinsic satisfactions that results may be simply too dear a price to pay. Somewhere in the grand scheme of things, I seem to recall a notion that sports and play can be done just for *fun* and nothing more. Or is that idea outdated?

The Stress Seekers

The motivational theories described thus far have provided us with several alternative ways of accounting for the processes by which we initially take up, or persist at, a sport. However, for a handful of sports and leisure-time pursuits, these theories fall short of providing completely satisfactory answers. For example, what would possess someone to take up rock climbing, white-water rafting, hang gliding, sky diving, or auto racing? Self-actualization or growth needs can be met just as easily in other, less risky sports. Surely, life and limb need not be imperiled in one's quest for optimal challenges to conquer. Numerous other demanding but nonhazardous sports exist for the expression of intrinsically and extrinsically motivated behavior, so why would one be attracted to sports that are seen to involve a high degree of personal danger? The answer, in part, is to be found in the work of Samuel Klausner (1968) on the stress-seeking personality and Zuckerman's (1979, 1983) model of sensation seeking.

Stress has been a popular topic for research since World War II. Typically, stress has been thought of as an unpleasant state; the ideal condition, in contrast, is one that lacks anxiety or tension. The natural state for people, then, is thought to be one of peace and tranquility with departures from that state setting in motion processes that act to restore the former equilibrium. This homeostatic process is seen in the effects of vigorous exercise. Body temperature rises and we "break into a sweat"; sweat, in turn, acts to cool the body down toward preexercise levels. People, too, seemingly strive for a peaceful resolution of any personal or group conflict in which they may have become embroiled. That island in the South Seas with the gently swaying palms and salubrious climate looks very attractive to most of us. But is it equally appealing to all people?

Klausner (1968), among others, has observed that some people on occasion act to increase rather than minimize the stress in their lives. In effect, some people quite deliberately seek out situations that expose them to tension-producing conflicts or risks. For example, women identified as "sensation seekers" (cf. Zuckerman, 1979) may act in ways that prolong or even intensify developing conflicts, for example, by dominating and being unwilling to oblige others (Pilkington, Richardson, & Utley, 1988). This tendency toward stress seeking is defined by Klausner (1968) as "behavior designed to increase the intensity of emotion or level of activation of the organism" (p. 139). Recent evidence consistent with this view (J.H. Kerr & Svebak, 1989) indicates that when individuals are given a free choice of sports they would like to participate in, those choosing a risky rather than a safe sport scored *low* on a measure of "arousal avoidance." Furthermore, despite their attraction to risky sports, these activities are not taken up thoughtlessly or without due regard for the possible consequences. In short, we cannot describe risk takers as impulsive or reckless.

There is a variety of means by which people can experience increases in arousal. Sports offer individuals a wide choice of often demanding and/or dangerous challenges. The stress seeker can accept the physical challenge of rafting a treacherous stretch of white water or ascending a peak by a new route. Still others may experience high levels of negatively toned arousal through their actions in provoking others to interpersonal conflict. The attraction of such experiences for the stress seeker lies not in the heightened arousal that accompanies such experiences but in the "drop" that follows at the conclusion of the activity. It is this *arousal jag* (Berlyne, 1960, pp. 197–200), a jump in arousal followed by a quick return to former levels, that is pleasurable for the stress seeker. Although the activity itself may be aversive, its attraction is in the relief that is felt when the negative emotional state ends. For stress seekers, then, the attraction of a dangerous sport lies not simply in the aversive experiences of fear, pain, or distress but in the relief that comes with the end to their discomfort. Berlyne brings home to us the overriding importance of relief in an illustration suggesting that "if mountaineers were habitually suspended over abysses for days on end instead of for a few minutes at a time, their number might well be smaller than it is" (pp. 198–199).

What characteristics set the stress seeker apart from his or her less adventuresome peers? Klausner (1968) identifies three general characteristics: *rationality*, *egocentricity*, and *repetitiveness*. First and foremost, stress seekers are rational and, despite appearances, are not deliberately tempting fate. They exhibit an ongoing interest in perfecting their skills and an intense concern with safety. Klausner's own work with sport parachutists provides the example of jumpers "constantly practicing the reach for the rip cord on an emergency parachute" (p. 143).

Egocentricity also marks the stress seeker. As Klausner observes, "they may demand center stage" (p. 144). For example, sport parachutists go to considerable lengths to have themselves photographed in flight. Finally, there is an obsessive quality to their behavior that sees stress seekers returning again and again to the stress-producing sport. Parachutists typically attempt incrementally more difficult maneuvers, jump from greater and greater heights, and increase the complexity of their soaring patterns. Further insights into the actual experience of jumping are provided in Speaking Tangentially 1.2.

****

Speaking Tangentially 1.2: The Agony and the Ecstasy
What are the dynamics of making a parachute jump? Is the emotional experience of veteran jumpers different from that of novices? Epstein and Fenz (1965) sought an answer to these and related questions in a study of sport parachutists. Their subjects were two groups of parachutists: 33 beginners with 1–5 jumps to their credit and 33 experienced parachutists each with over 100 jumps.

A somewhat surprising feature of their results is that the point of greatest fear is *not* that moment at which the parachutist leaps into space. Although the moment when one leaves the plane is objectively the time of greatest danger, Figure 1.2 shows that neither group experienced their highest level of fear at that point. In fact, for the *experienced* chutists, it marked the lowest level of subjectively experienced fear across the entire week leading up to their jump. Their fear peaked on the morning of the jump, declining thereafter to the point of leaving the plane. Even for the *novice* jumpers, the point of greatest fear occurs slightly before the actual jump. Their moment of peak fear occurs at the "ready" signal following a steady increase during the week.

A further feature of the data for experienced jumpers should be pointed out. After the parachutist exits the plane, fear increases with the opening of the parachute and continues to increase well after the landing. The authors favor an explanation suggesting that anxiety (fear) is inhibited in the interests of a smooth performance during the jump sequence. Thereafter, when the inhibition of fear no longer serves a purpose, it is released.

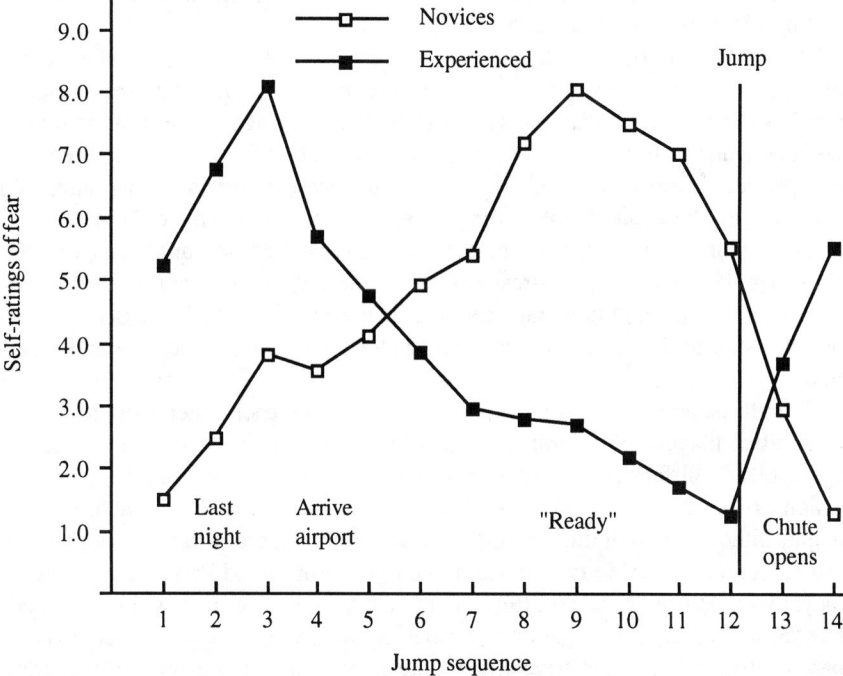

FIGURE 1.2 Chutists' fear during jump sequence (adapted from Epstein & Fenz, 1965).

A recent comparison of novice and experienced German parachutists has revealed a different pattern of results across the jump sequence (Schedlowski & Tewes, 1992). Although novices reported higher "arousal" levels than experienced chutists overall, changes in physiological processes (e.g., heart rates) ran parallel to each other. Interestingly, the authors also found that the moment of peak arousal occurred *just prior to deployment* of the chute. Differences in the findings of these two studies invite some interesting speculations.

****

Bruce Ogilvie (Johnsgard, Ogilvie, & Merritt, 1975; Ogilvie, 1974; Ogilvie & Pool, 1974) and several associates used a more direct approach to assessing the personality of stress seekers. They administered several of the more popular measures of personality to athletes who had already classified themselves as stress seekers by virtue of their participation in exceptionally stressful sports. In one study (Johnsgard et al., 1975), outstanding male athletes in car racing, sport parachuting, and football completed the Sixteen Personality Factor Questionnaire (16-PF), the Minnesota Multiphasic Personality Inventory (MMPI), and the Edwards Personal Preference Schedule (EPPS). (The evaluation of personality tests is discussed in chap. 7.) Each of the three personality measures involves a large number of subscales, allowing for an enormous number of possible comparisons among athletes in the three sports. Hence, I will attempt to convey only a few of the highlights of this exploratory study.

The authors are quick to dispel the preconceived ideas that many of us might already have formed regarding the sorts of people who fling themselves out of airplanes and drive cars at high speed. They find no evidence that these individuals "are neurotic, self-destructive, uncontrolled, or stupid" (p. 167). All three elite groups were found to be highly intelligent (the race-car drivers "remarkably so") and high in achievement motivation with energy and drive to match. Johnsgard et al. (1975) further characterize their subjects in terms very similar to those used by Klausner (1968) to describe stress seekers. Their athletes "are rather exhibitionistic, enjoy change, and have rather strong heterosexual needs. They don't like to be told what to do, are a bit disorderly, and are somewhat expedient and rebellious" (p. 167).

Overall, parachutists and race-car drivers resemble each other more than they do football players. The demands and risks, perceived and actual, of the former sports clearly differ from the latter. Both parachuting and racing require great precision and control; football, less so. Moreover, the risk of death in football is slight, although debilitating injuries are common. Whereas parachuting carries more than a measurable risk of death, the figures for Grand Prix race-car drivers may, by one estimate (Daley, 1963), approach 50% among those who remain active on the circuit for six years. Considering the greater stress and demands on parachutists and race-car drivers, they likely represent a purer form of the stress seeker.

Johnsgard et al. (1975) characterize the athletes taken together in these two sports as self-sufficient and independent free spirits who are not inclined to be strongly influenced by group pressures. While outwardly friendly, their relationships are superficial. They give little indication that they seek deep personal involvement with others. Finally, the race-car driver stands still further apart from the other two groups of athletes. The researchers describe him as "even more motivated, more intelligent, and more tough-minded" (p. 168).

Those Magnificent Men in Their Flying Machines

One other group of athletes from this series of investigations merits our attention if for no other reason than that their psychological profile appears to further distance them from race-car drivers. These are the aerobatic pilots who thrill their audiences with precision flying in performing loops, spins, and rolls. Although these daredevil pilots share many of the traits of the elite sportspeople mentioned above (i.e., parachutists and race-car drivers), they give evidence of a combination of additional characteristics unique to those in their sport (Ogilvie & Pool, 1974).

Similar to race-car drivers and parachutists, aerobatic pilots appear to be well adjusted though somewhat more cool, reserved and critical. Although not alone in this regard, they, too, tend to be exhibitionistic. Furthermore, they are highly independent, self-reliant, and tenacious in pursuit of goals. Finally, these pilots show themselves to be emotionally detached nonjoiners who do not require the emotional support of others around them. Ogilvie and Pool (1974) single out emotional detachment, strong achievement needs and abstract reasoning as the characteristics that most clearly separate these athletes from their stress-seeking counterparts in other sports.

And Females?

This curious admixture of fearful and pleasurable elements in situations that most of us carefully avoid holds an obvious attraction for some. However, because risk taking is commonly thought of as a male prerogative, I am in danger of giving you the impression that only males are stress seekers. Quite the contrary. A small percentage of women are also to be found participating in sports that appeal to stress seekers. As Bernard (1968) suggests, "there is . . . no reason to believe that women are naturally any less stress-seeking than men" (p. 39). She further points out, however, that the number of stress-seeking outlets is limited for women generally and that "excitement has to be sought in different channels" (p. 39).

One subset of female stress seekers has been profiled by Campbell (1967) in a study of beautiful women. Analyses of vocational interest data provided by 100 topflight fashion models from Paris, New York, and Minneapolis revealed what he describes as the James Bond syndrome. In Campbell's own words, the syndrome "includes preferences for exciting, adventuresome activities, including those with the abstract feel of danger, such as Criminal Lawyer and Secret Service Woman" (p. 970). The late Ian Fleming's portrayal of beautiful women as "swingers" was not too far off the mark! Their pattern of dislikes includes an aversion to routine, organized work schedules, and anything to do with mathematics and science, both of which demand accuracy, persistence, and precision. In characterizing these women in the most general terms, Campbell concludes, "These girls are pretty, they know it, and they prefer activities that allow them to take advantage of their beauty" (p. 969).

Campbell's (1967) profile of fashion models is interesting additionally in the fact that it anticipates many of the components of Zuckerman's (1979) theory of sensation seeking. In particular, the models' dislike of routine and their attraction to adventuresome activities have their counterparts in Zuckerman's description of people he has chosen to call sensation seekers. It is this latter approach to understanding the attraction of some people to arousing and/or risky experiences that follows.

Sensation Seeking

Our efforts to understand the behavior of those who seek out risky activities and experiences have been furthered by a second approach to the question, one that is complementary to that of Klausner (1968). The extensive work of Zuckerman

(1979, 1983) in developing both a model of *sensation seeking* and psychometrically sound scales to assess the trait offers an alternative view of those who are drawn to risky sports. Zuckerman's (1979) theoretically based definition of sensation seeking involves "the need for varied, novel and complex sensations and experiences and the willingness to take physical and social risks for the sake of such experience" (p. 10).

In developing a profile of the sensation seeker, Zuckerman recognizes four distinct elements. These dimensions have been consistently identified and are described in the following abbreviated form (cf. Zuckerman, 1983, p. 286):

1. *Thrill and adventure seeking (TAS)*: This aspect of sensation seeking simply identifies a preference on the part of individuals for risky activities.
2. *Experience seeking (ES)*: The dimension reflects attempts by the individual to obtain mental stimulation through a range of means, for example, music, travel, and associations with unconventional people.
3. *Disinhibition (Dis)*: Sensation is sought through activities such as gambling, partying and sexual experimentation.
4. *Boredom susceptibility (BS)*: This dimension reflects the fact that sensation seekers find routine repetition in work and social settings to be generally aversive.

Studies using Zuckerman's (1983) scale have yielded results that generally confirm aspects of the model as well as broaden our understanding of the sport selection process, sex differences, and the persistence with which people participate in a chosen activity. As predicted, sportspeople involved in hang gliding, auto racing (W.F. Straub, 1982), and rock climbing (Levenson, 1990; D.W. Robinson, 1985) scored higher on sensation seeking than nonparticipant comparison groups. However, other motives may also underlie the activities of risk takers.

Levenson's (1990) study marks an important reference point in his having recruited groups of adventurous, antisocial, and prosocial risk takers in comparisons of their respective personalities. The three types of risk takers were rock climbers, convicted felons, and heroes (i.e., policemen and firemen decorated for bravery). Our immediate interest is in his finding that the heroes scored *lower* on measures of general sensation seeking and experience seeking than the climbers and felons and, more important, lower than the norms of the general population. Although the heroes exposed themselves to extreme physical risk, their motives clearly did not include sensation seeking; altruism was far more likely a motive. Perhaps the most important lesson to be drawn from this study is that we should not lump all risk takers into the same category. Risk taking is a complex phenomenon that "may involve physical or social action, it may be premeditated or impulsive, prosocial or antisocial. It may also be governed by a relative lack of fear or by courage based on qualities other than fearlessness" (Levenson, 1990, p. 1079).

Other studies have examined the role of sensation seeking in the choices people make and their persistence with sports activities. For example, Rowland,

Franken, and Harrison (1986) have established that although high sensation seekers become involved in a greater number of sports than low sensation seekers, they leave each sport sooner than lows. They almost appear to hop from sport to sport in search of what Rowland et al. characterize as "new and varied experiences" (p. 219). In an interesting extension that incorporated several of the characteristics noted above, namely, the reluctance of sensation seekers to persist and their susceptibility to boredom, Babbit, Rowland and Franken (1990) predicted that women participating in aerobic exercise classes would generally be *low* on sensation-seeking tendencies. The routine and repetitive nature of the activity would presumably hold little appeal for the sensation seeker. In a comparison with nonparticipants of the same age, this was precisely what was found.

Of course, the foregoing provides little more than a sketch of the motivational processes underlying the behavior of those who seek out physically and socially risky experiences. Perhaps what is more important to the topic of this section is the recognition of additional motivational models that have direct applications to a number of sports and activities for which traditional motivational theories seem less than adequate to account for their appeal.

The first section of this chapter dealt with a small sample of motivational theories that began with Maslow's early views. Achievement motivation, equity theory and cognitive evaluation theory were then shown, in turn, to offer answers to some of the basic questions associated with sports participation and performance. Moving beyond the motivational question, we consider in the next chapter some of the social factors present in the performance domain that can affect the athlete's ability to excel in a sport or even to perform well on a given occasion.

Suggested Readings

Apter, M. (1992). *The dangerous edge: The psychology of excitement.* New York: Free Press
   The attraction of some people to activities (e.g., sky diving, driving at high speeds) that provide considerably more excitement than most of us care to experience is explained within a psychological framework.

Deci, E.L., & Olson, B.C. (1989). Motivation and competition: Their role in sports. In J.H. Goldstein (Ed.), *Sports, games, and play: Social and psychological viewpoints* (2nd ed., pp. 83–110). Hillsdale, NJ: Erlbaum.
   The authors present a review of cognitive evaluation theory with specific application to sports.

McClelland, D.C. (1987). *Human motivation.* New York: Cambridge University Press.
   This book offers a high level treatment of this fundamental aspect of human interaction.

Roberts, G.C. (in press). Motivation in sport: Understanding and enhancing the motivation and achievement of children. In R.N. Singer, M. Murphy, & L.K. Tennant (Eds.), *Handbook on research in sport psychology*. New York: Macmillan.

This chapter is an up-to-date scholarly review of achievement motivation with a focus on its development in children.

2

Performance and Social Influence

In the sections to follow, the performance of athletes will be shown to be subject to some degree of influence by virtually everyone present in the performance setting. Even those most intimately involved with the development of the athlete's skills (e.g., trainers, coaches) can unwittingly contribute to the success or failure of their students merely through the "expectations" they hold for the performance of each individual. Not to overlook those who pay the bills, fans, too, influence athletic performance, although not always for the better. A theory that attempts to account specifically for the strength of spectator influence (i.e., social impact) will be examined in regard to its implications for athletic performance. The support or lack of overt support shown by spectators can similarly affect the caliber of athletic performance. In this regard, explanations for the home (field) advantage are considered alongside evidence that playing before hometown fans is not always a blessing. Finally, the effects of crowd size on performance are considered along with the influence of active spectators and those who just quietly observe.

The Relative Age Effect

> Not tonight, honey, it's too early in the year.
> *Ottawa Citizen*, November 7, 1990

An Anecdote

This section begins with a little story, one that illustrates that not all research ideas spring from theory or are extensions of previous research. A substantial number of hypotheses result from astute observations of everyday circumstances. The birth of the relative age hypothesis is a case in point.

The story begins on a January evening in 1983 when psychologists Roger and Paula Barnsley attended a Lethbridge Broncos hockey game. During an extended lull in the action, Paula began reading the program to relieve her boredom. Something in the biographical sketches caught her eye. The players' birthdates were concentrated in the earlier part of the year, that is, January to April. Relatively few of the players appeared to have been born during the remaining months of the year. A coincidence? Perhaps! But coincidence or not, the Barnsleys, in collaboration with Gus Thompson, embarked on a series of archival investigations testing the generality of Paula's original observation. They were rewarded with confirming evidence supporting the existence of what is known as the relative age effect (Barnsley, Thompson, & Barnsley, 1985).

As you might already have guessed, the reason for the disproportionate number of hockey players with birthdays during the first few months is the January 1 cutoff date used throughout the sport. The effect itself arises from the practice of grouping children by age according to a deadline for their participation at various levels of a sport. Those starting out in minor hockey who meet the registration requirement of having reached their sixth birthdays before the January 1 deadline will ensure a homogeneous age group of 6-year-olds. However, within the group, those youngsters born in January will be almost a full year older (relative age) than their peers born in December. This fact provides a considerable relative age advantage to those born in the early months of the year. Not only are they more socially and emotionally mature, but their physical development is also advanced. They can be expected to be larger, stronger, and better coordinated. In a sense, those born in the autumn are behind before they even begin. The question then arises, Does all of this matter in the long run? In fact, it matters a great deal.

The dramatic impact of the relative age effect on achievement is seen in the birthdates of those playing at the higher levels of their sport. Figure 2.1 shows the month of birth of soccer players competing in the Under-20s World Tournament (Barnsley, Thompson, & Legault, in press). Whereas the distribution of live births nationally remains fairly level, players born during the first few months of the "activity year," beginning in August, outnumber those born late in the playing year by a margin of approximately four to one. The examination of player records from baseball (Thompson, Barnsley, & Stebelsky, 1991) has also revealed a relative age effect.

The implications of the Barnsley and Thompson research are profound and far reaching. With a cutoff date determining "success" in a sport for some and something less than success for others, we are required to recognize the fact that the native talents of many able young athletes are never fully developed. Two major reasons are suggested for this state of affairs (Barnsley & Thompson, 1988). First, those born late in the year may simply drop out of organized sports at a faster rate than others. Playing alongside larger and better coordinated peers, they predictably experience less success and fewer rewards. Other sports where they can perform on an equal footing may, as a consequence, hold more appeal. Second, those benefiting from a relative age advantage are more likely to be named to all-star teams that, in turn, provide superior coaching, better competition, and more playing time. The result is a greater development of their talents.

A Word to Coaches

The relative age effect poses a problem for the governing bodies of several sports, a problem for which there are no easy solutions. However, coaches and managers are in a good position to counteract or neutralize many of the negative experiences of those in age-grouped sports. The coach who is fully aware and sensitive to the struggles of late-born children can do much to offset the disappointment and setbacks they encounter. Encouragement, equal coaching time, and "progress" evaluated by

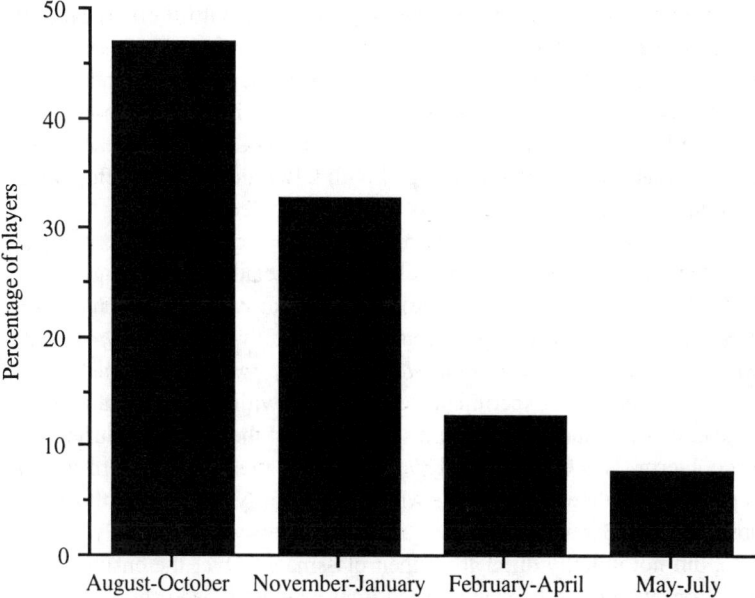

FIGURE 2.1 Players' birth quarters (adapted from Barnsley et al., in press).

comparisons with same-age peers may go a long way toward neutralizing the effect. Finally, do we really need all-star teams in children's sports that serve to widen the gap in abilities and leave behind many with equal, although underdeveloped, talents?

The Role of Expectations

During the decade of the 1960s, Robert Rosenthal, a Harvard psychologist, embarked on a research program investigating the potentially biasing effects of the researcher's own expectations regarding the outcome of an experiment on his or her data. At the risk of oversimplification, experimenters expecting particular results unwittingly convey those expectations to their subjects in such a way that the subjects often confirm the experimenter's predictions (Rosenthal, 1969). The influence process itself is *interactional,* involving an exchange of subliminal cues such as gestures, facial expressions, voice inflections, postural changes, and so on. The most important point to note is that the experimenter is unaware that his prophecies are being fulfilled through subtle changes in his own behavior that elicit corresponding and confirming changes in the subjects' behavior.

The actual process by which expectancies can influence the development of athletic skills is illustrated in the following example. A coach of two beginning and equally able gymnasts has found reason to expect exceptional progress from one of the youngsters (i.e., she is the daughter of a former Olympian). Thereafter, the likelihood is that the coach will unknowingly interact with the two girls in subtle but critically different ways. His expectations regarding the Olympian's daughter will find expression in the cues and reinforcements he unconsciously provides for correctly executed aspects of her routine. She, in turn, responds with a greater effort and mastery of elements in her performance. Ultimately, the coach will have his expectations confirmed. The girl with Olympic genes develops into the better gymnast; her teammate has a less impressive career.

Researchers and coaches are not the only prophets in society. All of us as parents, students, sports enthusiasts, and educators alike hold expectations regarding the behavior of those with whom we interact. Easily the best-known publication arising from Rosenthal's work on expectancy effects is his book *Pygmalion in the Classroom: Teacher Expectation and Pupils' Intellectual Development* (Rosenthal & Jacobson, 1968). Teachers in this experiment were provided with false expectations regarding improved performances they would see in some of their students during the upcoming school term. This was achieved by sharing with the teachers the results of a bogus test purporting to identify students who would shortly blossom forth academically. Those students identified by the test as late bloomers were randomly chosen and, of course, did not initially differ from their classmates. Over the ensuing year those students from whom teachers anticipated improvement indeed showed major gains in academic performance. The superior performance of the late bloomers was established by teacher evaluations, subject tests, and, most convincingly, externally standardized achievement tests. By any of these measurement standards, those expected to perform at a high level rose to confirm their teachers' expectations.

Pygmalion in the Pool

Clearly, one could generalize with considerable confidence on the basis of this extensive research literature alone and see expectancies at work as youngsters acquire sports skills and newfound self-esteem (Koocher, 1971) under the guidance of teachers and coaches. However, it may not be necessary to generalize from nonsports settings. Evidence of expectancy effects occurring specifically in sports has been provided by John Burnham (1968) in a model master's thesis. The setting for his field investigation was a swimming program conducted as part of a summer camp experience for boys and girls ages 7 to 14. As in Rosenthal and Jacobson's (1968) Pygmalion experiment, expectations were provided to the swimming instructors by letting them see the results of a bogus personality test that identified a (randomly assigned) group of youngsters as psychologically ready to learn to swim. Although these learners were the equals of their fellow campers, they developed into decidedly better swimmers over the 2 weeks of daily instruction. The criterion for determining the children's level of ability was their performance on the 21 graduated subtests of specific skills that they must pass in order to receive a Red Cross beginning swimmer's card. Finally, bear in mind that the swimming instructors did not knowingly favor any of their young charges. Rather, they unconsciously interacted with those from whom they anticipated success in subtly different ways, ways that provided reinforcements and encouragement for mastering the correct elements of a swimming stroke.

Burnham's (1968) results also revealed a major sex difference. Among the youngest campers (7 to 9), it was the girls whose performance was most affected by the expectancy manipulation. Among the 10- to 14-year-olds, the greatest gains were made instead by the boys. As Burnham suggested, the likelihood that the youngest group of girls received more instruction from males than their older sisters — a "given" in the camp's organizational structure—could account for their greater susceptibility to an expectancy effect. Additionally, Burnham points to an intriguing line of research in suggesting that girls below age 10 may be especially "attuned to the covertly communicated cues of father figures," that is, their male swimming instructors (p. 29).

In a number of sports, the measure of one's performance is provided by a panel of judges. However, the judges themselves are subject to expectancy effects. This potential for biased judgments is seen clearly in the context of a female gymnastics competition (Scheer & Ansorge, 1979). It is common practice in the gymnastics world for coaches to order the appearance of their gymnasts in a competition from the poorest to the best. The expectations of judges, then, is that the most skillful gymnasts will appear last, an expectation firmly established by tradition. Scheer and Ansorge arranged for videotaped performances to be scored by nationally and regionally certified female judges. However, the tapes were edited such that for one half of the performances the gymnasts normally appearing in first and fifth positions were reversed. Although the routines in both orders were identical overall, those seen fifth in the order were given higher scores than those who led off. Moreover, the strength of this expectancy bias was not equal across all members of the panels. The judges most susceptible to expectancy effects were found to be those with a belief in an external locus of control (i.e., luck, chance, or fate). From this perspective, outcomes are thought to be largely the result of external factors rather than due to the individual's own efforts (Rotter, 1966). A more detailed discussion of this personality variable and its relationship to sports appears in chapter 7.

Summary

The sections above have thus far described the operation of two powerful variables not commonly recognized as playing an important part in the learner's attempts to achieve mastery in a sport. Whether as a result of an accident of birth (i.e., the relative age effect) or the private expectations of a coach, one implication is that aspiring youngsters with equal and sometimes greater native talents than others are being shunted from the mainstream of advancement. The ideal of all participants being afforded equal opportunities to fully develop their skills is frequently compromised by the operation of these subtle but nonetheless effective factors. Similarly, elitist sports programs designed to identify and train topflight athletes in a sport have undoubtedly fallen short of the mark for some of the same reasons. It is safe to conclude that other Chris Everett Lloyds and Nolan Ryans exist but are presently doing other things, such as clerking, driving a truck, or pursuing their studies. We are not seeing the "best" in sports performances.

A Theory of Social Impact

Before examining the specific ways that athletic performances can be affected by those in attendance, we might first consider the actual impact that audiences exert on performers. Social impact theory (Latané, 1981; Latané & Nida, 1980) addresses this question in the context of the various settings and conditions under which people perform. It does not, however, deal with the quality or direction of influence but rather focuses solely on the impact that audiences have on performance. By impact is meant

> any of the great variety of changes in physiological states and subjective feelings, motives and emotions, cognitions and beliefs, values and behavior, that occur in an individual human or animal as a result of the real, implied, or imagined presence or actions of other individuals. (Latané & Nida, 1980, p. 5)

Three basic components make up social impact theory, namely, social forces, marginal impact, and multiplication/division of impact.

Social Forces

The impact of social forces on the target performer is, in turn, determined by three factors whose joint effects are illustrated in Figure 2.2.

Strength

The first of these, *strength* of the sources, is represented by the area of the circles in Figure 2.2. Strength includes "the salience, power, importance, or intensity of a given source to the target—usually determined by such things as the source's status, age, socioeconomic status, prior relationship with the target, or future power over the target" (Latané & Harkins, 1976; Latané & Nida, 1980, p. 7). For example, the large figure "Scout" might be the representative of a professional team whose attendance at a junior game has been noticed by the players. The impact of his presence on those players looking to pro careers will be considerable.

Immediacy

The second term, *immediacy*, takes into account how close the sources are in space or time to the target. Immediacy is decreased, however, as barriers (parti-

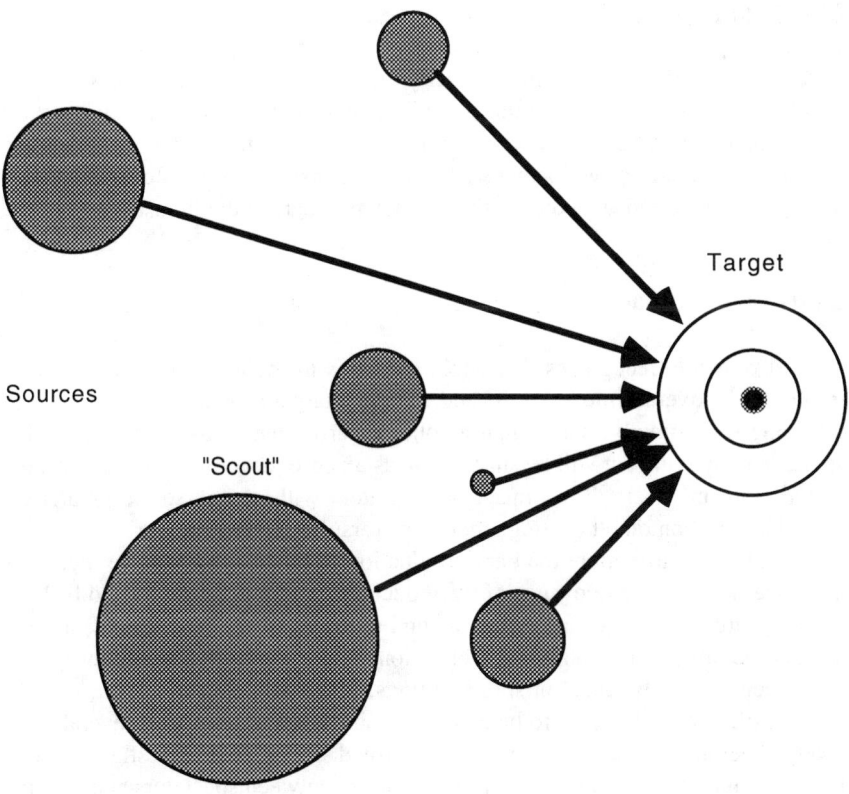

FIGURE 2.2 Multiplication of impact (adapted from Latané & Nida, 1980).

tions, screens, fencing, glass, etc.) are put in place between sources and the target. For example, spectators at basketball games generally can sit at floor level with little between them and the players. In contrast, at some soccer venues fans are kept behind steel fencing, a cordon of police officers, or sometimes a moat.

Numbers

The third contributing factor to social impact refers to the sheer *number* of sources present—in Figure 2.2, six (e.g., Latané & Harkins, 1976). Impact then, is a multiplicative function of all three factors. Hence, I = f(SIN), where S = strength, I = immediacy, and N = the number of sources. With regard to the formula, note that if the value of any of the terms is zero, the overall impact of the sources will also be zero.

Marginal Impact

As the second of three principles underlying social impact theory, marginal impact takes into account the fact that as additional people are added as sources their impact on the target diminishes proportionately. That is, increasing the size of an audience from one to two persons results in a considerably greater impact than adding one person to an audience that already numbers in the thousands.

Division of Impact

A third principle recognizes that while increases in the number of people contribute to the overall impact of the audience, the target of their influence may, at the same time, involve more than a solitary performer. Thus, in the case of a sports team, the impact will be shared and, as a consequence, be felt less by individual team members. The impact of spectators will, of course, be greater on some players than on others (e.g., the "star" versus a second stringer).

The above is little more than an introduction to this comprehensive theory of audience impact. The relevance of the model and its applications should be kept in mind through discussions of the upcoming topics of the home (field) advantage, crowd influences, and social facilitation. While some variables of the model have been indirectly tested in sports settings, for example, crowd size (Russell, 1983a), there would appear to be a need for simultaneously testing several variables in the same research design. Perhaps crowd size could be investigated jointly with immediacy variables such as the distance between spectators and athletes at different sports venues. It might also be possible to evaluate the "strength of sources" variable by comparing the performances of the more talented, professionally minded athletes during regular league games with those occasions when scouts are known to be in attendance.

The theory, however, is not without its critics. Mullen (1985) conducted a review of the effects of source strength and source immediacy. Based on meta-analyses, Mullen concluded that the effects were "weak" and "inconsistent," and hence seriously undermine the explanatory value of social impact theory. Jackson (1986) has risen in defense of the theory and has engaged Mullen in a vigorous and continuing exchange (Mullen, 1986). Whatever the direction and outcome of future research on the theory, Latané and his colleagues have thus far provided an insightful accounting of the dynamics of audience impact with the promise of a greater understanding of this topic in the future.

The Home (Field) Advantage

One is merely reaffirming an article of faith in observing that an individual athlete or team generally performs better on the home field. This view, shared by gamblers, sportscasters, and spectators alike, recognizes that "playing at home" is often a decisive factor in determining the outcome of a contest. Most are quick to credit the motivating influence of supportive fans with creating this advantage for the local athlete or team.

Studies based on sports records have consistently supported the reality of the home advantage across several cultures and a variety of sports (Courneya & Carron, 1992). One of these archival investigations has shown that the phenomenon dates back to the 19th century. Pollard (1986) found that a home field advantage has occurred continuously in English First Division soccer since 1888. In fact, there is every indication that the margin of advantage was actually greater prior to World War II.

Two additional points deserve mention. First, the advantage of competing at home may be less pronounced in high school sports than at the college and professional levels. McCutcheon (1984) found relatively minor margins of wins among high school teams competing at home in football, basketball, and cross-country. Second, the home advantage is more in evidence in some sports than in others. The most pronounced effects are to be found in soccer (Pollard, 1986), basketball (Altman, 1975; Hirt & Kimble, 1981; Schwartz & Barsky, 1977; Silva & Andrew, 1987; Varca, 1980), and ice hockey (Gayton, Matthews, & Nickless, 1987; Russell, 1981b, 1983a; Schwartz & Barsky, 1977). Cricket (Pollard, 1986) and football are likely intermediate in the magnitude of an advantage they provide home teams, whereas baseball appears to offer only the slightest edge to teams playing in their own stadia (Edwards, 1979; Hirt & Kimble, 1981; Mann, 1979; Schwartz & Barsky, 1977). However, the home team in baseball may enjoy a substantial edge when the sport is played at the college level (Courneya, 1990). One of the more intriguing questions surrounding this topic is that which seeks an explanation of the phenomenon. Five interpretations are described and evaluated on the pages to follow.

Origins

An Ethological Explanation

The ethological concept of territoriality (Lorenz, 1966) "is one of the most hallowed concepts of animal behavior" (Moyer, 1987, p. 169). It has also served as an attractive explanation for some writers (e.g., Edwards, 1979) attempting to account for the home field advantage. Originating with the influential European tradition of observing the behavior of lower organisms in their natural surroundings, the concept of territory is but one of a number of useful concepts used by ethologists to describe and understand regularities observed in the behaviors of infrahuman species. Thus, for example, a Thompson's gazelle will establish a specific range within which its grazing and breeding activities take place. Males competing for food and/or females are intercepted at the urine-marked boundary and, in most instances, driven off. It is worth keeping in mind that many species, indeed even some herd animals, are not territorial (see, e.g., Barnett, 1988). Despite its inconsistent application among lower animals, the concept has nevertheless found its way into everyday conversation and has been adopted as an explanation for a variety of human behaviors, from gang wars to international conflict. Due in part to the engaging writings of Robert Ardrey (*The Territorial Imperative*, 1966), many have been persuaded that the territorial behaviors exhibited by some species are also displayed by humans, even symbolically, for some of the same reasons of group or team survival. Indeed, references to the local sports facilities as the "home grounds" or our "turf" seem implicitly to affirm an acceptance of an ethological explanation. However, before uncritically accepting the proposition that athletes excel at home because they must of evolutionary necessity turn in a superior performance in defense of their territory, several points should be noted.

Evaluation

The adequacy of an ethological explanation of the home advantage can be evaluated from two perspectives, one philosophical and the other empirical. In our attempts to understand social phenomena through a scientific approach, social scientists favor the more parsimonious explanation for any established relationship. One wields Occam's razor, as it were, in cutting away complex, remote explanations in favor of those more simple and immediate. In the present instance, it makes little sense to reach far down the phylogenetic scale to embrace a concept applicable to only some species and unreservedly apply it to the human level to account for the margin of wins by sports teams playing at home. Other explanations are straightforward and closer at hand.

The empirical basis for discounting a territorial explanation follows from a summary of comparisons of the aggression displayed by home and visiting teams (Russell, 1981b). Among territorial creatures, it is commonly observed that the defender of a territory is more vigorous and savage in its defense than the interloper. The defender is also more likely to win, even against a larger adversary who, in other settings, may be a more competent fighter. The tiny cichlid fish, for example, will fairly consistently drive off a larger intruder. Indeed, from an evolutionary perspective, such must generally be the rule if the species is to survive. It follows, then, that if athletes are defending the ethological equivalent of their territory they could be expected to be more aggressive than invaders. Such is not the case. With few exceptions (e.g., Kelly & McCarthy, 1979), there are no discernible tendencies for teams in a variety of sports (i.e., basketball, football, hockey, soccer) played in several countries to exhibit any more or fewer aggressive infractions than their visitors (Russell, 1981b). The lack of support for this direct and clear prediction undermines the validity of a territorial explanation for the companion prediction of superior performances by teams playing at home. Moyer (1987) summarizes a substantial body of scientific opinion in concluding that whereas "the construct is of dubious value in understanding animals, it may be even less useful in understanding humans" (p. 182). It appears, then, that we must look elsewhere for an answer.

Travel-Related Explanations

A set of more immediate factors associated with travel might provide an edge in performance for the home team. Visitors can reasonably be expected to suffer from the debilitating effects of travel itself, changes in diet, and sleeping in unfamiliar surroundings. Furthermore, the obligatory separation from family and friends during extended road trips may also undermine the athlete's ability to perform well. Certainly, it is not idle speculation to suggest that one's performance can be adversely affected by fatigue, dietary, and sleep factors. The question, however, is whether these travel factors operate with sufficient effect to produce more than trivial decrements in the performance of highly trained young athletes.

Evaluation

Schwartz and Barsky (1977) have provided an indirect test of the contribution of travel-related factors to the home advantage. These researchers note that while professional baseball players spend the greatest amount of time on the road, it is baseball that shows the weakest home field advantage among several major team sports. Furthermore, they reason that insofar as fatigue tends to be cumulative, the home advantage should become greater as the season wears on. Comparisons between the first and second halves of the season in five sports failed to provide support for the hypothesis. A similar study of minor league Double A baseball records also failed to provide support for travel as an explanation for the home field advantage (Courneya & Carron, 1991). Thus, such evidence as is available suggests that the disruptive effects arising from travel-related factors are not sufficiently strong in the general case to measurably impair athletic performance.

Learning

Those writing about the home advantage appear to be unaware of an extensive literature on learning that offers an entirely plausible explanation for the phenomenon. An important principle derived from learning research recognizes that skills are performed better in the setting in which they were originally learned as opposed to a new or novel situation. The term applied to the phenomenon is *context-dependent memory* (Hall, 1971, pp. 467–469). Insofar as athletes in many sports train and practice in the very facilities they later compete in, they would be expected to enjoy some margin of advantage. Moreover, teams competing in league play are usually at home in that original learning setting for half of their games.

Evaluation

A number of experimental investigations have firmly established that one performs better on a variety of tasks in the original learning setting. The field experiment that perhaps best illustrates the research findings in the area of context-dependent memory is that of Scottish psychologists Godden and Baddeley (1975). They had scuba divers learn word lists both on land and underwater, at a depth of 20 feet. The diver-subjects were then asked to recall words from the lists, again, both on land and underwater. Support for context-dependent memory would be forthcoming if the recall and learning of words in the same environment (i.e., learn on land, recall on land; learn underwater, recall underwater) were superior to conditions where the learning and recall took place in different environments (i.e., learn on land, recall underwater; learn underwater, recall on land). That is precisely what was found. Lists learned on land were best recalled on land; lists learned underwater were best recalled underwater. This clever and novel experiment is consistent with the overall pattern of findings on this question and offers one explanation among several for the home field advantage.

Officiating

Being but mere mortals, contest officials frequently fall short of perfection in the performance of their duties. As well trained, conscientious, and experienced as officials may be, their ability to provide valid and reliable judgments is open to question (see chap. 7). To be sure, their ability to render accurate and consistent decisions is dictated in large measure by the structure of the task set for them by the requirements of a sport. However, as with any measuring device, be it a spring scale or stopwatch, judges, referees, and umpires, too, are subject to *instrumentation effects* (Campbell & Stanley, 1966). The error introduced by such effects might originate, for example, with fatigue-induced inattention. Contest officials are also subject to expectancy effects whereby their expectations of success or failure, and aggression or nonaggression on the part of athletes and teams are unwittingly reflected in their own calls or judgments (e.g., Frank & Gilovich, 1988; Scheer & Ansorge, 1979). Additionally, where judges are called upon to make impartial calls yet at the same time are affiliated with one of the parties to a contest, their decisions are apt to be biased.

Evidence on the latter point is best seen in an early communications study by Rosnow (1965). Democrats and Republicans were asked to dispassionately judge the quality of performances by John F. Kennedy and Richard M. Nixon in the famous presidential debates of 1960. Despite the subjects' conscientious efforts and experimental instructions urging them to be objective in their assessments, they literally failed in their task. Subjects with a commitment to either party saw their candidate skillfully refuting his opponent, scoring the most debating points, and moving ahead in the debate. Even with the best of intentions, then, people are sometimes unable to suspend their allegiances in the interests of being impartial.

Those officiating in sports contests may be contributing to the home advantage for yet another reason, that of the social influence of crowds. It would be naive to assume that officials are somehow able to completely insulate themselves from abusive and hostile fans. Insofar as they are frequently the target of the crowd's wrath (Greer, 1983; Russell, 1983a) and, indeed, see crowds to be the major source of the hostility they attract (C.L. Phillips, 1985), it is reasonable to assume that some measure of influence is reflected in their decisions.

Evaluation

A strong case for officiating bias contributing to the home field advantage has been found in the 1984–1985 season records of the Los Angeles Lakers of the National Basketball Association. Lehman and Reifman (1987) reasoned that bias favoring the home team would most likely be seen in fewer penalties being called specifically against the "star" players on the home team. Partisan fans and officials alike recognize that it is the stars on the team who are best able to produce a victory. In a test of their hypothesis, players identified as stars were compared to nonstars in terms of the numbers of fouls awarded both at home and away. The nonstars were called for an equal number of fouls on their home court and on the road. By contrast, the stars drew fewer fouls at home than they did at away games. A major rival explanation for their findings was ruled out when the authors determined that the star players had equal amounts of playing time in their home and away games.

Is the unthinkable, thinkable? For the most part, I think we can assume that where officials are biased in their decisions, they unknowingly favor the home team. However, in a few instances the bias is undoubtedly deliberate. Whether for reasons of enhancing national prestige or lining one's pockets, officials have been known on occasion to stray from their role as impartial enforcers of the rules of play. An analysis of the records of international cricket test matches played from 1877 to 1980 reveals a strong nationalistic bias by home umpires (Sumner & Mobley, 1981). Although the authors attribute some of the margin of bias to different playing conditions in the competing nations, the remainder appears to be willful. For example, on one occasion "Pakistani umpires resigned alleging that they had been coerced by their Cricket Board to 'see' things the way of their own team" (p. 29). Clearly, in contests of any importance, in cricket as elsewhere, it would be in the best interests of a sport to appoint neutral officials. While officiating bias may still occur for reasons of fan pressures, expectancy effects, and so on, the assignment of contest officials without ties or allegiances to either party would be a step in the right direction.

Crowd Influences

The most popular explanation for the home advantage shared by the media, promoters, and the public alike is fan support. It is commonly assumed that supportive fans are able through their applause and cheers to spur the home team to an above-average performance. As promoters are quick to point out, the greater the turnout of fans for a contest, the better the home team can be expected to perform. However, we might pause to consider how spectators actually behave. Clearly, a full range of supportive as well as negative behaviors can be seen across audiences. For example, those attending bowling, curling, golf, and gymnastics typically applaud a good performance or effort irrespective of an athlete's origins and do nothing to disrupt a performance. Other crowds show less courtesy and sportsmanship toward competitors. In sports where witnessing superior athletic skills is clearly subordinated in the interests of "winning," spectators cheer the home team and direct hostility at the visitors, in some cases to the point of attempting to directly interfere with an athlete's performance. However, these observations beg the question of whether abusive fans can successfully disrupt an athlete's performance.

Consideration of this question is preliminary to an understanding of the relationship between crowd influence and performance. The most convincing evidence that abusive spectators can indeed interfere with a performance was provided by Laird in 1923 (see also Silva, 1979). Pledges subjected to "razzing" by a group of fraternity men were thoroughly disrupted in the performance of a series of lab tasks. Not surprisingly, they were also angered by their treatment.

The effects of crowd influence, then, should be seen as two distinct processes. In the case of basketball, hockey, football, and so on, fans act to support the home team and hinder the visiting team. It might be presumed that the combination of these influences acts to create a performance margin favoring the home team. What is the evidence?

Evaluation

Greer (1983) conducted a study of the effects of sustained booing on the performance of basketball players. Trained observers recorded aspects of the play for 5 minutes of running time (equal to approximately 2 minutes of playing time) following each 15-second period of continuous spectator protest. Some 15 such episodes of extended crowd abuse were recorded during two seasons of play. Using multiple measures of performance (i.e., scoring, turnovers, violations, and a composite index), Greer's analyses yielded results consistent with both officiating and crowd influence interpretations. The effect of sustained booing was to further widen the performance gap that already favors the home team during periods of normal crowd activity. However, as Greer notes, "most of the performance differences between home and visiting teams during the postprotest periods was accounted for by the deterioration of visiting team performance" (p. 257).

Similar results were obtained in a second study of basketball performance. Using the 1971–1981 records of the Atlantic Coast Conference, Silva and Andrew (1987) sought to identify the source of the home (court) advantage. Do home teams play better than usual, or do visitors play worse, or both? Using a criterion of coaches' performance standards, the records revealed substandard performances by visiting teams in the categories of field goals, turnovers, and personal fouls.

The results of another study of crowd influences, this time in hockey (Russell, 1983a), led to a similar conclusion. Inasmuch as larger and larger crowds should produce increasingly stronger effects on performers, a positive correlation between crowd size and the performance (i.e., goals) of the home team would be predicted. However, over a full season of play the relationship was nonsignificant. There was instead a negative relationship between crowd size and the performance of visiting teams. Thus, as the numbers of spectators in attendance rose, there was a corresponding deterioration in the play of visiting teams. It would appear from these studies that partisan spectators do little to improve the performance of the home team but rather disrupt the play of visitors to a significant degree.

Three studies (Greer, 1983; Russell, 1983a; Silva & Andrew, 1987), then, confirm the importance of crowd influences as a contributor to the home advantage, although the processes creating the advantage differ from those espoused by popular belief. At the same time, learning, officiating, and perhaps travel-related factors remain as viable explanations for the home field advantage. The relative contributions of these factors in favoring home teams is clearly not fixed. Their impact can be expected to vary widely from sport to sport and with the circumstances and structure of competitive play.

An Exception

Is the Home Field Always Advantageous?

Is the home field always advantageous? Apparently not! In the case of a do-or-die championship game, the home team is more likely to die. The circumstances in which enthusiastic and supportive hometown fans actually bring about the downfall of their athlete(s) appear confined to that final performance that determines gold or silver, the green jacket at Augusta, or the champions of whatever for 1992. These paradoxical effects have been the focus of a research program by psychologist Roy Baumeister of Case Western Reserve University. In a series of investigations (e.g., Baumeister, 1984, 1985; Baumeister & Steinhilber, 1984; Tice, Buder, & Baumeister, 1985), Baumeister and his colleagues have demonstrated that skilled performances may be seriously impaired in circumstances where enthusiasms and expectations for success on the part of the home crowd run high.

A preliminary point should first be noted. Audience pressures are not felt equally by all performers (cf. Latané & Nida, 1980). It appears that those who characteristically focus their attention away from the self and toward the external environment are more susceptible to audience influence. For these *low self-conscious* competitors, audience sentiments are more salient, and consequently they stand to be more easily affected (Heaton & Sigall, 1991).

Sports, of course, are rife with stories of the hometown hero who, even with the backing of his fans, choked under pressure. Not only did Casey strike out before his loyal supporters in Mudville, but so, too, do players in final championship games in baseball and basketball (Baumeister & Steinhilber, 1984). However, the phenomenon is not confined to team sports. An analysis of the records of play in the British Open Golf Championship revealed that the play of British golfers deteriorated more than that of the foreign entrants from the first to the final rounds of the tournament (Wright, Jackson, Christie, McGuire, & Wright, 1991).

Data from team play yields similar findings. Using the records of World Series baseball performances during the period 1924–1982, Baumeister and Steinhilber (1984) found that although home teams tended to win the first two games of a series, they tended to lose the last game. As can be seen in Figure 2.3, the home field *disadvantage* is even more pronounced when the analysis is restricted to the seventh and defining game.

Which Team Creates the Gap?

Does the home team choke in the decisive game, or do the visitors rise to an outstanding performance? Analyses based on fielding errors suggest that the home team chokes. During the first two games of a series, the visitors commit more errors, whereas the home team makes more errors in the seventh game. Further analysis shows that the number of fielding errors by visitors remains constant throughout the series, whereas those of the home team increase significantly in the seventh game. A similar conclusion was reached using the number of error-less games as a measure of performance. Again, flawless play is far more likely to be exhibited by home teams in the opening games of a series, with a reversal occurring in the seventh.

Underlying Causes

What causes the deterioration in play by home teams in the decisive game? Baumeister and Steinhilber (1984) found an answer to this question by examining the outcomes of Game 6 in seven-game series. Each team in this game faces a different type of pressure. For one team a loss means final defeat; for the other there is an opportunity to clinch final victory. An analysis of outcomes in Game 6 revealed a disproportionate number of wins by the home team when it faced elimination but a tendency to lose when it was on the brink of a final victory. The authors also found a similar pattern in the records of the National Basketball Association. By this line of reasoning, choking when success appears imminent rather than the alternative explanation of avoiding defeat seems a more plausible description of the underlying dynamics.

A further question remains unanswered. Specifically, what process is involved in the choking phenomenon when success is at hand? There are several possibilities. Briefly, it may be that the heightened self-awareness produced by a supportive and expectant crowd diverts the local athletes' attention away from the cues essential to a superior performance. These "self-presentation" concerns (see Baumeister, 1984, pp. 85–86) are greatest for the home players inasmuch as the home crowd is especially sympathetic and supportive of their efforts. Thus, a lo-

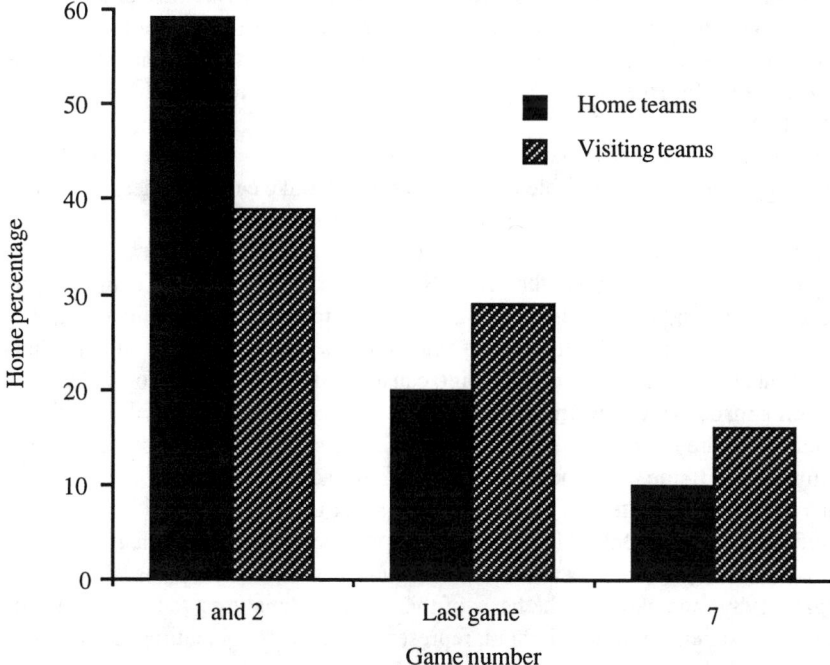

FIGURE 2.3 World Series game winners 1924–1982 (adapted from Baumeister & Steinhilber, 1984).

cal high jumper prematurely visualizing herself on the top step of the victory podium during her preparation for her final jump may misjudge her approach. Rather than claiming her long-sought *identity* as gold medalist, she must instead graciously settle for silver.

An alternative model would see the heightened self-awareness causing the competitor to focus on the components of an already well-tuned and coordinated sequence of motor responses with disruptive results (Baumeister, 1984). The local golfer playing in the final threesome of his club's regional tournament may begin to analyze the swing that has taken him to the top of the leader board through earlier rounds, again with disastrous results.

More recently, a third explanation has been suggested. Whereas home teams poised on the brink of success in the final game of a championship series seemingly choke for reasons of self-presentational concerns and self-attention, Heaton and Sigall (1989) additionally propose that they come up short as a result of *fearing failure*. The imminent possibility of a new and unwanted identity, that of "loser," earned in the presence of one's most ardent supporters is a frightening prospect, one that leads to choking in the defining game. Support for Heaton and Sigall's hypothesis was sought in the World Series records covering the same time period used by Baumeister and Steinhilber (1984). However, Heaton and

Sigall compared Game 7 with Games 1 through 6, whereas Baumeister and Stein-hilber compared Game 7 only with Games 1 and 2. Interestingly, home teams in Game 7 lose only marginally more often ($p < .10$) than they do in the first six games. Thus, by Heaton and Sigall's analysis, the championship choke is some-what less striking.

Let me emphasize that Game 7 is totally different from all earlier games in the series. Recovery is not possible if things go badly. Unlike earlier games, there is no "next time"; one is either a champion or a loser. Heaton and Sigall (1989) reasoned that a fear of acquiring a negative identity causes choking. Such a fear is justified for a team falling behind in the score. Specifically, as a team falls behind in the seventh game and the prospect of losing becomes more of a reality, the possibility that the players may shortly assume identities as losers becomes salient. Self-attention concerns increase at this point, causing a disruption in performance.

Being made acutely aware of an impending negative identity by falling behind, home teams are far less likely than visitors to regain the lead, in the seventh game. Fully 46% of home teams never recover from relinquishing the lead in contrast to only 12% of visiting teams. However, the first six games in a World Series reveal a different pattern. Only 24% of home teams failed to regain the lead, whereas 35% of visiting teams were unable to overcome an early deficit. Thus, Heaton and Sigall (1989) conclude, on the basis of this and other analyses, that a fear of fail-ure, made salient by falling behind, represents a further explanation of the cham-pionship choke. As a consequence, both impending failure (Heaton & Sigall, 1989) and impending success (Baumeister & Steinhilber, 1984) can lead to chok-ing, albeit for quite different reasons.

However, a word of caution: One may not be able to freely generalize these findings to all sports. Gayton et al. (1987) were unable to find evidence of a home ice disadvantage in hockey using the records of Stanley Cup championship play from 1960 to 1985. They suggest that the demands on hockey players are such that they only rarely have opportunities to adopt the narrow internal focus of attention thought to facilitate self-presentation concerns. Thus, our local high jumper and golfer (above) had ample time to reflect on the implications of the moment, where-as the structure of hockey requires players to attend constantly to external de-mands. In effect, self-presentation concerns may not be activated in some sports with the result that the predicted margin of disadvantage fails to materialize.

Is the championship choke a fading phenomenon? This intriguing question was raised by Heaton and Sigall (1989). The difficulties experienced by home teams in performing well in championship games initially stems from the extra pres-sures brought to bear by the live presence of enthusiastic and supportive fans. In contrast, the visitors' fans are, for the most part, geographically distant. However, Heaton and Sigall point out that through the miracle of television the visitors' own distant fans and millions of others are in some sense right there with them in the stadium. As television coverage of championship games expands to include more viewers and additional sports, these distant audiences will increasingly find their way into the consciousness of athletes. More and more visitors, too, will be playing in front of supportive audiences. They, too, will begin to experience the pressures previously reserved for home teams. Perhaps, as Heaton and Sigall suggest, the next generation of sports psychologists will look back on the championship choke as something of a historical curiosity. While much remains to be learned about the effects of audiences on performers in sports and in other areas of human endeavor, the research of Baumeister and his colleagues has given us an exciting beginning.

Crowd Size and Performance

Active, Partisan Spectators

In considering the impact of crowd size on performance, it is important to maintain a distinction between the experiences of local and visiting athletes. Most of the evidence, scant though it is, derives from major team sports in which expressive audiences attempt to influence the emotional states and skill of athletes. Generally speaking, encouragement is provided the home team, whereas the efforts of visitors are met with derision and hostility. The effects of "razzing" have already been shown to be extremely disruptive in Laird's (1923) fraternity study as well as in other investigations (e.g., Silva, 1979).

Two archival studies conducted specifically in sports settings have produced somewhat conflicting results. Paulus, Judd, and Bernstein (1976) sought to assess the relationships between attendance and performance in the American and National baseball leagues using the records of a full season of play. The results of their initial analysis were largely uninterpretable. However, when they combined the data from both leagues, runs by the home team and errors by the visitors were found to be negatively related to crowd size. Similar results were obtained by Kerr and Yukelson (1977) in their analysis of basketball records. For teams on the road, better free-throw performances were found to be associated with larger crowds. One of the factors likely producing these counterintuitive relationships is the caliber of visiting teams. That is to say, larger crowds turn out when the better teams come to town. Against generally better teams, the home team is predictably less apt to do well.

A somewhat different set of results was obtained in a study of crowd size in relation to hockey performance (Russell, 1983a; see also Greer, 1983). In this regard, a number of writers have suggested that crowd *density* rather than the sheer numbers of spectators in attendance may exert the stronger effects on athletes (e.g., Mann, 1979; Paulus et al., 1976). Certainly, the suggestion has merit. The 5,500 screaming spectators who fill my local arena would scarcely be noticed, much less influence the athletes, when scattered about the Houston Astrodome. As noted above in conjunction with the home advantage, crowd size was unrelated to goals by home teams but negatively related to goals by visitors. Interestingly, crowd density was negatively related to the *combined* goal performance of home and visiting teams, whereas the relationship between density and goals by visiting teams fell short of significance ($p < .10$). However, in the interests of providing some perspective on the practical importance of the variables of crowd size and density, their power to predict performance was determined overall to be quite weak (Russell, 1983a).

Passive, Neutral Spectators

Of course, sports are not always performed in the presence of boisterous spectators. Many sports and recreational pursuits involve a solitary performance, often with no one present. At other times a coach and/or a few observers may be looking on. Certainly, athletes putting in those long hours of arduous training for their event attract little or no attention from the general public. However, as social creatures, we are not oblivious to the presence of others. A question of long-standing interest to social psychologists has been the influence of bystanders on human performance (e.g., Meumann, 1904, cited in Cottrell, 1972). To be sure, the question has implications for a wide range of endeavors, from the stage, to the workplace, to seminar presentations, to the diving platform. The topic is generally referred to as *social facilitation* and pertains to those settings in which one performs a task in the presence of generally passive onlookers.

Early research on this question yielded a mixed and perplexing set of results. Some investigations showed performance increments; an almost equal number showed decrements in the presence of passive spectators (Cottrell, 1972; Geen, 1980). Research waned until Robert Zajonc published a major paper in 1965 in which a successful theoretical resolution of the previously conflicting findings in this area was achieved.

Briefly, spectators are seen as a source of drive arousal. This heightened state of arousal is presumed to facilitate the performance of well-learned or simple skills. However, if a skill is not well-learned or complex, the increase in arousal will interfere with its performance. The underlying notion is that an increase in drive arousal favors the emission of the performer's dominant responses. In the case of a polished performer, her dominant responses are presumed to be largely "correct" ones. Her performance stands to be improved with an audience present. In a case where the performer is still struggling to master a skill, incorrect responses are present in abundance and are thereby presumed to be dominant responses. As a consequence, onlookers can only worsen the performance of a beginner. Hence, the performer's level of skill and the complexity of the skill itself will determine whether an audience helps or hinders a performance.

Support for the model's basic assumption that the presence of others is a source of arousal has generally been forthcoming. Latané and Harkins (1976) have shown that the presence of an audience produces tension in a performer, tension that increases with the size of the audience. The amount of tension created for a performer is further influenced by the makeup of the audience. For university-age subjects, audiences in their late 30s produced two to three times more tension than did teenage audiences. On the other hand, male audiences generated only somewhat greater tension than those comprised of females. The next logical question is, How can we account for social facilitation?

A number of explanations for social facilitation have been advanced, and for each there is some evidence to support the view. One long-standing issue centers on whether the source of the drive is innate (Zajonc, 1965, 1980) or learned (Cottrell, 1972). More specifically, one view holds that the mere presence of others is sufficient to increase arousal (see Zajonc, 1980, on this point).

An alternative to the innate model proposes that the presence of others induces *evaluation apprehension*; that is, the performers feel that they are in some way being judged or evaluated by the observers, and anxiety is increased as a result. Comprehensive reviews of these positions and the relevant research have been provided by Geen and Gange (1977) and Guerin (1986); and a meta-analysis has been provided by Bond and Titus (1983). Instead of pursuing the relative merits of this and other issues on social facilitation, it may be more instructive for present purposes to first consider several tests conducted in sports.

The studies to follow did not yield uniform results. This is perhaps fitting insofar as it is an accurate reflection of the broader set of investigations conducted in athletic settings (cf. Bell & Yee, 1989). A field investigation by Tice, Buder, and Baumeister (1985) points up the critical importance of subjects' ages in social facilitation research. Their study was conducted in a video arcade using three groups of skilled players, namely, children (under 12), adolescents (14–19), and adults (20 and older). Children showed improved performance in the presence of an attentive observer, whereas the performance of adolescents suffered markedly. Adults showed only a modest decline from the alone to the observer conditions. The variable of age, then, is an important directional determinant and should be taken into account in the design of research on social facilitation as well as in comparisons across studies.

An Australian squash center served as the setting for an interesting study by Forgas, Brennan, Howe, Kane, and Sweet (1980). The presence of an audience produced a general deterioration in the quality of play across the conditions of the study. However, within pairs of expert and novice players, the expert members showed performance decrements, whereas their novice partners showed improved performances with an audience present—just the opposite effects of those predicted by Zajonc's (1965) theory! While the authors acknowledge that any of several explanations could be offered for their results, their preference is a cognitive one. In the absence of an audience, the play is a competition with both players making every effort to excel. However, in the audience condition players interpret the situation as one calling for them to be seen as part of a smoothly functioning unit. As a consequence, the caliber of their play drew closer together. This subtle *automatic matching* process favored by Forgas et al. has much to recommend it and further highlights the role of cognitions in mediating the effects of an audience on athletes.

Social facilitation effects have also been examined on a *simple* sports task (Strube, Miles, & Finch, 1981). This time, the setting was the field house at the University of Utah and the subjects were a contingent of recreational joggers comprised of students, faculty, and staff. The joggers were unobtrusively timed as they ran alone or before inattentive and attentive male/female spectators. Only attentive observers, irrespective of gender, were associated with faster running times. The authors interpreted their results as arising from the conflict created when one attempts to attend to the task at hand *and* to interested spectators. This conflict produces drivelike effects (R.S. Baron, Moore, & Sanders, 1978) that in the present case enhanced the joggers' performance.

A major study in this sample of sports investigations of social facilitation examined the performances of gymnastic students on a floor exercise routine (Paulus, Shannon, Wilson, & Boone, 1972). This study deserves special mention insofar as a truly "alone" condition was created by means of a video camera filming from a concealed position. With the experimenter absent, subjects performed alone or before a group of 17 of their fellow students, who watched passively. One of the principal findings was a performance decrement among subjects, especially those more highly skilled, in the audience condition. The authors proposed a modification to the Zajonc (1965) model in which dominant responses approach a ceiling such that under increasingly higher levels of arousal, the probability of subordinate (i.e., incorrect) responses being emitted now increases. This extension to the model posits an inverted-U curve to describe the relationship between arousal and performance on well-learned complex tasks. Interestingly, the highest levels of arousal were apparently created for the gymnasts by giving them advance knowledge that they were to perform in front of their peers.

Earlier it was mentioned that there are sharp differences of opinion on whether social facilitation arises from the mere presence of another person (Zajonc, 1965) or from the subjects' apprehensions that they are being evaluated in some fashion by that person (Cottrell, 1972). In a carefully designed experiment, Schmitt, Gilovich, Goore, and Joseph (1986) have convincingly demonstrated that evaluation apprehension is not a *necessary* condition for social facilitation effects to occur. Subjects in all three of their conditions (alone, merely present, evaluative) were asked to enter their name and a code on a computer before the experiment ostensibly got under way. Subjects in the *mere presence* condition found themselves in the company of a confederate who was otherwise occupied and who wore a blindfold and earphones. Those in the evaluation apprehension condition entered their names and codes into the computer with the experimenter looking over their shoulder. The experimental task required subjects to enter their names in the computer (simple task) and, for coding purposes, also to enter their names backward with the letters interspersed by ascending numbers (complex task). At this point, the subjects were suddenly debriefed and thanked for coming out. It could be said that this experiment was over before it even began.

The pattern of results was perfectly consistent with social facilitation theory. Those performing the simple task with the confederate either merely present or in a position to evaluate them were faster than those assigned to the alone condition. For the complex task, the opposite was found. Subjects were slower in the merely present and evaluative conditions. Both viewpoints, the merely present and evaluation apprehension, thus draw support from this experiment as they have from numerous other investigations. It is not a matter of having to choose. As Schmitt et al. (1986) conclude,

> These two rival interpretations are perfectly harmonious. No advocate of the mere presence hypothesis, for example, would deny that evaluation apprehension is an important variable that can indeed increase people's general arousal level and thus further facilitate their dominant response tendencies. (p. 246)

Indeed, subjects performing the simple task under evaluative conditions were faster yet again then their counterparts in the mere presence condition. Presumably, the presence of the experimenter peering over their shoulders produced an additional measure of arousal that improved their performance even further.

Summary

To conclude, the truly social side of our nature is revealed in the foregoing sections. Our performance can be profoundly influenced by others regardless of whether they are active in their role as spectators or merely quiet observers. Indeed, as private a matter as the expectations of another can determine one's success in mastering a sport. This is a matter of some importance inasmuch as predictions based on theoretical models and lab results sometimes fail for support in sports settings. Hypothesis testing in sports not only can increase the generalizability of laboratory findings but, in turn, often reveals the need for modification of existing models (e.g., Forgas et al., 1980; Paulus et al., 1972). A social experimental lab approach and field investigations in sports, as elsewhere, are complementary and stand to enrich each other while furthering our understanding of social influence.

Suggested Readings

Barnett, S.A. (1988). *Biology and freedom.* New York: Cambridge University Press.
   An entertaining and authoritative assessment of the ethological view.

Schmitt, B.H., Gilovich, T., Goore, N., & Joseph, L. (1986). Mere presence and social facilitation: One more time. *Journal of Experimental Social Psychology,* 22, 242–248.
   An excellent example of the application of scientific reasoning and the clever application of experimental design in pursuit of answers to the long-standing issue of "mere presence" effects.

Snyder, M. (1984). When belief creates reality. In L. Berkowitz (Ed.), *Advances in experimental social psychology* (Vol. 18, pp. 247–305). New York: Academic Press.

The powerful and often unrecognized role of self-fulfilling prophecies in influencing human affairs is demonstrated in a variety of social situations.

3

Social Theory and Performance

This chapter will feature coverage of *attribution* and *self-efficacy* theories. Both theories have emerged in recent years and have already provided valuable insights and enriched our understanding of sport and recreational processes. While they have been shown to have applications to a wide variety of fields, our immediate interest lies primarily with those studies that have tested aspects of the theories within sports settings. Our choice of studies on the pages ahead will, of course, reflect that interest.

Attribution Theory

Our need to understand the reasons for our own behaviors and those of others is part of an ongoing process by which we hope to be able to predict and, to some extent, control those situations in which we find ourselves. What caused me to bowl 40 points below my average in the company bowling tournament? Was it an unusual number of headpins? I do recall feeling poorly for most of the day. Why did our basketball team lose last Saturday's game? Was it because of biased officiating, or did those injuries to two of our key players cause the loss? It is this fairly complex process of obtaining information about our own or another's behavior and assigning (causal) responsibility for those actions that is at the heart of attribution theory.

Attributions abound in sports. Following an athletic contest of any consequence, the coaches, players, fans, sportscasters, and armchair quarterbacks analyze and try to arrive at some understanding of the reasons for the outcome. Irrespective of whether the team (or player) won or lost, the explanations that are given can be classified as either *internal* or *external* in origin. In the case of losses, internal attributions might, for example, include a lack of ability or effort by the athlete; external attributions might be made to poor officiating or bad luck. Similarly, success can be attributed to internal or external causes. When we win it is because "our team has a surplus of talent" or "our team was better prepared for the game" (internal). Alternatively, we could say "Lady Luck was on our side" or, "Our fans were great, they made the difference" (external).

A theoretical framework proposed by Kelley (1972) has proven particularly effective in predicting whether our observation of another person and his or her circumstances will prompt us to attribute that person's behavior to internal or external causes. In particular, we attend to three important factors in making a determination of the locus of causality: consensus, consistency, and distinctiveness. *Consensus* refers to the degree to which others would be expected to react in a fashion similar to that of the person we are observing. *Consistency* relates to whether the person we are observing has reacted in the same way in this situation on previous occasions. *Distinctiveness* refers to the extent that the person we are observing reacts in a similar fashion to other, *different* situations.

According to Kelley's (1972) theory, it is the combination of high or low conditions on each of these three dimensions that guides us in making either an internal or an external attribution. To illustrate, we are likely to attribute another's behavior to *internal* causes under the conditions of low consensus, high consistency, and low distinctiveness. In contrast, where the situation involves high consensus, high consistency, and high distinctiveness, we are more apt to attribute another person's behavior to *external* causes. Of course, these combinations provide the clearest predictions. Other combinations may yield a mix of internal and external attributions. Perhaps a simple example will clarify how the theory works in practice.

Your friend is a ranking tennis player in your region and has invited you along to see her play in the third round of a major tournament. Midway through the first set, you and most of the other spectators are shocked to see her storm off the court, forfeiting the match, after a series of close calls by one of the linesmen went against her. Her attitude toward the official was accusatory and her language abusive. What could have caused her outburst? Is the linesman actually inept or showing favoritism, or is your friend just ill-tempered? Consider now the circumstances of your friend's behavior in relation to Kelley's (1972) three dimensions. First, other players have not been challenging the calls of this particular linesman (i.e., low consensus). Second, you recall that your friend stomped off the court last year when this same linesman was officiating (i.e., high consistency). Finally, you have seen her do something very similar when things don't go her way in golf and bridge games (i.e., low distinctiveness). Chances are that you would be drawn to the conclusion that her behavior originates with internal causes. In all likelihood, you would decide that her outburst was the result of her immaturity and lack of self-control.

In contrast, your friend's unseemly behavior might be interpreted quite differently with different dimensional information available to you. For instance, you are aware that a number of other players in the tournament have had occasion to challenge this linesman's calls (i.e., high consensus). Moreover, there have been other occasions when your friend angrily forfeited her matches with this linesman assigned to her court (i.e., high consistency) and, indeed, has shown nothing resembling this behavior in the other activities in which you share an interest (i.e., high distinctiveness). Under this set of circumstances you would likely find yourself leaning toward an external attribution for your friend's behavior, such as that the linesman is myopic or biased, or both.

The general framework described above is, however, subject to several modifying principles. First and foremost, the two principles of *discounting* and *augmenting* are seen to operate when we are aware of several potential causes of another's behavior. Let us suppose that your friend is taking his final test for a Red Cross lifesaving certificate. The judge, who is known to have exacting standards, fails him. How would you explain your friend's poor showing? In all likelihood, you would attribute the cause of his failure to the judge who has such unreasonable expectations. However, suppose you also know that your friend has spent more time in the pub than in the pool in recent weeks. Given this additional information, either cause, the demanding judge or your friend's lack of preparation, would be given less weight and be seen as less important in bringing about your friend's downfall. Thus, consistent with the attribution of discounting, the availability of multiple explanations tends to lessen the certainty with which we attribute behavior to any single cause.

We might now envision another scenario in which your friend trained properly and passed his test. Now the principle of augmenting comes into play. You would be extremely confident that your friend's ability and hard work saw him through the test, especially as he had to overcome the added obstacle of a tough examiner. When a factor working against a performance is present along with a factor working for a performance, we give extra weight to the factor facilitating the performance; that is, our friend's ability is now seen as a *very* important factor in his success.

While attribution theories are generally useful in helping us understand the actions of ourselves and others, they are at the same time open to a number of sources of bias. The first of these is the *fundamental attribution error,* whereby observers tend to adopt a dispositional (internal) attribution at the expense of situational (external) causes. To illustrate, we learn from a news broadcast that the quarterback of our local team has admitted taking a bribe prior to last Saturday's game. No details are available. At this juncture, most of us would be likely to attribute his actions to a character flaw (e.g., dishonesty, greed). Other plausible explanations do not come to mind as readily. However, he may have acted as he did in order to pay for an operation on his critically ill child! (Admittedly, I am reaching.) In other words, the fundamental attribution error involves the tendency to attribute another person's behavior to some relatively enduring trait, that is, to emphasize the disposition of the person and largely ignore plausible explanations that might arise from the circumstances.

Another major source of error is the *self-serving bias* (sometimes called a hedonic bias). A consistent finding of attribution research is a general tendency for people to attribute their successes to internal causes and to make external attributions for their failures (Miller & Ross, 1975). For example, consider your friend's transparent explanations for having *won* at the Friday night poker game. Are you not more likely to hear him say "Actually, I've always been pretty good at poker; I'm not surprised that I won $10.00" (internal attribution) rather than "It was just pure luck that I won" (external). In contrast, his explanation following a *losing* night at the table is more likely to be along the lines of "I just wasn't getting the cards" (external) rather than "I bet foolishly all evening" (internal). A self-serving bias, then, points to the fact that we are quick to take personal credit for our success but reluctant to take responsibility for our shortcomings. Instead, we tend to see our failures as being the result of bad luck or other external factors.

It follows from the above that a self-serving bias would be strongest among those individuals who are the most centrally involved in an athletic performance, namely, the athletes. Among those less centrally involved (i.e., coaches, fans, and media representatives), the bias would predictably be less strong. The intense commitment and involvement required of those competing at the highest levels of their sport would similarly lead one to predict a greater use of self-serving attributions than would be found among those competing at lower levels of their sport. Several of the studies discussed below address these very points.

Bird and Brame (1978) provide a clear illustration of the operation of a self-serving bias in women's basketball. Winning players were found to give greater credit to a team effort (internal) for their victories than did losers. These same players more frequently implicated luck (external) as a contributing factor when they suffered a loss. Other sports studies, however, have yielded mixed results.

Alpine skiing provided a setting for testing a self-serving bias under conditions that might be presumed to represent increasing degrees of ego-involvement (Riess & Taylor, 1984). Skiers are rated by the United States Ski Association according to a fivefold classification system ranging from state level competitions (Levels 1, 2, and 3) to regional and national levels (4 and 5). Inasmuch as races officially increase in importance from Levels 1 through 5, it was assumed that the racers themselves would, as a consequence, be more personally involved in their performances at the higher levels. The authors further reasoned that topflight skiers would, as a result, be more likely to resort to self-serving explanations as a means of preserving their self-esteem. However, the racers' degree of involvement was unrelated to the attributions they made for successful and unsuccessful performances. Generally speaking, the racers overall were found to credit internal factors when they performed well (i.e., ability, effort). This tendency to enlist a self-serving explanation following success did not, however, extend to those skiers whose best efforts met with failure. Their attributions were evenly divided between internal (e.g., strength, concentration) and external reasons (e.g., weather, course conditions, wax).

The degree to which attributions are stable (i.e., a permanent versus a temporary cause) and controllable (i.e., by the player or anyone else) has also been examined in conjunction with a self-serving bias (Mark, Mutrie, Brooks, & Harris, 1984). Studies of squash and racquetball players revealed that winners provided attributions that were more stable and controllable than those offered by their vanquished opponents. However, support for a self-serving bias was not forthcoming; winners and losers did not differ in terms of ascribing the outcomes of their performances to internal causes. While not dismissing other findings of a self-serving bias in sports (e.g., McAuley & Gross, 1983), Mark et al. conclude that "stability and controllability differences may be more prevalent in sports settings than locus of causality differences" (p. 193). Their conclusion draws support from a recent study of basketball players, coaches, and spectators that produced a similar pattern of findings (Grove, Hanrahan, & McInman, 1991). Again, both winning and losing outcomes were attributed to internal factors. Additionally, winners again offered attributions that were more stable and controllable.

There may be good reason that it has proven difficult to consistently demonstrate a self-serving bias in sports. Scanlon and Passer (1980) suggest that both the norms surrounding many individualized sports and the sports setting itself do not make it easy for losers to attribute their failure to external sources. For example, the standardized and homogeneous conditions of play in squash and racquetball (e.g., temperature, lighting, court, ball, absence of a referee) leave little by way of an external attribution available to the loser (e.g., Mark et al., 1984). The *attributional dilemma* facing the athlete, then, may to a large extent be predetermined and resolved in favor of an internal locus. In essence, there may be little else to blame but oneself.

Media Attributions

Attribution theory has also been tested in a series of archival investigations (Lau & Russell, 1980; Peterson, 1980; Watkins, 1986). Richard Lau and Dan Russell set about to test attribution predictions in the sports section of our daily newspapers. Their analysis of 107 newspaper accounts of football and baseball games yielded 594 explanations offered by players, coaches, and sportswriters for the outcomes of the contests. As shown in Figure 3.1, there was a tendency for both the athletes and their coaches, and the even more peripheral sportswriters, to attribute wins to internal causes. However, following a loss, players, coaches, and writers alike are equally likely to attribute the outcome to internal factors. In fact, the explanations offered for failure by both groups did not differ in their locus of attribution (i.e., internal versus external). The latter finding is in agreement with the general pattern of results in attribution research (e.g., Miller & Ross, 1975). That is to say, a self-serving bias is generally evident following success and, although predicted, does not consistently occur following failure. Such was the case in the present instance and in the earlier study of alpine ski racers (Riess & Taylor, 1984).

A replication of the Lau and Russell (1980) study was undertaken using sports stories appearing in two major New Zealand newspapers. Watkins's (1986) analysis was based on 105 stories that offered explanations for successful and unsuccessful performances in a variety of sports ranging from cricket to huskie racing. As in the earlier studies, attributions were again mostly internal following wins (81%) and, to a lesser extent, also internal following losses (58%).

The third study in this archival series revealed clearer support for attributional predictions. Peterson (1980) found that over a full season of National Football League play coaches and players consistently made internal attributions for victories. As would be predicted (Miller & Ross, 1975), external attributions were made for losses but only during the early part of the season. Attributions became increasingly internal as the season progressed. This trend was apparent regardless of whether the teams were enjoying a successful or a losing season. Perhaps players and coaches alike recognize that external attributions (e.g., luck, biased officiating) have a shorter shelf life than do internal attributions and feel increasingly pressured to acknowledge that their shortcomings may have more to do with a lack of ability, effort, or preparation. In short, after a time external attributions begin to sound more like lame excuses and less like believable explanations.

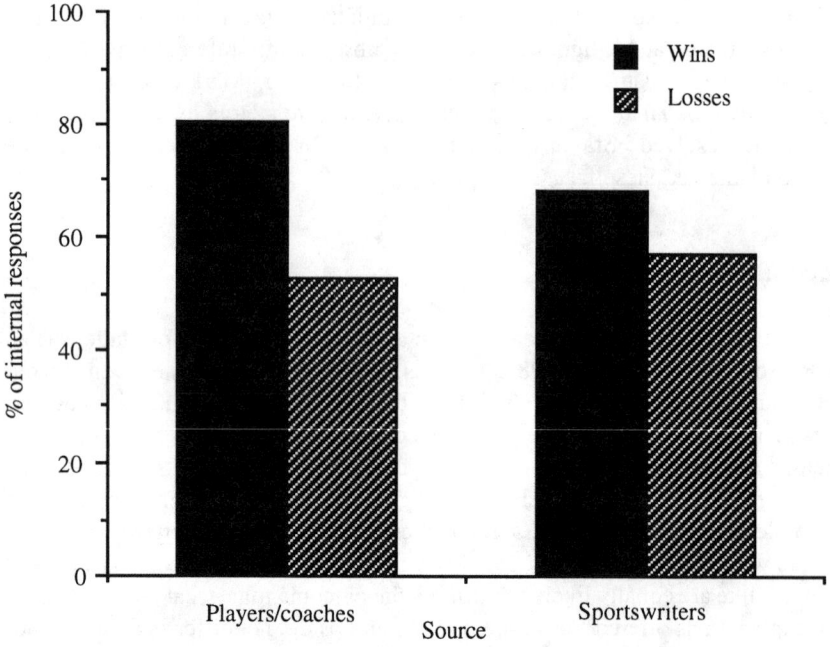

FIGURE 3.1 Attributions for wins and losses (adapted from Lau & Russell, 1980).

Alternatively, Peterson (1980) suggests that increased attempts at coping may follow from the expression of internal attributions for past performances insofar as such statements may represent an assertion of personal efficacy. (Self-efficacy is an upcoming topic in this chapter.) He proposes a "wait until next year" effect whereby increased self-efficacy coupled with an expectation of control over future events conveys the promise of a better result in the future.

The critical reader may already have noticed that several "social" factors have been overlooked in the studies described thus far. One might ask, as Zaccaro, Peterson, and Walker (1987) did, whether self-serving attributions would differ for athletes in individual as opposed to team sports. Might attributions not also differ between team sports that are strongly interdependent (e.g., basketball and football) and those where the skills of team members are not interdependent (e.g., bowling)?

As regards individual versus team performances, it is generally recognized that as a group increases in size there is a diffusion of responsibility among the members for outcomes resulting from their joint efforts. This fact alone would suggest that fewer self-serving attributions will be offered in the team situation. Also, as overall team performance increasingly relies on the harmonious integration of members' playing skills (i.e., more interdependent), less by way of individual member attributions for success would be predicted. After all, to claim the credit for success at the expense of teammates is to indirectly detract from their contributions.

In the main, these predictions were confirmed. Zaccaro et al. (1987) found that self-serving attributions for success were clearly more common among solo performers than among team performers. Also, the locus of attributions differed in a comparison of explanations offered for success in relatively independent sports compared to highly interdependent sports. Following success in independent team sports, players and coaches made more "member-internal attributions than group-internal attributions" (p. 261). In team sports where group performances are more interdependent, success was likely to be explained by group-internal causes, for example, "We really came together as a team tonight." This tendency to make group-internal attributions possibly serves the interests of improved team performance through enhancing the self-esteem of individual members and increasing group cohesiveness.

The operation of a self-serving bias may explain some team failures. In particular, a case can be made for a self-serving bias having a potentially disruptive effect on team harmony. To take the simplest case of "doubles" play, each player tends privately to take credit for whatever success the pair enjoys. When the team loses, there is an equally strong tendency for both players to place responsibility for their failure on their partner (an external attribution). To the extent that a self-serving bias is operating and fault attributed to a teammate, the stage is set for an increase in tensions, if not open conflict.

An additional factor that can affect attributional judgments is whether the outcome of a competition was expected or unexpected (Feather & Simon, 1971). This expectancy view holds that anticipated outcomes, be they a win or a loss, will tend to be attributed to internal causes (e.g., ability, hard work). On the other hand, unexpected wins or losses will result in people offering more external explanations (e.g., playing conditions, luck). However, this view has been buttressed mainly by the results of lab investigations; support has not been forthcoming when the predictions have been tested on the pages of the sports section. As mentioned previously (Lau & Russell, 1980), wins were followed more often by internal attributions than were losses; at the same time, there was no indication that expected or unexpected outcomes differentially affected the locus of attributions. This finding was echoed in the results of Watkins's (1986) analysis of New Zealand sports stories. However, both the Watkins study and that of Lau and Russell reveal that players, coaches, and writers alike provide a greater *number* of explanations for unexpected outcomes. It is generally the case that people are more likely in practice to make attributional judgments following the unusual or unexpected. We are not disposed to engage in thoughtful causal analyses of outcomes that were predicted or commonplace.

A further feature of the attribution model (Weiner, 1979), noted previously in this chapter, makes a distinction between *stable* and *unstable* explanations. In the context of Lau and Russell's (1980) study, explanations that make the same prediction now and in future games (e.g., opposing a better team) were regarded as stable. If attributions were made to factors that are not constant in their effects on performance (e.g., effort), then the researchers classified them as unstable. The model predicts that stable attributions will be made for both expected wins and expected losses. Although the generalizability of findings stood to be increased in shifting from the laboratory setting that previously provided support for the hypothesis (e.g., Feather & Simon, 1971; Weiner, Frieze, Kukla, Rest, & Rosenbaum, 1971) to the sports newsroom, the results proved disappointing. The prediction failed for support.[1] Of additional interest is the finding that fully two thirds of all attributions made to the press were classified as unstable, a result also seen in the New Zealand data (Watkins, 1986). The ubiquitous attribution of *effort* is evident in their results and once again highlights "the strong preference for explanations involving effort (such as great concentration or making a spectacular play) on the part of their team or the other team by attributors" (Lau & Russell, 1980, p. 35).

Through Rose-Colored Glasses: Fans' Attributions

One might anticipate that the close emotional ties observed between devoted fans and their team (Cialdini et al., 1976) would likely give rise to biased performance attributions. This is clearly the case (e.g., Hastorf & Cantril, 1954; Mann, 1974; Winkler & Taylor, 1979). A pattern of attributional bias is seen in a(n) (air)field study by Winkler and Taylor, conducted in part aboard an airliner en route from Chicago to Seattle. Passengers who were enthusiastic supporters of either the Dallas Cowboys or Pittsburgh Steelers football teams were recruited and asked to make causal attributions relative to the 1976 Superbowl championship. Pittsburgh had defeated Dallas by a score of 21 to 17. In addition to providing ratings of the strength of their respective teams, the subjects were also asked to attribute the outcome to good/bad play factors and to situational factors (e.g., luck). A further question asked subjects if their team would be likely to repeat the favorable and unfavorable aspects of their game were a rematch to be held.

The results were straightforward. Credit was taken by fans for the successes of their team; at the same time, they gave less credit to the opposing team for successful aspects of its play. Moreover, events favorable to their team (e.g., a series of quarterback sacks) were thought likely to recur in a rematch, whereas unfavorable events (e.g., a series of pass interceptions) would be unlikely to happen in any future game with their Superbowl opponents. Finally, fans of both football squads felt that outcomes favorable to the other team and outcomes unfavorable to their own team could have been prevented with better play and tactics.

Sports fans are generally outspoken. They are more than willing to comment on the overall quality of play and to offer their analyses; also, they seem especially sensitive to dirty play or inept officiating. Again, the question is whether their loyalties predispose them to see things any differently than rival fans do. After all, they are watching the very same event. Mann (1974) asked spectators leaving Australian Rules football matches in Melbourne about the event they had just wit-

[1] $p < .09$.

nessed. Fans supporting the losing team saw dirtier play and felt the winning team was helped more by penalties and benefited from poor officiating. Supporters of the losing side also tended to make external attributions for the outcome (e.g., luck, poor officiating), whereas fans of the winning team attributed their victory to internal factors (e.g., good play). Mann has aptly characterized these various perceptual responses to defeat as mild *sore loser* reactions. Fans' bitter reactions to a loss will be mentioned again in chapter 10 in connection with the suggestion that they play a role in certain types of sports riots.

Several points of disagreement among the foregoing studies should be noted. Winkler and Taylor (1979) were unable to find evidence that the losing Dallas fans saw dirtier play by the Pittsburgh Steelers, nor did they see officiating as biased against the Cowboys. Furthermore, contrary to Mann's (1974) results, losers did not judge the game to be of lower quality. In fact, it was the neutral, nonpartisan airline passengers who thought the Superbowl game was of inferior quality. One suggestion would point to cultural and between-sport differences as an explanation for these conflicting findings. Alternatively, subjects' memories of media interpretations of the game may have faded in the six-week interval until Winkler and Taylor gathered their data. In any event, fans who strongly identify with a team in a very real sense see a *different* game than do rival fans or even neutral observers (e.g., Hastorf & Cantril, 1954). The game, like beauty, is in the eye of the beholder.

The caliber of athletic performances can also be misjudged for reasons that have nothing to do with team or player loyalties. Spectators with some regularity credit an individual athlete with a truly exceptional performance when in fact it is nothing out of the ordinary or nothing that would not be expected by chance alone. The point is made in Speaking Tangentially 3.1.

Attributions may also influence our decision to attend a sports event in the first instance. Our initial decisions are, in part, guided by the attributions we make for the recent performances of the teams scheduled to play each other (Iso-Ahola, 1980). Potential (student) spectators were given hypothetical descriptions of upcoming football games in which the home and visiting teams were credited with either a winning or a losing record. It was further stated in the pregame publicity that the previous success or failure of the contending teams could be attributed to either internal (i.e., ability and effort) or external causes (i.e., luck and difficult opponents). The influence of these variables on the likelihood of subjects' attendance can be seen in Figure 3.2.

For home teams, external attributions for the team's losses and internal explanations for their wins were associated with an increased probability of attendance. In the case of visiting teams, only the reasons for their previous failures had a bearing on the decision to attend. That is, when the visitors' losses were attributed to external factors (e.g., bad luck or their having faced difficult opponents), subjects expressed a greater likelihood of attending the game. Iso-Ahola's additional finding that expectations of attendance also increased overall following recent wins is consistent with the results of other studies showing that winning streaks are, indeed, good box office (Noll, 1974; Russell, 1986).

****

Speaking Tangentially 3.1: The Hot Hand
Basketball players, coaches, and fans alike share in the recognition that during some games an individual player may have "a hot hand." That is, a player hits on successive shots from the field or on certain occasions has a hot night on the court. Whichever of the overlapping terms "hot hand" or "streak shooting" is applied, the assumption is that the player's performance surpasses what might be expected from his overall record. Gilovich, Vallone, and Tversky (1985) have sought evidence for these commonly held beliefs in the shooting statistics of the Philadelphia 76ers of the National Basketball Association (NBA).

To illustrate their research, consider the question of whether, having just hit on their last shot (or a series of shots), players then make a higher percentage with their next shot than they do following a miss or series of misses. In fact, their results show that the probability of a hit being followed by a hit is actually slightly lower than a hit following a miss. Similarly, comparisons of hits following runs of two or three hits with hits following two or three misses revealed trends in the opposite direction to that predicted by a hot-hand hypothesis. Yet another analysis examined the question of whether players' shooting percentages across games deviated sufficiently from their overall shooting percentages to justify speaking of "hot" or "cold" nights. They do not.

Consider further these same questions at the free-throw line where the player has been awarded two shots. A preliminary survey of basketball fans revealed that a 70% free-throw shooter was expected to hit on 74% of his shots after a hit and 66% following a missed first shot. Two seasons of free-throw statistics for the Boston Celtics of the NBA served as the basis of the analysis. Once again, "there is no evidence that the outcome of the second free throw is influenced by the outcome of the first free throw" (Gilovich et al., 1985, p. 304). I might add that there is also no evidence to indicate that success in the first of two back-to-back games increases the likelihood of winning the second; in fact, teams winning the first are more likely to lose the second (Mizruchi, 1991).

In sum, a powerful cognitive illusion is seen to operate among basketball players and their following. The implications for improving team performance are straightforward. It is a common tactic to pass the ball to the player who is "hot." The opposing team also recognizes the hot hand at work and guards the player more closely than usual. Another player, equally skilled and now less closely guarded, would in fact have a better chance of scoring. Thus, an unfounded belief in the "hot hand" may occasionally work against a team's best interests.

****

The Value of a Wooden Leg: Self-Handicapping Strategies

An outgrowth of attribution theory that has direct implications for coaching practices as well as understanding performance is the expanding literature on self-handicapping strategies (E.E. Jones & Berglas, 1978) and its variant, excuse theory (e.g., Mehlman & Snyder, 1985). The central importance of the topic for athletic training is seen in the observation of Jones and Berglas that "self-handicappers are legion in the sports world" (p. 201). At the heart of self-handicapping strategies is an attempt by the athlete to *predetermine* the nature of the interpretation or attribution that will be made by others in the event of failure.

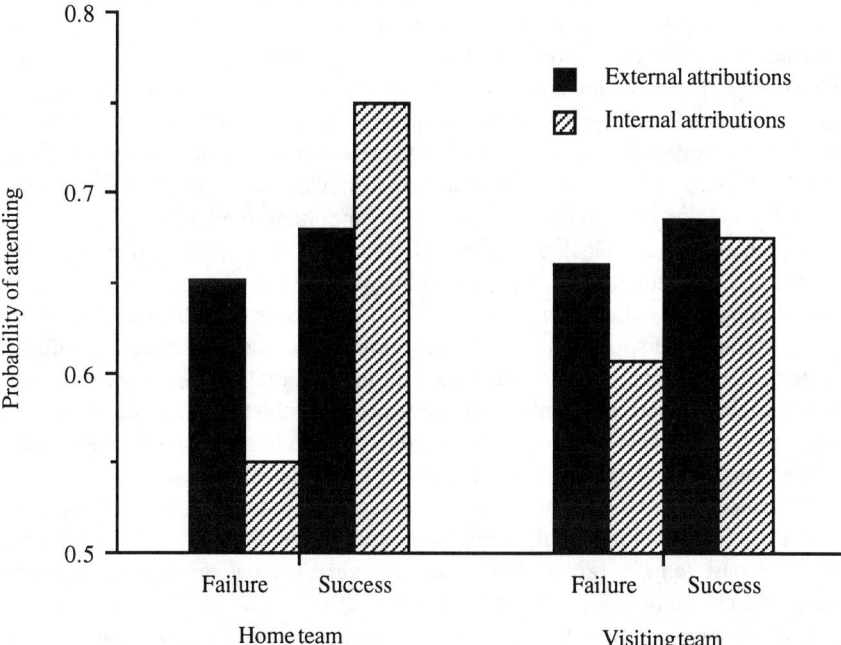

FIGURE 3.2 Attendance as a function of previous performance (adapted from Iso-Ahola, 1980).

How does it work in practice? Specifically, self-handicapping allows the individual, win or lose, to benefit from the attributional principles of discounting and augmenting. For example, the athlete who chooses to party instead of resting on the eve of her event stands to minimize a loss of self-esteem resulting from a poor showing the next day. The principle of discounting is seen to work to her advantage when observers later credit her lack of preparation with having caused her poor performance. Her partying (an external attribution) led to her downfall; her athletic ability need not be seriously questioned. But what if she should somehow be victorious despite her lack of preparation? Now the internal attribution to her ability is augmented. The plucky little lady has won despite having to fight through a hangover. Truly, an amazing athlete!

The use of self-handicapping strategies among competitive athletes is seen in two field studies by Rhodewalt, Saltzman, and Wittmer (1984). In the first of these, the researchers assessed the use of a number of behaviors that could serve self-handicapping ends for intercollegiate swimmers (e.g., effort in practice sessions, physical ailments, outside distractions). A substandard performance, especially at an important meet, could seriously undermine one's self-esteem. Swimmers scoring high on a measure of self-handicapping tendencies reported no appreciable increase in their effort in practice prior to important, and hence potentially threaten-ing, competitions. By contrast, swimmers who scored low on the measure in-creased their efforts in the days leading up to important meets. As seen in Figure 3.3, ratings of actual attendance provided independent confirmation that highs at-tended practice less frequently than lows prior to important swim meets. A second, parallel assessment was conducted on data provided by a sample of professional golfers. Golfers who use self-handicapping behaviors were also found to spend fewer hours in practice in the week preceding important tournaments.

Incidentally, while a lack of practice effort served as the preferred esteem-sav-ing tactic, it is noteworthy that health problems were not used as a self-handicap-ping strategy by either type of athlete. The authors make a further important point. Members of sports *teams* may have a limited number of strategies available to them. Condemnation by teammates for slacking off in practice or for com-plaining about their academic load may threaten athletes' self-esteem just as much as a team loss. Put another way, athletes in individual sports may have a greater range of self-handicapping options at their disposal.

Of course, self-handicapping strategies can take many forms. One common strategy is to remind others of, or otherwise accentuate, the traumatic experiences of one's past (e.g., a broken home, an impoverished background, an old war wound). For example, college coeds faced with the prospect of taking a test of "social intelligence" were found to emphasize the adverse effects arising from the negative experiences of their earlier years (DeGree & Snyder, 1985). Any result-

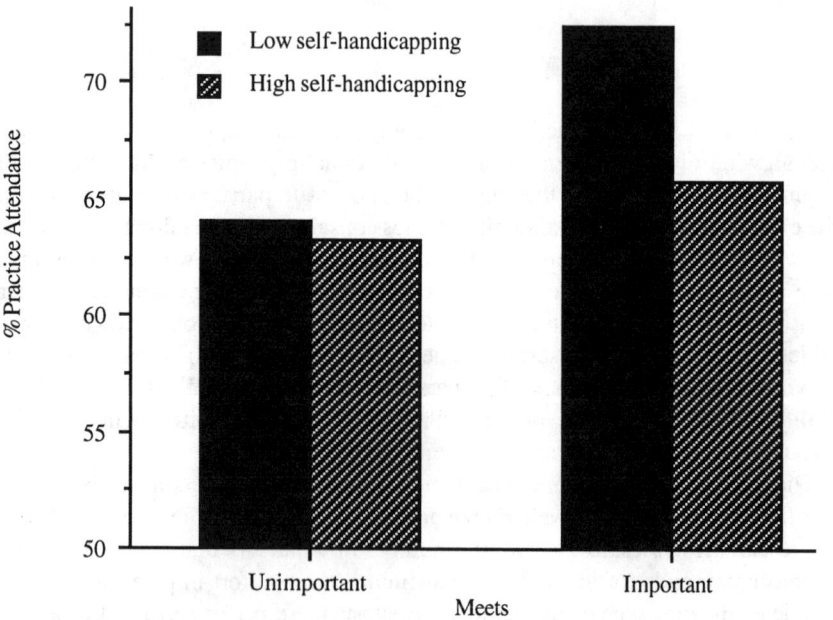

FIGURE 3.3 Practice attendance and meet importance (adapted from Rhodewalt et al., 1984).

ing shortfall in social IQ could thereby be at least partly attributed to an external cause over which they had little or no control.

A second example falls even closer to home. The self-handicapping strategy is that of invoking symptoms of test anxiety. Among a group of test-anxious university women, there was an increased reporting of (state) anxiety symptoms during an interval between the administration of two halves of an extremely difficult test of intelligence (Smith, Snyder, & Handelsman, 1982). However, this result occurred only under conditions where others might later conclude that "anxiety" was the cause of a poor performance. For subjects in another experimental condition, the situation was structured such that test anxiety symptoms could not be used in this self-protective manner. Here anxiety symptoms were simply not reported. Instead, test-anxious subjects reverted to an alternative tactic, that of making less of an effort. Thus, they could take comfort from the knowledge that if they did badly, a greater effort in the future would bring a better result.

To conclude, various self-handicapping strategies can be enlisted by athletes in the interest of preserving self-esteem. Some preevent tactics, such as reduced effort and partying, have obvious implications for the quality of athletic performance. One might suggest that tactful and supportive counsel by coaches will lead some athletes to develop insights into their behavior and to gradually abandon their use of self-defeating strategies.

Excuses, Excuses!

> And oftentimes excusing of a fault
> Doth make the fault the worse by the excuse.
>
> Shakespeare, *King John*

Excuse theory (C.R. Snyder, Higgins, & Stucky, 1983) represents an offshoot of attribution theory in recognizing the role of excuses in shielding the individual from failure and the loss of self-esteem that often accompanies failure. In this regard, it is my impression that athletes as a group make excessive use of excuses. The reasons perhaps lie with the structure of the typical training program. Athletes come under intense and continual scrutiny in evaluative situations where any shortcomings are a cause for immediate concern. The athlete's progress is closely monitored by the athlete and her coach. Within this setting, she is repeatedly called upon to explain aspects of her performance, especially those that are unsatisfactory. Because the reasons for observed deficiencies are usually jointly determined by coach and athlete, it is essential for continuing progress that both understand the part that excuses can play in biasing their conclusions. Clearly, modifications to a training program that are introduced on the basis of invalid excuses may be ineffective at best, harmful at worst.

The short-term advantage of managing others' impressions of an inferior performance by invoking external reasons is easily recognized in its simplest form. By attributing the cause to an external factor (e.g., bad luck, an injury, environmental conditions), the athlete weakens the implication that she, and she alone, is responsible for a substandard result. However, more subtle attributional processes are frequently at work.

From the work of Mehlman and Snyder (1985), it appears that following failure people often manipulate one or more sources of information as a means of externalizing the reasons for their poor showing (cf. Kelley, 1972). Specifically, these investigators found that subjects who were given feedback indicating "failure" on a bogus test of intelligence invoked explanations that were distinctiveness-raising (e.g., they would do better on *other* similar tests of intelligence) and consistency-lowering (e.g., they would do better if they were to retake the test at a future date). The further prediction that subjects would engage in consensus-raising (e.g., other subjects also did poorly on the test) was not supported. Perhaps, as the authors suggest, the fact that the researchers actually had such information in hand made such an excuse too transparent.

Excuses for failure are usually offered for the benefit of an audience. For an excuse to be credible, and thereby somewhat effective in managing one's self-image, the knowledge or expertise of the audience must be taken into account. It would be a lame excuse indeed that is given to an audience that is knowledgeable about the performance domain and recognizes the inadequacy of the excuse as an explanation for failure. Thus, the excuse maker faces the ever present danger of being exposed by an all-knowing audience. This prospect creates an increase in negative mood state. On the other hand, excuses accepted by an uninformed audience can reduce negative emotional states; in effect, the individual feels better at least for the time being (Mehlman & Snyder, 1985).

Coaching can be successful only to the extent that it is based on accurate information about the athlete's progress or lack thereof. An understanding of the athlete's state (e.g., her moods, motivation, physical condition, experiences) results from a joint undertaking in which her self-reports and explanations constitute the initial and basic inputs to coaching decisions. The coach with an understanding of excuse theory should be better able than others to disentangle ego-protective excuses from the authentic reasons offered by an athlete for dismal training or competitive outcomes.

"I'll Start Training...uh, Tomorrow, Perhaps!"

Whereas excuses may be offered for a poor performance, they are also offered for performances not even begun. Some of us would rather not deal with those oftentimes taxing and difficult responsibilities we all face preferring instead to put them off to another day. Others buckle down and do what has to be done. In an article entitled "At Last, My Research Article on Procrastination," Clarry Lay (1986) defines procrastination in the context of the coaching relationship. Procrastination involves

> deviations between what the athlete and his coach judge to be the most important training projects, on the one hand, and rated adequacy of time

spent by the athlete on such projects, on the other. Spending less than adequate time on important projects is deemed to be procrastination. (p. 494)

Preliminary work designed to identify some of the personality and behavioral correlates of procrastinatory behavior is well under way (Ferrari, 1991; Lay, 1986). One of the early findings is that students who procrastinate do not differ in either achievement motivation or actual academic achievement (GPA) from those who do not procrastinate (Lay, 1986). Additionally, procrastinators differ from others in their preferences for "projects," that is, those activities or obligations they have undertaken to accomplish. Subjects scoring high on a procrastination scale chose projects involving hobbies and a consideration of career choices as preferred activities. Compared to nonprocrastinators, they gave family obligations and home maintenance responsibilities a low priority. As a project category, sports were nominated with equal frequency by high and low procrastinators. Finally, true to form, procrastinators approached in an airline terminal and given a letter to mail from their travel destination took longer to do so than their more organized fellow travelers. The measure of procrastinatory behavior was, of course, the date on the postmark.

The common tendency to procrastinate has been linked to several personality variables in the work of Ferrari (1991). Procrastinators generally score higher on measures of social anxiety and need for social approval than do nonprocrastinators. They are further marked by low self-esteem and a lack of self-confidence.

Ferrari (1991) has also established an important connection between procrastination and the topic of the previous section, self-handicapping. Procrastinators use self-handicapping strategies more readily than do nonprocrastinators, seemingly as a means of protecting their already low levels of self- and social esteem. Their self-handicapping seems to be limited to (1) the public performance of tasks that are nonevaluative of their abilities and (2) privately performed tasks that provide an evaluation of their abilities. Procrastinators do not self-handicap when the task is diagnostic and in the public realm, or when nondiagnostic tasks are privately undertaken.

Ferrari's (1991) conclusions are based on results obtained with female subjects tested under laboratory conditions. As intriguing as his findings are, it remains to be determined whether athletes with procrastinatory tendencies are also led to use self-handicapping strategies when comparable conditions arise in the sports world.

It is probably too early in the development of research on this topic to offer more than tentative suggestions to coaches and others on how to minimize or otherwise alter procrastinatory behavior. One promising suggestion comes from a recent study of students' exam preparations. Procrastinators intend to begin studying later than do nonprocrastinators, although each group plans to put in the same number of hours. However, by the time exam day arrives, procrastinators have actually studied for *fewer* hours overall (Lay & Burns, 1991).

If something very similar happens with athletes who procrastinate, they might be persuaded to plan an earlier start for their training program irrespective of what they intend as a total work load leading up to a competition. As Lay and Burns (1991) suggest, this "may help them close the gap between their intended and actual hours of" training (p. 21). The emphasis of that advice "would be on planning to do at least something for a greater number of days" (p. 21). The results could be beneficial. Although the topic has thus far received little attention from sports researchers, I would hazard the guess that Lay's ground-breaking work will shortly stimulate a fresh new line of applied investigations.

Self-Efficacy

Why do some athletes excel in their sport while others, equally skilled and able, baffle and perplex their coaches with mediocre performances? Why does an athlete excel on one occasion only to perform badly, without any apparent reason, on others? A good part of the answers may be found in Albert Bandura's (1977, 1982, 1986) theory of *self-efficacy*. As one facet of self-knowledge, personal efficacy allows a person to organize subskills from within his or her behavioral, cognitive, and social repertoires into workable modes of action. Those who are plagued with doubts may abandon their efforts at mastery early on. Indeed, a challenging task may not be taken on in the first instance; if it is attempted, the individual low in perceived self-efficacy will likely expend less effort on the task.

Self-efficacy is not a relatively enduring feature of one's personality. Unlike stable traits, self-efficacy is situation-specific: a person may feel highly efficacious in one situation, much less so in other circumstances. Also, the construct of self-efficacy should not be confused with self-confidence. I am supremely confident in my belief that I will not take up bungy-jumping in the foreseeable future. While this statement is an expression of my confidence, it does not convey any indication of my feelings of self-efficacy for the activity. Expressions of confidence indicate the strength of one's belief without specifying its direction. On the other hand, self-efficacy refers to one's belief that one has the capabilities to attain a designated performance.

Self-efficacy underlies the successful performance of a full range of human endeavors including, of course, recreational activities and sports competition at all levels. There is often little difference among the topflight athletes in most sports. Innovative training methods and burgeoning technologies have produced pools of elite talent that are relatively homogeneous. In competition, the difference between first place and finishing out of the money frequently comes down to a brief lapse in concentration; a momentary hesitation; or, to use the present terminology, a weak sense of self-efficacy. It is the high efficacious athlete who performs well under extreme competitive pressures that is the joy of coaches everywhere.

Sportspeople are well aware that a surfeit of capability does not guarantee an outstanding performance. Followers of a sport usually know of one or more highly motivated athletes who, despite their best efforts, consistently fall short of what would be predicted for them on the basis of their informal performances in practice. Other outstanding athletes experience seemingly inexplicable slumps. Still others never quite regain their former standing in a sport long after their recovery from an injury or a "close call." What many of these athletes have in common is, among other things, self-doubts regarding their capabilities. We catch a glimpse of the importance of self-efficacy when less able but self-assured athletes outperform their more talented but doubting rivals. The athlete's self-judgment regarding his or her capabilities, then, is frequently a determining factor mediating the talent of an individual and its enactment in formal competition.

A formal definition may be in order, particularly as it becomes important at this point to distinguish between *self-efficacy* and *response-outcome expectations*. Bandura (1986) defines perceived self-efficacy

> as people's judgments of their capabilities to organize and execute courses of action required to attain designated types of performances. It is concerned not with the skills one has but with judgments of what one can do with whatever skills one possesses. (p. 391)

Thus, self-efficacy is one's personal assessment of whether one possesses the wherewithal to achieve a designated level of performance. By contrast, "an outcome expectation is a judgment of the likely consequence such behavior will produce" (p. 391). To illustrate, if a high school miler believes that she can run the mile in a record-setting time, then that belief is an efficacy judgment. The acclaim, the personal satisfaction, and the offers of track scholarships that she anticipates will follow her performance are outcome expectations.

The distinction between self-efficacy and response-outcome expectations is seen in a further example that is closer to the day-to-day experiences of many of my student readers. Most professors are aware that numerous undergraduates go to extraordinary lengths to avoid taking statistics and seminar courses beyond what is absolutely required for their major. Even though individually they have expectations that such courses will enhance their later marketability or improve their chances of admission to graduate and professional schools, self-doubts abound about their ability to understand all those squiggly symbols and/or to present their views to classmates. The sad result is they do not act consistent with their outcome belief. Their behavior speaks to low self-efficacy. Other courses are taken, and consequently for them their degree represents something less than what it might otherwise have been. Both they and society are the poorer for their having taken a path of lesser resistance.

As a predictor of performance, self-efficacy overshadows outcome expectations. The strong dependency of outcome expectations on judgments of personal self-efficacy essentially relegates outcome expectations to a lesser role in predicting behavior. As a consequence, investigations have typically revealed that self-efficacy bears the stronger relationship to various performance criteria. Barling and Abel (1983) report on two studies that provide comparisons of the relative strength of their roles in predicting sports performance. In the first of these, self-efficacy was related to tennis performance, whereas response outcome was not. In the case of a physical fitness program, self-efficacy proved to be a better predictor of perseverance in the program than the factor of outcome expectations. More precisely, participants' perceptions of both their self-efficacy and outcome expectations were related to their attendance. However, the former was considerably stronger in its relationship to their staying in the fitness program.

One additional point should be noted. Recent evidence (Fitzsimmons, Landers, Thomas, & van der Mars, 1991) suggests that self-efficiacy may not be a uniformly strong predictor of sports performance. Among *experienced* weightlifters, for example, their past lifts were a strong predictor of performance: A measure of self-efficacy was found to be only weakly predictive, especially near the end of a series of training sessions.

The Sources of Information

There are four major sources from which we derive information regarding our efficacy: performance attainments, vicarious experiences, verbal persuasion, and our physiological states (e.g., Bandura, 1986). The most influential of these is the information (i.e., feedback) that comes to us as a result of our successful or unsuccessful performances. Obviously, success produces a number of positive effects, not the least of which is an increase in self-esteem (Koocher, 1971). In addition, however, success fosters a belief in personal self-efficacy; a series of failures reduces efficacy. Efficacy strengthened by repeated successes may in turn allow an individual to weather occasional failures with little noticeable effect on his or her self-assessed abilities. Furthermore, a strong sense of efficacy in one performance domain often generalizes to other, similar performance domains. A strong sense of personal efficacy derived from success in fielding baseballs may prompt an individual's participation in other ball sports.

Our observation of others and the success or failure they experience also acts as a basis for judgments of our own self-efficacy. Although not generally as strong an influence as direct performance attainments, vicariously experiencing the activities of others may confirm sensed inadequacies if the model fails or enhance efficacy when successes are observed (e.g., Lirgg & Feltz, 1991). However, the direction and magnitude of modeled performances will, to a large extent, depend on the amount of the observers' prior experience and their past success or failure in performing the task.

A third means of inducing a stronger sense of efficacy is to convince the self-doubting athlete that he or she possesses the capabilities to perform successfully. However, a caution is in order. *Unrealistic* appraisals of capabilities open the door to failure, with an attendant lowering of efficacy. At the same time, the athlete's trust in his or her coach is apt to be seriously undermined. Although a common tactic of coaches, persuasion per se may be of limited value in effecting lasting increases in self-efficacy except as the athlete is persuaded to take a more positive view of his or her capabilities and thereby makes a greater effort. If success follows the stronger effort, then performance attainments may increase self-efficacy in a more decisive fashion.

Our physiological state serves as a fourth source of information regarding our capabilities. Pain cues, fatigue, soreness, and so on are interpreted by the athlete as signs of physical inefficacy. Indeed, the coaching tactic of dissociation (described below) involves redirecting the athlete's thoughts toward external cues and away from those internal cues that can prove debilitating through a lowered sense of physical efficacy.

The effects of self-efficacy on performance are seen in an experiment by Weinberg, Gould, and Jackson (1979). Feelings of either high or low self-efficacy were induced by an experimental confederate with whom each subject was paired. High self-efficacy was created when the confederate was heard to say that he had strained knee ligaments and subsequently demonstrated less leg strength than the subject. A low self-efficacy condition was created when the confederate instead identified himself as a member of the track team who regularly lifts weights to develop leg strength. He also ostensibly outperformed subjects on a leg-strength apparatus. With high and low self-efficacy conditions established, subjects competed twice with the confederate on a leg-extension task; that is, the contestants were seated and attempted to keep their leg elevated in a horizontal position for as long as possible. The confederate's leg was unobtrusively supported, ensuring that all subjects lost on both trials. The results of this interesting experiment, later replicated (Weinberg, 1986), can be seen in Figure 3.4. Clearly, high efficacious subjects outperformed low efficacious subjects. Moreover, following their defeat on Trial 1, the performance of lows declined sharply, whereas that of highs showed a

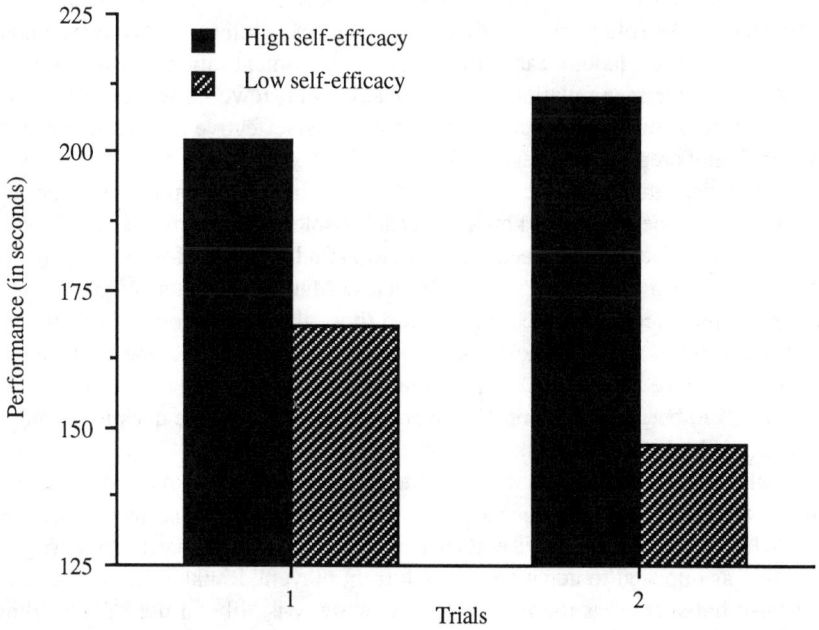

FIGURE 3.4 Efficacy and performance following failure (adapted from Weinberg et al., 1979).

slight improvement. In the face of adversity, then, those who are high in self-efficacy show persistence and increased effort; those low in self-efficacy exhibit a sharp drop in persistence.

Two cognitive strategies, *dissociation* and *positive self-talk,* have been proposed as effective strategies for mediating the self-efficacy/performance relationship. Dissociation requires the athlete to focus her thoughts on external cues during her performance (e.g., an afternoon at the beach). By ignoring those cues that arise internally and signal pain and/or fatigue, the athlete is insulated from thoughts of physical inefficacy (Bandura, 1982, p. 127). The effectiveness of dissociation is seen in a study of cross-country runners. Those who closely attended to external cues recorded generally faster times than did other competitors who were not encouraged to adopt a dissociative strategy (Pennebaker & Lightner, 1980).

The alternate cognitive strategy of positive self-talk involves repeating statements of encouragement to oneself (e.g., "I can do it," "I can finish," etc.). For the athlete, the effects of these statements of self-encouragement may include an increase in self-efficacy brought about by a strengthened belief that he or she can successfully perform the requisite behaviors. It should be borne in mind, however, that simply reiterating an optimistic statement that one can do something may not lead to a *belief* that it can be done. The belief may be quite unrealistic in the face of available evidence to the contrary. Saying, then, is not necessarily believing.

As a performance strategy, self-talk draws support from an experiment by Weinberg, Smith, Jackson, and Gould (1984). Subjects using positive self-talk were able to enhance both their muscular strength and their endurance. As effective as these and other cognitive strategies appear to be generally, Weinberg's (1986) test of the role played by these two cognitive strategies introduces a note of caution. The results of a carefully designed experiment failed to reveal any interaction with the manipulation of self-efficacy. Thus, it would seem that the specific conditions under which cognitive strategies are effective in influencing self-efficacy beliefs remain to be established.

The practical matter of increasing self-efficacy in athletes remains to be addressed. More specifically, what is the coach's role in developing self-efficacy? Traditionally, coaches have seen their role to include the use of various means to instill a sense of optimism in their athletes. Many of the techniques shown through experience to be effective are also those that would logically follow as recommendations from efficacy theory. Has experience shown some strategies to be more effective than others? Have some been adopted while others are largely ignored? Weinberg and Jackson (1990) sought answers to these questions among the ranks of high school tennis coaches.

All of 13 self-efficacy enhancing strategies were used to a moderate degree, and all were judged by the coaches to be above the mean of a scale of effectiveness. The most effective and frequently used technique was that of encouraging "positive as opposed to negative self-talk from player." Ranked fifth in frequency of use but second as the most effective strategy is "liberal use of rewarding statements." Although coaches believe it to be very effective as a means of increasing self-efficacy, I would remind the reader of the caveat to its use noted in regard to cognitive evaluation theory (chap. 1). Briefly, preliminary evidence (Baumeister, Hutton, & Cairns, 1990) suggests that although effort may be increased by praise, skilled performance may be impaired. Praise, then, should be used sparingly with an eye to the type of performance that the athlete is attempting to master.

A further answer to the question of how to increase self-efficacy lies with mastery training. Here, the coach's task is to structure circumstances such that the athlete experiences success most of the time. The goals or standards set are only incrementally more difficult with the result that setbacks are few and far between. However, occasional mild setbacks are important to the development of self-efficacy. Success that comes too easily does not equip one to cope with failure. The lesson to be drawn from failure is that one's best efforts must be sustained in order to realize success. Efficacious athletes, then, are better able to bounce back from adversity and to steadily improve their skills in an environment tailored to their level of performance and rate of development. It would be an unwise move for any coach to prematurely put a talented but untested rookie into a crucial, pressure-packed game. The possible short-term gain is far outweighed by the risk of crippling the rookie's sense of self-efficacy. The implementation of mastery training, then, demands considerable skill on the part of a coach in maintaining and modifying a graduated series of incrementally more challenging goals. The long-range returns on that effort, however, can be considerable.

A novel but untested means of increasing self-efficacy has been described by Feltz (1982). The Soviets reportedly showed their elite athletes films of their best performance. However, the films were carefully edited to show an incrementally better performance. This tactic was intended to change the athletes' performance beliefs and cause them to progress beyond what they might see as their limits for an event.

Summary

To summarize, recent years have seen a flurry of research activity testing self-efficacy predictions in an athletic context. The predicted relationship between self-efficacy and performance appears to be well established (e.g., see a review by Wurtele, 1986) across an assortment of sports. For example, J. Taylor (1987) reported self-efficacy to be related to performance in alpine and nordic skiing, basketball, cross-country running, tennis, and track/field. Self-efficacy predictions have also been confirmed for gymnasts (McAuley & Gill, 1983) and marathon runners (Gayton, Matthews, & Burchstead, 1986). Gayton et al., for example, found self-efficacy scores to be related to runners' predictions of their times as well as their actual finishing times. Feltz (1982), however, found only partial support for self-efficacy theory in her study of back-diving performance. The theory did predict success on the first attempt to learn the dive. Thereafter, the level of success on the first dive became the better predictor of success on later dives. In sum, the initial promise shown by the concept of self-efficacy and the questions raised by much of the early research ensures the concept a central and continuing role in a developing psychology of sport.

Suggested Readings

Bandura, A. (1990). Perceived self-efficacy in the exercise of personal agency. *Journal of Applied Sport Psychology, 2,* 128–163.
    The current status of self-efficacy theory is reviewed with specific applications to athletic performance.

Higgins, R.L.; Snyder, C.R.; & Berglas, S. (Eds.). (1990). *Self-handicapping: The paradox that isn't.* New York: Plenum.
    An advanced reference source by contributors who are active researchers in this field.

McAuley, E., & Duncan, T.E. (1990). The causal attribution process in sport and physical activity. In S. Graham & V.S. Folkes (Eds.), *Attribution theory: Applications to achievement, mental health, and interpersonal conflict* (pp. 37–52). Hillsdale, NJ: Erlbaum.
    The authors provide an overview of attributional research in sports and exercise that concludes with a valuable section recommending future directions for research.

Mullen, B., & Riordan, C.A. (1988). Self-serving attributions for performance in naturalistic settings: A meta-analytic review. *Journal of Applied Social Psychology, 18,* 3–22.
    This article provides a large-scale review of studies that were conducted beyond the social science laboratory in naturally occurring situations.

4

Group Dynamics

Throughout the course of human history, people have come together in groups as a means of achieving common goals. Their aims have been varied and far too numerous to document. Consider the purposes of such diverse groups as Jesus and his disciples, the Flat Earth Society, a student union, Greenpeace, the Women's Christian Temperance Union, and the National Rifle Association. Within sports, one sees owners', players', and referees/umpires' associations, supporters' clubs, recreational and leisure time organizations, and of course, a countless number of teams at all levels of sports.

Sportspersons may band together for a variety of purposes that include attaining economic, political, social, health, and competitive goals. While a group may be formed with one or more goals in mind, there is a common assumption that most purposes can more easily be served through a group rather than an individual effort. In general, this assumption appears to be correct.[1] A players' association has more clout than any one of its members can muster and is more likely to gain concessions from management on matters of concern to its membership. A pole vaulter may be better able to develop his skills and compete as a member of a track and field organization that can provide assistance with equipment, facilities, and travel. Of course, groups are not always successful in achieving their purposes; they may achieve all, some, or none of their goals.

But what distinguishes a *group* from a cluster of people standing at the curb waiting for a traffic light to change or the two dozen people in the pool for a noon-hour swim? Although numerous and varied definitions have been proposed during the course of social psychology's long-standing interest in group processes, only three will be noted here. Each emphasizes somewhat different aspects of the group.

> A group is a social unit consisting of a number of individuals who stand in role and status relationships to one another, stabilized in some degree at the time, and who possess a set of values or norms of their own regulating their behavior, at least in matters of consequence to the group. (Sherif & Sherif, 1969, p. 131)

> Two or more persons who are interacting with one another in such a manner that each person influences and is influenced by each other person. (Shaw, 1976, p. 11)

---

[1] For a challenge to this assumption see Buys's (1978) thought-provoking article "Humans Would Do Better Without Groups."

Two or more interacting persons who share common goals, have a stable relationship, are somehow interdependent, and perceive that they are in fact part of a group. (cf. Paulus, 1989)

As mentioned above, groups are not always successful in achieving their objectives or, I would add, even in maintaining themselves. While some groups persist in the face of adversity, others begin to break apart with even minor setbacks. Disillusioned members of a team no longer pursue their common interests, effort lags, and some members start to drift away from the group. Simply put, some groups are tightly knit, others are only weakly held together. It is this internal dynamic of the group process, *cohesion,* that constitutes the subject of the section to follow.

Group Cohesion

Probably all of us at one time or another have experienced something special about a group to which we belonged. Whether it was a fish-and-game society, a badminton club, or a cheerleading squad, we felt an attraction to the other members and valued our membership. Had our group been criticized or otherwise come under attack, we would have felt obliged to come to its defense. Indeed, in the very act of defending our group, our feelings of solidarity or esprit de corps would in all likelihood have been intensified. In contrast, other groups are marked by looser ties. The members are only weakly attracted to one another and would make little effort to defend the integrity of their group. It is this central feature of groups, *cohesion,* that is generally assumed by coaches to be an important requisite for team success.[2] To be sure, coaches are not alone in this assumption.

Politicians, industrialists, and the military know well the importance of group solidarity and camaraderie to the success of their efforts. For example, political incumbents have long recognized the gains to be made by raising the specter of an attack from a neighboring country or by a foreign ideology on the eve of an election. The electorate consistently rallies to the support of its embattled leader.

Cohesion was also seen to develop quickly in response to an external threat in the Robber's Cave experiment (see Sherif & Sherif, 1969, chap. 11). In a matter of days, two groups of young campers who were previously unknown to each other developed close in-group bonds. Strong "we" versus "they" perceptions sprang up between the Rattlers and the Eagles. At the same time, hostility grew between the two groups. Although they had little love for their rivals, within each group bonds of friendship and intense feelings of loyalty were soon apparent to the camp personnel.

In general terms, research from a number of disciplines converges to support a conclusion that internal group cohesiveness is increased in the face of external

---

[2] This is not to say, however, that cohesion is a *necessary* condition for team success. There is the celebrated example of the German rowing team that won Olympic gold despite internal conflicts (Lenk, 1977).

conflict (Stein, 1976). However, two conditions must first be met. The external conflict must pose an equal threat to all members, and the group itself must at the outset be somewhat cohesive and possess an effective leadership structure. When these qualifying conditions are met, we have every reason to predict an increase in group cohesion.[3]

In describing group cohesion, I have knowingly used a variety of terms interchangeably (e.g., attraction, camaraderie, esprit de corps, solidarity, etc.) to describe the underlying dynamics of the cohesion process. This problem of finding common ground for a satisfactory definition of cohesion has been especially troublesome over the years. As one reviewer has been prompted to observe, "The history of research into group cohesiveness has been dominated by confusion, inconsistency, and almost inexcusable sloppiness with regard to defining the construct" (Mudrack, 1989a, p. 45). The importance of reaching some level of agreement on a definition, and how that definition might best be represented as a measure in research, became apparent in the aftermath of an early review of cohesion-productivity studies.

Stogdill (1972) reviewed some 25 investigations, essentially concluding that there was *no* support for "the view that high group cohesiveness leads to high productivity" (p. 37). The impact of this influential review was such that systematic research on the topic was drastically curtailed. Mudrack (1989b), in a critical review of the topic, makes two telling points: (1) "no two studies referenced by Stogdill operationalized group cohesiveness in exactly the same way," and (2) over 40% of the studies do "not appear to be concerned with anything remotely resembling cohesiveness" (p. 775). However, in contrast to Stogdill's early conclusion, it should be noted that a small-scale review of more recent studies is substantially more supportive of a cohesion-performance relationship (Evans & Dion, 1991).

Clearly, the use by researchers of a few common and valid measures of cohesiveness would greatly facilitate comparisons of findings across studies, as would a common definition. I find myself in agreement with Mudrack (1989) in recommending a definition proposed by Carron (1982), one that captures the essential elements of cohesion, namely, "a dynamic process that is reflected in the tendency for a group to stick together and remain united in the pursuit of its goals and objectives" (p. 124). Carron's definition would seem a good starting point for those interested in pursuing the topic in a sports context.

As reviewers have previously noted (e.g., Mudrack, 1989a), anyone venturing into the traditional research literature on group cohesion is quickly engulfed by inconsistent and often contradictory findings. The confusion arises in part from the use by researchers of a wide variety of definitions and methods of measuring the construct. For many years, cohesiveness was seen to be reflected in the attraction of the group's members for one another (Festinger, Schachter, & Back, 1950; Lott & Lott, 1965) or to the group itself. In retrospect, the concept seems to have

---

[3] For a description of the social chaos that can result when these conditions are *not* met, see Hammerschlag and Astrachan's (1971) amusing account of the Kennedy Airport "snow-in."

been too narrowly defined inasmuch as only a single dimension of a multidimensional concept was usually being assessed. Also troublesome is the fact that evidence of the psychometric properties of the measures themselves was generally lacking. Of the measures used, few had been established as *valid,* that is, as in fact measuring "cohesion" as defined by the particular researcher. By the same token, evidence of their *reliability* (i.e., consistency of measurement) was seldom reported. An important step has more recently been taken in an attempt to rectify many of these shortcomings.

Carron, Widmeyer, and Brawley (1985) have undertaken a careful reconceptualization of group cohesion that takes its complexity into account. Equally important, an impressive start has been made on laying the psychometric groundwork for an instrument that measures four major dimensions thought to underlie the concept. Carron and his colleagues make an initial conceptual distinction between *group integration* and *individual attractions to the group.* Their model further subdivides each of these two categories into *social-* and *task-focused* player perceptions. The resulting four constructs are labeled and illustrated as follows:

—Group Integration–Task (GI-T); for example, an all-star team is formed with a view to winning a postseason tournament.
—Group Integration–Social (GI-S); for example, a recreational bowling league is formed with a view to improving social relations among the company's employees.
—Individual Attractions to Group–Task (ATG-T); for example, an inner-city woman joins a revolver club to learn skills she hopes will ease her fear of intruders.
—Individual Attractions to Group–Social (ATG-S); for example, a young man joins a square-dance club in hopes of improving his social life.

The Group Environment Questionnaire (GEQ)

The 18-item Group Environment Questionnaire (GEQ) provides a measure of cohesion based on four subscales that represent each of the dimensions described above. Subjects are asked to make ratings on nine-point scales of the extent of their agreement with statements reflecting each dimension of group cohesion. A sample question from the individual attractions to group–task (ATG-T) is, "This team does not give me enough opportunities to improve personal performance" (Carron, Widmeyer, & Brawley, 1988, p. 130). The measure, then, provides for a more complete mapping of the cohesion process. Equally important, however, are demonstrations of the instrument's success in testing cohesion predictions in sports groups.

The GEQ in Practice

Several investigations have been undertaken in sports settings using the GEQ. The results thus far have been encouraging. For example, Carron et al. (1988) administered the GEQ to groups of elite athletes (e.g., track, basketball, badminton, etc.) and others engaged in a variety of fitness classes. Their prediction was that the GEQ would successfully discriminate between those who would persist in a program and those who would quit prematurely. The rationale, of course, was that individuals feeling strong ties to a program, at a group or an individual level, would be less likely to fall by the wayside. Among elite athletes, three of the four GEQ scales (ATG-T, GI-S, and GI-T) proved to be powerful predictors of who would remain in the sport and who would drop out. Somewhat different findings emerged among those enrolled in fitness classes. In this case, the cohesion measures ATG-T and ATG-S successfully discriminated between the two types of participants.

Carron et al. (1988) also reasoned that lateness to or absenteeism from a group provides a further indication of its cohesiveness. Adults competing in recreational leagues over a summer completed the GEQ. Attendance records were also kept. For both males and females, the GI-S scale served to distinguish absentee and tardy players from their more reliable teammates. Two additional relationships with GEQ deserve mention. Using volleyball teams competing in the English National League, Davids and Nutter (1988) report a relationship between GI-T scores and clubs' percentages of wins. Also, teams ranked higher in this elite league scored higher on both GI-T and ATG-T, suggesting the importance for success of task- over social-related cohesion at this level of play.

One further point deserves mention. Until recently, evidence for a cohesion-performance relationship in *coacting* team sports was generally lacking. In coacting sports (e.g., rowing, golf), team success is determined by a tally of each member's independent performances. Williams and Widmeyer (1991) tested the strength of a cohesion-performance link using women golfers competing on NCAA Division I university teams. Their analyses of GEQ responses revealed that task cohesion (ATG-T and GI-T) successfully predicted performance outcome. In other words, the more (task) cohesive teams generally played better. At the same time, social cohesion (ATG-S and GI-S) bore only a negligible relationship to golf scores. Certainly, a causal relationship between team cohesion and performance cannot be assumed. However, as Williams and Widmeyer point out, coaches who nonetheless wish to make an inferential leap of faith with a view to improving their team's performance would at the very least be advised to channel their energies into fostering task rather than social cohesion.

Group Size and Cohesion

Cohesion can also be looked at in a more fundamental way, that is, as it relates to the *size* of the group. Sport teams generally are restricted to a size that is dictated by the rules of the sport. This is not to say, however, that the size mandated by any set of rules is necessarily optimum for fostering a cohesive unit. Widmeyer, Brawley, and Carron (1990) recently extended the question to sports in providing an extended test of the group size–cohesion hypothesis. The relationship was tested in a 10-week, three-on-three basketball league and in a series of recreational volleyball games. In both tournaments team size was varied (i.e., 3-, 6-, or 9-person basketball squads and 3-, 6-, and 12-person volleyball teams). Their prediction was confirmed. As the size of teams was increased, there was a corresponding decrease in cohesion. Equally interesting is their finding that *enjoyment* of the activity also decreased as the size of teams was increased. Cohesion, then, may be a more elusive goal in those sports played with larger rosters.

There are, however, circumstances where the traditional finding of increasing group size leading to decreasing cohesiveness does not apply (e.g., with mixed-sex groups). J.E. Marshall and Heslin (1975) used measures that represent earlier definitions of cohesion (i.e., a desire to remain as a member of the group; cf. Festinger et al., 1950) in their examination of the question. As predicted, *same*-sex groups expressed a greater desire to remain with smaller rather than larger groups. However, the pattern of findings was much different with *mixed*-sex groups. Females expressed a greater attraction to larger rather than smaller groups, whereas males found large and small mixed-sex groups equally attractive. The factors of size and sexual composition, then, would appear to be critical determinants of the success of teams and activity groups in holding a continuing attraction for members. As a consequence, the overall effectiveness of co-educational sports or recreational programs is likely to be enhanced by taking findings such as these into account.

To summarize, a fresh beginning has been made by Carron and his co-investigators in providing an expanded model of group cohesion. The GEQ has already been demonstrated to discriminate effectively among a number of behaviors having important implications for athletic performance as well as the design and promotion of a wide range of programs. Research thus far makes clear that the predictive importance of the subscales will vary with the type of sport or activity, level of competition, and possibly gender and culture.

Loyalty

Player Loyalty

Organizational loyalty is a close relative of cohesion. Strong attachments to a team or its coach often develop and allow the group to persist in times of adversity and, perhaps, to excel in competition. Although many organizations are successful in fostering loyalty among their members, only a handful of human groups develop truly *intense loyalties*. In addition to some sports teams, intense loyalty can be seen to develop in such groups as police tactical squads, elite military units, surgical teams, and religious cults.

Patricia and Peter Adler (1988) undertook a ground-breaking five-year investigation of intense loyalty in the context of a major college basketball program. The Adlers defined organizational loyalty as follows:

a bond formed either to an organization or to some person or group within it that can be either individually or collectively forged. It consists of feelings of attachment, of belonging, of strongly wanting to be part of something; it involves the readiness to contribute part of one's self; it incorporates trust, the voluntary alignment of self with the group, and a willingness to follow faithfully the leadership or guidelines of the organization. (p. 401)

Using a participant-observation technique, several classes of students playing on a nationally ranked team were closely followed over the course of their college careers. An analysis of the observational data revealed five elements fundamental to the development of intense loyalty: *domination, identification, commitment, integration,* and *goal alignment.* Briefly, domination refers to the extraordinary power vested in the office of coach and the pervasive influence and control that coaches exert over all aspects of their players' lives. The subordinated athletes are resocialized, a process in which newcomers are deliberately subjected to experiences in which they are shamed, embarrassed, and intimidated in what might be called rites of degradation (Trice & Beyer, 1984). These stripping-down rituals jar the athletes loose from their self-centered attitudes and prepare them for the lessons of team loyalty.

Identification is cultivated both with the program and with the coach. Players are encouraged to internalize the goals and ideals of the overall enterprise and to reflect those ideals both on and off the basketball court. The coach himself develops a paternalistic relationship with his players. Informal social evenings are held at the coach's home during which players get to know their coach and his family on a more personal level. These visits are punctuated with frequent reminders that the coach is always there to help with problems. The players, in turn, are led to understand the reciprocal nature of the relationship and must themselves "be there" when the coach needs their help.

Another key element in fostering feelings of intense loyalty is commitment to the program. The act of signing with a school, although not totally binding, is treated with the utmost seriousness. As part of the rites of passage (Trice & Beyer, 1984), the occasion is usually a media event staged with considerable fanfare and the traditional donning of a team sweater. The ceremonial signing, "a symbolic loyalty oath" (Adler & Adler, 1988, p. 410), establishes an initial bond to the program.

Integration of players into a cohesive, smoothly functioning team may be achieved in several ways. To be sure, athletes may become strongly united under a domineering, dictatorial, and hated coach (cf. Stein, 1976). More commonly, however, team solidarity is enhanced through common living arrangements and effectively isolating the team members from the rest of the student population. Additionally, senior players sponsor new arrivals, introducing them to college life and guiding them around potential pitfalls on campus.

The final element involves aligning the players' personal goals (e.g., having fun, graduating, receiving pro offers) with that of the organization (i.e., winning).

Players are made to see that their secondary goals are more likely to be realized through achieving success on the court.

The model further recognizes that feelings of loyalty fall along a continuum of intensity. The most intense bonds develop when all five components of loyalty are operating in an organizational setting. Although organizational units in general are seldom found to involve intense loyalties, the few that do may be more prevalent in sports than elsewhere. The highly competitive circumstances that frequently surround certain team sports (e.g., basketball, football) may be especially conducive to the forging of these extraordinarily strong bonds.

Additionally, it may be the case that intense loyalties facilitate the emergence of leaders seen to have charismatic qualities. Although the concept is admittedly elusive, there is a recognition that contextual factors play an important role in fostering the emergence of charisma (Conger & Kanungo, 1987). Possibly, intensely loyal groups provide the very setting in which charismatic qualities are most likely to be attributed to the successful leader. In effect, the combination of a particular set of leader characteristics displayed against the background of an intensely loyal following may lead to a perception of charismatic leadership. It does seem that football and perhaps basketball have produced more than their share of charismatic leaders, from Rockne to Lombardi to Wooden and so on. Of course, these are also the very sports in which the process of intense loyalty, as described by Adler and Adler (1988), is so carefully cultivated. However, it remains to be determined how loyalty is related to group longevity, player satisfaction, and team performance. Any comprehensive understanding of group processes in sports is more likely to be realized by taking into account the concept of loyalty. The Adlers have given us a good start.

Fan Loyalty

For the most part, our formal and informal memberships in groups are meaningful and important to us. Whether as an official team member or as one of a more diffuse group of team supporters, we want to see our group realize its objectives. In the case of a team's fans, individual members who strongly identify with the cause may feel personally threatened when their group encounters setbacks or failures (e.g., their team loses on the field of play). The interpersonal dynamics operating within a group generally see in-group members judging and treating each other more favorably than out-group members. There are, however, exceptions. There is, for example, good reason to believe that the in-group member with questionable loyalties may be judged especially harshly by other members when things go badly.

Branscombe, Wann, and Noel (1991) examined the role of several factors, including loyalty, that might be expected to influence the evaluations by sports fans of one of their number. Students who strongly identified with the University of Kansas men's basketball team were asked to read a newspaper account and commentary of a game against the University of Oklahoma. (A number of versions

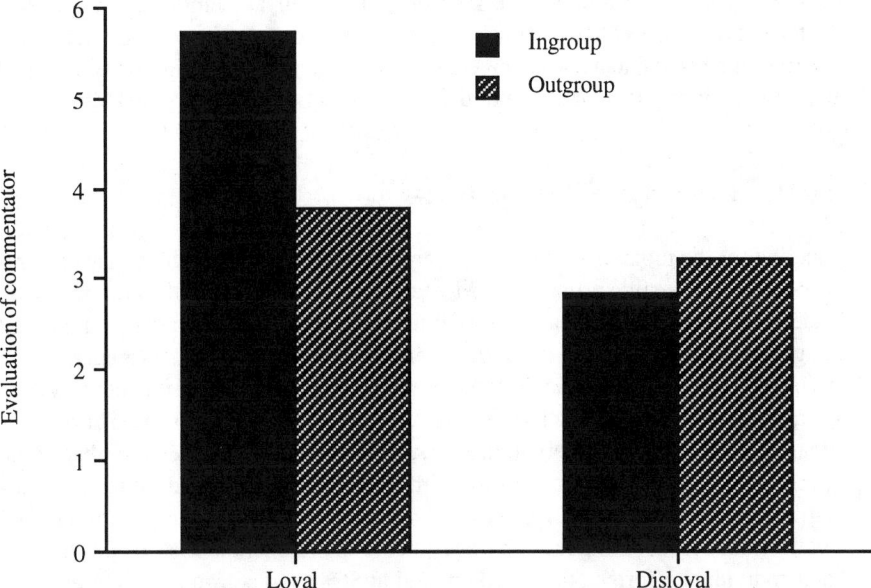

FIGURE 4.1 Evaluation of commentator following a Jayhawk loss (adapted from Branscombe et al., 1991).

were created.) The article was ostensibly written by a journalism student who let it be known in the commentary either that he was a Kansas "Jayhawk" fan or a fan of Oklahoma. Within both versions, the commentator indicated either his strong loyalty to the team or only a weak sense of loyalty that wavered with the team's most recent performance. In one version, the game was won in overtime by Kansas; in the other by Oklahoma. Next, the Kansas fans provided an evaluation of the journalism student, that is, of his knowledge and journalistic abilities as well as their liking for him.

The pattern of findings shown in Figure 4.1 was consistent with the authors' predictions regarding the importance of loyalty in determining the evaluation of a group member, in this case the commentator. The particular version used was that of a game with Oklahoma in which Kansas was defeated, an outcome that threatened the social identity of Kansas fans. The first point to note is that, among dedicated fans, loyalty is a highly regarded attribute. When the commentator was described as wavering in his commitment (disloyal) to either of the teams, he was rated less favorably overall. Moreover, the disloyal Jayhawk member drew a surprisingly strong reaction from his group in the aftermath of the loss to Oklahoma. That is, the disloyal in-group commentator was rated far more negatively than the commentator described as loyal to the Jayhawk cause.

In the eyes of those who value their membership in a sports group, be it fans, a team, or an executive board, individual loyalty is clearly an important determinant of how a person will be evaluated. When the group suffers a defeat or some form of failure, it poses a threat to members' identity. The disloyal member similarly represents a source of threat to that same identity. In order to maintain or even enhance the worth of their social identity, members reject or in some way diminish the stature of those who might act to dissociate or distance themselves from the group's failure.

Social Loafing: When 2 + 2 = 3

Imagine for the moment a tug-of-war competition in which one team has been replaced by a powerful spring scale. Most of us would assume that as members are added one by one to the team the total team force would increase by an amount roughly equivalent to what the added member alone could exert. Just such an experiment was conducted in France by Max Ringelmann over a century ago (Kravitz & Martin, 1986). The results are intriguing. As the team size was increased to two, to three, to eight, the *average* force exerted by each member of the team fell dramatically. That is to say, with increases in the number of people sharing in an effort, each person makes correspondingly less and less of a personal contribution. In the Ringelmann experiments, pairs exerted 93% of the total of their individual efforts, a threesome pulled at 85%, and a group of eight expended only 49% of their individually combined efforts. This shortfall of effort has been given the name *social loafing* (Latané, Harkins, & Williams, 1980). Incidentally, the original reports of Ringelmann's pioneering research, long thought to have been lost or unpublished, were discovered a few years ago and reported on by Kravitz and Martin (1986).[4]

The Ringelmann effect has been demonstrated with a variety of tasks that include sprinting (Huddleston, Doody, & Ruder, 1985), brainstorming (Harkins & Jackson, 1985), clapping, shouting, typing, detecting signals, evaluating poetry (Latané, Williams, & Harkins, 1979), and cheerleading (Hardy & Latané, 1988). Of immediate interest is an investigation of social loafing conducted in competitive swimming (Williams, Nida, Baca, & Latané, 1989). Within the swimming fraternity there is a common assumption that performances on the relay team are generally superior to those recorded in individual competition. If this were true, laboratory findings on social loafing would not square with at least one aspect of social reality. Confirmation of the assumption that relay swimmers are faster was sought in the records of a Big Ten intercollegiate swim meet. Significantly faster times were indeed found in the relay events, that is, differences of .77 and .74 seconds for the 100/400-yard and 200/800-yard individual and relay events, respectively. However slight these differences are in absolute terms, they can easily spell the difference between first place and an "also-swam" finish.

---

[4] Although a variety of sources credit Triplett (1898) with having conducted the first social psychological investigation having relevance to sports, his work was, in fact, preceded by Ringelmann's series of experiments carried out from 1882 to 1887. However, credit goes to Triplett for first *publishing* the results of his work; Ringelmann's results did not appear in print until 1913.

While these results ostensibly show a group effort to be superior to that demonstrated individually, several factors may be at work to create the difference. Williams et al. (1989) point out that three of the four swimmers on a relay team use a "flying" start and can initiate some movement prior to the start of timing. This advantage is itself sufficient to account for the faster times in the relay events. Moreover, the performance of each individual team member is not "lost" in the total team effort as it is, for example, in the tug-of-war. Individual lap times are recorded and shouted to swimmers by timers, thereby publicly identifying them with a measure of their performance. High or low identifiability, in turn, was thought to be a major variable influencing the degree of social slacking occurring in group efforts.

The setting chosen for a test of these ideas was the 50-meter pool at Ohio State University, where members of the swimming team served as subjects. Williams and his colleagues staged a simulated meet that included prizes, an audience, and both individual and relay events at the 100- and 200-meter distances. Lap times were either announced *or* withheld from individual and relay swimmers, thus creating high and low identifiable conditions. The design further called for *all* swimmers to compete in each of the individual and relay events.

The major finding is shown in Figure 4.2, where an interaction between the variables of identifiability and event is apparent. Where swimmers could not be identified with their times, they swam slower as members of the relay team than they did in the individual event. However, under the condition of high identifiability, members of the relay team posted faster times than those recorded when they swam in the individual event. The authors attribute the faster times of relay team members in the high identifiability condition to the added pressure they felt

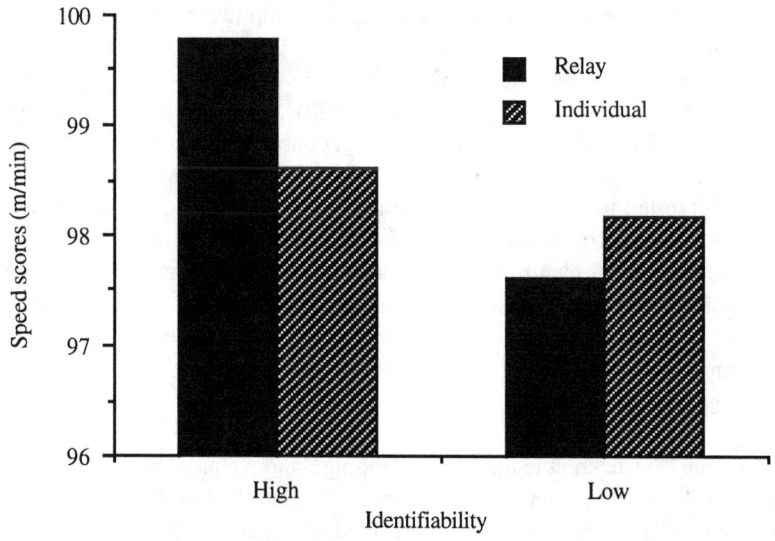

FIGURE 4.2 Relay and individual times as a function of identifiability (adapted from Williams et al., 1989).

from teammates expecting them to excel. Yet it is interesting to consider that despite their reporting that they felt greater pressure from teammates, the relay swimmers clocked the slowest times of all under conditions of low identifiability. The effects of team spirit are seemingly outweighed by a stronger tendency to expend less effort when one's performance makes a completely private contribution to the group's output.

Team sports, of course, vary greatly in the extent to which individual performances can be readily isolated and evaluated. Unlike team play in golf, where an individual's score for the round indicates how well he has played, the performances of individual members of a rowing team are not subject to public scrutiny. Latané, Harkins, and Williams (1980) cite the example of one Big Ten football coach who attempted to increase the identifiability of linesmen's play. His coaching staff routinely reviewed and evaluated film footage in which each player's performance was isolated. The results were also announced to teammates and to the press. Although unconfirmed, line play was likely improved.

Another investigation conducted in a real-life competitive situation attempted to determine whether social loafing was evident when groups perform tasks that are highly involving, intrinsically interesting, and seen by the participants to be important. Hardy and Latané (1988) chose a cheerleading camp for high school girls as the setting for their field experiment. The girls (blindfolded) performed in pairs and, through headphones, were led to believe either that they were shouting or clapping alone, or were performing with a partner. The young women gave it their all. The authors report the average shout measured 101 decibels, "louder than the sound of a New York subway train, as heard from the platform" (p. 111). However, as involving and meaningful as the task was to the girls, loafing was still in evidence. In contrast to their solo performances, those cheerleaders who believed they were cheering with another girl made only 94% as much noise.

It is important to point out that identifiability alone may not always reduce loafing (Harkins & Jackson, 1985; Kerr & Bruun, 1983). Subjects who participated in brainstorming sessions in which their individual contributions could be identified (number of uses for various objects, e.g., a knife) generated more ideas but only when they were led to believe their performance would be compared to that of their co-workers (Harkins & Jackson, 1985). It is not just identifiability that eliminates social loafing but identifiability *plus* an anticipated evaluation of one's output by means of comparisons with a standard or the performance of peers. At the group level, the prospect of an evaluation of the group's performance has also been shown to eliminate loafing (Harkins & Szymanski, 1989). The effect, then, appears to be robust both in the context of various team sports and the social laboratory.

Now, it must be acknowledged that clapping, finding uses for a knife, and watching for blips on a monitor are not the sorts of tasks that one can become deeply involved with; nor can it be expected that people will see their performance as having personal consequences in the future. Would social loafing occur to the same extent with tasks that are more personally involving? Apparently not! Brickner, Harkins, and Ostrom (1986) successfully replicated previous findings of loafing under conditions of low identifiability, but only with a task that did not have personal consequences for the subjects. The task itself solicited student opinions on the merits of introducing a senior comprehensive exam as a requirement for graduation. Some subjects were told that their school would adopt the proposal next year (high involvement); others were told that it would be adopted at another school (low involvement). In the case of highly involved students facing the prospect of a comprehensive exam, identifiability did not influence their performance. That is to say, under conditions of high and low identifiability the students produced an equal number of opinions. There was no evidence of social loafing. Personal involvement in the task, then, may act to reduce or even eliminate social loafing.

One might also anticipate that loafing could be eliminated by simply providing athletes with detailed information about the phenomenon prior to their performance. In a test of this suggestion (Huddleston et al., 1985), female sprinters competed individually and as members of relay teams in a 55-meter dash. Half of the teams were informed about social loafing and its likely causes. Contrary to expectations, providing information proved to be ineffectual in reducing loafing.

Loafing may, however, be eliminated under two other conditions. Harkins and Petty (1982) found that when individuals in a group can make *different* contributions to the assigned task rather than everyone making the same contribution, loafing disappears. The effect also vanishes when the task is *difficult* rather than simple. In short, when members of a group can make unique contributions and/or the task is challenging, a loafing effect may not be in evidence.

Explanatory Mechanisms

What factors might account for this general tendency to slack off when performing as a member of a team? One explanation holds that because the output of the individual members is often not apparent to anyone, no single individual can be held more than fractionally responsible for an overall inferior performance. Specifically, a *diffusion of responsibility* may induce individuals to expend less effort than they would otherwise, albeit under conditions where their actions cannot be monitored.[5] In this regard, we saw earlier that when people believe that their individual outputs can be measured, social loafing all but disappears (e.g., Williams, Harkins, & Latané, 1981).

A second explanation suggests that team members often have few opportunities to make a unique contribution to team goals. In such circumstances, individuals might understandably lack interest in the task at hand and be less than fully motivated to make a maximum effort (e.g., Harkins & Petty, 1982). However, whatever the explanation may prove to be, the implications for team sports are clear. De-

---

[5] A diffusion of responsibility has also been proposed as a contributory factor in some forms of riotous behavior by sports crowds (see chap. 10).

pending on the structure of a team's task and/or the availability of means to monitor and quantify individual efforts, social loafing may be assumed to adversely affect competitive outcomes (Harkins & Szymanski, 1989).

A Universal Truth?

Inasmuch as social loafing is a learned form of behavior, it might be anticipated that cultural differences exist. That is, social loafing may be less apparent in group-oriented societies where collective undertakings are stressed and valued by the culture. This hypothesis was tested in comparing the performance of U.S. and Taiwanese schoolchildren on an auditory tracking task (Gabrenya, Wang, & Latané, 1985). Whereas the American youngsters predictably exhibited social loafing, the Chinese children, by contrast, showed just the opposite behavior in the group setting. They performed better in groups than alone, a result the authors describe as *social striving*. A culturally fostered group orientation likely favors some nations in international team competitions. On the other hand, one might speculate that nations espousing an individualistic philosophy generally excel in individual events.

Let George Do It

An interesting offshoot of social loafing is seen in a similar reduction of effort when one's capable partner or teammates consistently experience success. If teammates' successful performances appear to ensure overall team success, there is a tendency for one to reduce one's own efforts. Interestingly, this occurs despite a strong social norm that deplores "letting George do it." This reduction in effort on *disjunctive* tasks (i.e., where the best performance defines success for a group) has been termed the *free-rider effect* (Kerr, 1983). Thus, for example, a cross-country meet may count only the top 10 finishers in calculating points to determine the overall team title. The slower runners on each team with little or no hope of finishing near the top may make less of an effort, leaving it to their speedier teammates to win the day.

The strength of free-rider effects has been shown to increase with the size of the group. In point of fact, however, nearly all of the research on free-rider effects has involved neither large groups nor group contributions to the public good. Strictly speaking, the "theory is concerned primarily with the provision of *public goods* by *large* groups, potential or actual" (Albanese & Van Fleet, 1985, p. 251). We will shortly turn for an example to an area of the sports enterprise where large groups are more common and where free-rider effects would, as a consequence, be stronger.

Thus far, the focus of this chapter has been almost exclusively on processes involved in the most visible and publicized of sports groups—athletic teams. It is all too easy to overlook the important contributions of other groups whose success or failure has implications for the performance and well-being of participants in sporting and recreational activities. The success of any group in which those involved seek a common goal usually requires the best efforts of all members. Whether it is a door-to-door fund-raising blitz, the organizing committee for a Special Olympics, or any of a number of management committees, the presence of free-rider effects can cause the group to fall short of its objectives.

By way of illustration, consider the case of a community-wide membership drive in support of local sports teams. The outstanding success of one or two members on the committee has made it seem likely that the target will be reached. At this point, other members may decide that their continued efforts are unnecessary and begin to coast. Any resulting shortfall experienced by the committee could, of course, jeopardize the success of the sports program they have undertaken to help. There are, however, a number of means by which free-riding tendencies can be minimized in sports organizations.

Toward Reducing Free-Rider Effects

Several suggestions for offsetting free-rider effects have been offered by Albanese and Van Fleet (1985). Insofar as the effects are stronger with larger groups, sometimes it may be useful to restructure larger groups into a number of smaller operating units. Similarly, emphasizing the unique aspects of the tasks assigned to individuals as well as the difficulty of their tasks can also reduce free-riding tendencies. The latter tactics are presumed to produce beneficial results through increasing the intrinsic satisfactions experienced by members. As was the case with social loafing, identifying the individual's contribution to the group effort can likewise stimulate a greater effort. Finally, free-riding tendencies may not develop under conditions where the activities of members are monitored. Clearly, the preferred suggestions for eliminating free-rider effects are those that prevent their development in the first instance. As Albanese and Van Fleet suggest, the creation among members of a strong commitment to the goals of the organization or group might represent just such an effective preventive measure. When individuals take pride in their joint efforts to achieve the public good, the likelihood of self-serving inaction is apt to be reduced.

Sucker Effects

A group member may also realize that his partner or other group members, although entirely capable, are deliberately slacking off in their efforts and that he is being left to carry the load. Playing the sucker role is not an attractive prospect for most people. As a consequence, we are likely to see a reduction in their effort in what has been called the *sucker effect* (e.g., Kerr, 1983). Interestingly, when men find themselves cast in this role they find the experience to be more aversive than do women and as a consequence make substantially less of an effort. On the other hand, we appear willing to carry an inept and failing partner who nonetheless makes an effort. However, that willingness does not extend to an able partner who willfully performs poorly and whose inferior performance thrusts the responsibility for team success on our shoulders. We are unlikely to sustain our efforts in these circumstances.

While free-riding and sucker effects have clearly been demonstrated on disjunctive tasks, purely disjunctive tasks in sports are few in number. Rather, team competitions tend to be more conjunctive; that is, the worst performance defines success for a group. Thus, for example, relay teams in track and swimming with one weak or unmotivated member may find that others on the team hold back on their efforts. The implications arising from this distinction are that highly able group members will show greater motivation losses than those who are less able on a conjunctive task. On the other hand, those members with low ability will show a greater tendency to free riding on a disjunctive task (Kerr & Bruun, 1983).

Summary

The topics of this section have dealt with similar types of motivation loss occurring in the group situation. Nonetheless, social loafing, free-rider, and sucker effects are each presumed to stem from different processes (e.g., Kerr, 1983). Social loafing originates with the group member's perception that her or his individual contribution to the group cannot be determined. On the other hand, free riding occurs as the individual notes that she stands to benefit personally from the superior contributions of other group members. Finally, sucker effects originate with yet another perceptual judgment. Here, a shortfall of effort results when a group member perceives that others are free riding in a situation where her superior contributions all but ensure that group goals will be reached. All three processes can potentially undermine a group performance whether it is a committee of management or an athletic team. Fortunately, ongoing research is suggesting steps by which the loss of motivation from these sources can be minimized and the full potential benefits of group endeavors realized.

In this section, we examined the major factors that influence group cohesion and the loyalty of members to a team. Other influences originating inside and outside the group were also shown to adversely affect our motivation to perform optimally in the case of social loafing and its close cousin, free riding. The upcoming topics of cooperation, competition, and rivalry examine concepts that derive their meanings from the attitudes of individuals, either singly or as members of groups. These basic attitudes in turn may determine the nature of interactions within the group or, alternatively, the group's interactions with other groups. It is equally important to note that the form interactions take (e.g., cooperation, competition) can also be determined by the structure of a sport or activity itself.

Competition Versus Cooperation

Competition is perhaps the most central and hallowed concept in the sports world. Its presence and influence are also felt throughout the business community, somewhat less so in education and scientific circles. There is general agreement that competition involves "two or more units, either individuals or groups, engaged in pursuing the same rewards, with these rewards so defined that if they are attained by any one unit, there are fewer rewards for the other units in the situation" (Berkowitz, 1962, p. 178).

That competition enjoys such widespread acceptance as the basis for interpersonal and intergroup dealings might lead one to the conclusion that it must therefore be a superior means of bringing out the best in people. What evidence is there, however, to support a belief that competition is superior to other modes of interaction, such as, say, an individualistic orientation or cooperation? Fortunately, a substantial amount of research is available to assist us in answering this question. Our answer will be drawn from investigations conducted primarily in education and industry.

D.W. Johnson and his colleagues (D.W. Johnson, Maruyama, Johnson, Nelson, & Skon, 1981) undertook a review of 122 studies published between 1921 and 1981 that compared the effectiveness of cooperative versus competitively structured tasks on achievement and performance. One of the major findings was that cooperation was clearly superior to competition in fostering achievement and productivity across a wide range of tasks, including *motor* tasks. Of 109 findings used in one analysis, 65 favored a cooperative setting, 8 favored competition, and 36 showed no advantage to either type of setting.

Competition has also fared poorly in other occupational contexts. A sample of 103 male Ph.D. scientists in a variety of fields (e.g., biology, engineering, etc.) completed the Work and Family Opinion Questionnaire (WOFO; Helmreich & Spence, 1978). This instrument was designed as a measure of achievement motivation. Three motivational subscales underlie the WOFO and include "Mastery (preference for challenging, difficult tasks), Work (enjoyment of working hard), and Competitiveness (liking for interpersonal competition and the desire to better others)" (Helmreich, Spence, Beane, Lucker, & Matthews, 1980, p. 897). The results were straightforward. The number of citations by others to the work of these scientists served as the measure of their attainment. The greatest number of citations was to the work of those who scored *high* on the Mastery and Work scales but *low* on the scale of Competitiveness (Helmreich, Beane, Lucker, & Spence, 1978). Similar results are found elsewhere. Using citations as the criterion, Mastery and Work scales were associated with high attainment among personality and social psychologists, and again those academics who were most competitive had the fewest citations to their published work (Helmreich et al., 1980).

High Mastery and Work scores in combination with low Competitiveness is additionally seen to be associated with higher salaries among businessmen and higher grade point averages among male and female undergraduates (Helmreich & Spence, 1978). This consistent pattern of motivational needs, as well as the literature review noted above (D.W. Johnson et al., 1981), strongly implies that other interactive modes are superior to competition.

Group experiences can play an important role in the emotional, physical, and social development of children. Groups provide opportunities for youngsters to experiment and learn a variety of physical and social skills, values, and appropriate behaviors. Of course, lessons that are not in the best interests of the individual child or society can also be learned in groups. However, it is generally recognized that common goals are more easily achieved through group efforts. For this reason alone, the development of a cooperative orientation through group experiences is desirable. Cooperative attitudes facilitate effective group actions that are generally to be preferred to the obstructive behaviors of the uncooperative group member.

Cultural Differences

The pervasive role of culture in fostering cooperative or competitive behavior in children is seen in two studies that used similar procedures (Miller & Thomas, 1972; Richmond & Weiner, 1973). Both used a board game in which two youngsters could work to obtain prizes cooperatively or competitively, with one child winning at the expense of the other. The two conditions were created by means of instructions (i.e., *group*-reward and *individual*-reward). Under group-reward conditions, the children were told that they both would receive a prize for jointly maneuvering a pen to either of two targets. In the individual-reward condition they were told that only one of them could be given a prize, and that for moving the stylus to the circle containing their own name. The direction of the pen's movement was under the control of both players, who pulled strings from opposite ends of the board.

Richmond and Weiner (1973) compared the performances of black and white children in Georgia, whereas Miller and Thomas (1972) used Indian children from the Blood reserve in Southern Alberta in a comparison with white children. Children in both studies were of approximately the same age (i.e., 7 to 9 years old). The analyses revealed that black and Indian children played more cooperatively than their white counterparts. Sex differences were not apparent in either study. The white children in the individual-reward conditions were so highly competitive that Miller and Thomas felt obliged to comment. A tug-of-war strategy intended to prevent the "opponent" from gaining an edge developed, with many of the youngsters complaining "that their hands were hurting from pulling so hard" (p. 1109). So determined were the white children to beat their partner that the researchers had to replace broken cords several times!

The authors of both investigations attribute the superior performance of the black and Indian children to the socialization experiences within their respective cultures. Where cultural themes of sharing, extended families, and the common good prevail, cooperation is more likely to be adopted as a means of interacting with others, to everyone's advantage. Recall that a similar cultural explanation was advanced to account for the *social striving* of Taiwanese students.

Sex Differences

The sexes differ sharply in their preference for a cooperative versus a competitive approach to social exchange. Women typically adopt a cooperative rather than a competitive stance in their interactions. Among men, a competitive orientation is far more common than a cooperative strategy (Knight & Dubro, 1984). With women perhaps taking the lead, we might do a surprisingly better job for our children and young athletes by striking out in a cooperative direction.

There is a critical distinction to be drawn between competition and rivalry. Although the words have distinctly different meanings, people frequently use them interchangeably in referring to the same activity. Rivalry is best seen as an attitude that is carried into competition. In the view of Thibaut and Kelley (1959) an association between rivalrous attitudes and competition is learned in the formative years. The attitudes of rivalry "appear in the form of personal intentions that go beyond merely doing well in competition and involve the goal of hurting the other person, perhaps going out of one's way to do so" (p. 228).

In the absence of rivalrous overtones, competition offers a wealth of benefits to competitors. It can be extremely satisfying to an athlete to have done well against some personal or externally established standard of excellence. One can take pride in having bettered one's previous mark in an event or performed well under the prevailing conditions of the competition. It matters little whether one finished 1st, 2nd, or 10th in the field of competitors. Finishing first may be nice and something of a bonus, but the importance of the competition lies with having acquitted oneself well irrespective of the "official" standings. The distinction, then, between competition and rivalry should not be blurred, and note should be taken of those instances when those writing about competition are in fact referring to competitive situations in which rivalrous attitudes prevail.

I would like to think that this brief review of cooperation has persuaded readers, if not already persuaded, that cooperative attitudes and behaviors are generally preferable to those that underlie competition, especially competition containing rivalrous elements. I say this fully recognizing that the preponderance of sports, and even recreational activities, are structured in the competitive mode. More than that, we in North America seem obsessed with winning, all too often by any means, fair or foul. In this regard, readers may be interested in Jeffrey Goldstein's (1979) description of how a preoccupation with winning robs spectators of the more enriching experiences that sports can provide. I think Goldstein has it right when he says,

> To the extent that nonskill factors rather than superiority determine outcome, then winning is not only *not* the only thing, it is hardly anything at

all. But it still matters how the game is played: It can be played with fi-
nesse, with grace, daring and beauty. . . . If the emphasis on winning is
diminished, there should be a corresponding increase in the intrinsic motivations and satisfactions inherent in sports. (p. 407)

The case for cooperative programs has been firmly established through empirical research and ably summarized in a number of sources (e.g., Orlick, 1978).
However, the implementation of a cooperative program is not always as straightforward and simple a matter as it might seem. This is especially true in instances
where the prevailing social climate has been one of competition.

As noted earlier, there is a strong tendency for competition to breed hostility between individuals and contending groups (Berkowitz, 1962, 1973; Gaebelein &
Taylor, 1971). Certainly, the summer camp studies of Sherif and Sherif (1969) in
Oklahoma and Diab (1970) in Lebanon demonstrate that competition can lead to
ill-will, if not outright aggression, between groups. It is also worth noting that the
intense antagonisms that sprang up were between groups that had an existence
only for the duration of the camp. The strength of this process is seen in Diab's
Lebanon study. Here, the boys squared off against one another on the basis of the
group to which they had been assigned rather than along religious lines. One
might have thought that any resulting conflict would have arisen between the
Moslem and Christian campers. Not at all. In this instance, their memberships in
centuries-old religions played no part in the hostility that developed. The conflict
was along the lines created by their temporary and "matched" assignment to
groups in the camp. Group memberships simply overrode religious differences.
The pitched battle that took place in the camp dining hall between the Rattlers
and Eagles (Sherif & Sherif, 1969) was more than matched by extreme manifestations of intergroup hostilities in the Middle Eastern study. So severe was the an-
imosity (a knife was brandished) that Diab was unable to proceed with a replication of the final phase of the earlier Oklahoma study, that of introducing *superordinate goals*.

A Cooperation-Attraction Hypothesis

Superordinate goals may be defined as "those goals that have a compelling appeal
for members of each group, but that neither group can achieve without participation of the other" (Sherif & Sherif, 1969, p. 256). The definition emphasizes that
neither group can by itself attain an attractive goal; rather, each group requires the
help of the other. The further implication is that other group goals may have to be
subordinated if the joint undertaking is to be successful.

The Oklahoma researchers staged several major emergencies as a means of
testing the proposition that the pursuit of superordinate goals by rivalrous groups
can lead to a reduction of hostilities and increased liking for one another. These
included a sudden breakdown in the waterline to the camp that had to be located.

On another occasion the boys were on a day trip to a lake when shortly before mealtime the truck that was to go for their food mysteriously developed engine failure. The truck could only be restarted by all of the campers pulling together on a tow rope. These "accidents" had potentially serious consequences for both groups of boys. It was further apparent that it was mutually in their best interests to cooperate with each other, as in fact they did. As a result of their cooperative efforts, there was a reduction in intergroup hostility and a parallel increase in liking for one another. The improvement in relations did not, however, occur overnight but took place gradually as a result of the cumulative effects arising from their series of joint efforts.

Those who have responsibility to develop or oversee childrens' activities may find a cooperative emphasis more to their liking and to be in the better interests of their charges. Indeed, as noted above, the comparisons of cooperation and competition made in a variety of research settings strongly suggest that society is better served by cooperation. However, whether or not the introduction of a cooperative program to a group setting proves successful will depend on at least two additional considerations.

Although it appears that competition is unlikely to foster an attraction between groups (e.g., Worchel, Andreoli, & Folger, 1977), and in some instances may instead create hostility (Diab, 1970; Sherif & Sherif, 1969), the conditions under which cooperation leads to liking are fairly specific. The key to a cooperation-attraction link is both the outcome of the cooperative task and whether the groups have previously interacted cooperatively or competitively. Previously competing groups that experience failure in their combined endeavors become less attracted to each other. Success, however, results in increased attraction. Groups with a history of cooperation present a different picture. Irrespective of whether their joint efforts meet with success or failure, intergroup attraction increases (Worchel et al., 1977). Thus, the simple introduction of cooperative tasks does not guarantee that intergroup conflicts will be resolved in every case. The history of group interactions and their success in joint undertakings will largely determine the effects of a cooperative program.

Group behavior will continue as a topic in chapter 5, although the spotlight will shift away from its internal workings to focus instead on an external influence on group performance, namely, the leader. Thus, we will move from discussing the interpersonal dynamics underlying cohesion, social loafing, and cooperation to consider groups as units subject to the influences of leaders in improving, or even occasionally worsening, the performance of their groups.

Suggested Readings

Arnold, A. (1989). *Winners*. North Pomfret, VT: Paladin.
A far-ranging and thought-provoking book that, among other issues, proposes that winners may be losers in disguise.

Harrison, A.A., & Connors, M.M. (1984). Groups in exotic environments. In L. Berkowitz (Ed.), *Advances in experimental social psychology* (Vol. 18, pp. 49–87). New York: Academic Press.
A review of findings from research conducted on groups operating in unusual environments ranging from submarines to space labs to stations in Antarctica. Topics include group composition, cohesion, leadership, and conflict.

Hinde, R.A., & Groebel, J. (Eds.). (1991). *Cooperation and prosocial behaviour.* Cambridge: Cambridge University Press.
A collection of chapters by international experts on the topics of cooperation and prosocial behavior. Cooperation is discussed at the interpersonal, inter-group, and international levels by scholars representing a variety of disciplines. This book will hold the attention of students, researchers, and recreational readers alike.

Johnson, D.W., & Johnson, R.T. (1989). *Cooperation and competition: Theory and research.* Edina, MN: Interaction.
A thorough and well-organized review of the research literature on cooperation.

Paulus, P.B. (Ed.). (1989). *Psychology of group influence* (2nd ed.). Hillsdale, NJ: Erlbaum.
This volume presents a collection of readings by leading researchers who highlight some of the newest developments in the rapidly expanding area of group psychology.

Worchel, S., Wood, W., & Simpson, J.A. (Eds.). (1991). *Group process and productivity.* Newbury Park, CA: Sage.
A state-of-the-art review of group processes by contributors actively involved in researching questions of cohesion, the quality of decision making, and group dynamics.

5

Leadership

Leadership Dispute Endangers Everest Expedition
Field Hockey Players Threaten to Resign if Coach Retained
Billy Martin to Manage Yankees, Again

Each of the above was a major national news story. In addition to calling attention to what might be called a crisis of leadership, these headlines also share an underlying assumption that formal effective leadership is essential if a group is to achieve its goals. The strength of this unquestioned and pervasive belief is seen in the regularity with which coaches and managers of losing teams are replaced at all levels of sports. The wisdom of replacing the coach with a faltering record will be evaluated later in this chapter.

Leadership can be seen whenever people assemble for some common purpose and collectively face a significant challenge or obstacle to the attainment of their goal. People riding together on an elevator scarcely constitute a group and certainly don't require leadership from anyone to reach their floor. However, if the elevator becomes stuck between floors, leaders quickly emerge to perform needed functions, one perhaps comforting the more distraught passengers, another seeking outside help.

Leadership can also be seen to arise almost spontaneously in a group that assembles for a common activity. For example, children gathering on a sandlot after school will quickly structure their interrelationships to reveal leadership patterns. One or more of the youngsters will step forward to organize the activities, appointing himself captain; choosing sides; and, if enough boys are present, announcing that girls can't play. The basis of his leadership generally stems from some aspect of status or power such as physical stature, superior playing skills, or the fact that he owns the only available bat and ball. Thus, leadership can emerge somewhat democratically from within the membership to assist a group in reaching its goals, or, alternatively, a leader may be imposed on the group by a powerful external source. To continue with our sandlot example, a parent may arrive on the scene "to help out" and proceed to appoint team captains from among those assembled. Determining leadership in this way, that is, selection by an external source of authority (boards of directors, owners, the parent, etc.), appears to be typical of how leaders come to office in most organized sports.

Leadership has been a topic of interest to social groups throughout most of human history, whether the groups are religious, political, military, or business organizations. Few subjects have received more attention from social scientists working in a variety of disciplines, each bringing his or her own specialized research techniques and theoretical perspectives to bear on the topic. However, despite a half-century or more of vigorous research and theoretical speculation, it is fair to say that the success of those efforts has been limited. Our understanding of the leadership process to date is incomplete. Throughout this chapter, I will attempt to outline successive historical views of leadership, sketch several theoretical approaches to the topic, and highlight research findings on a number of practical issues specifically related to sports leadership.

Definitions

While it may be comforting to a reader to be presented at the beginning of a chapter with a single definition of the concept under discussion, it would at the same time be misleading. In the present case, offering the reader my preferred definition of leadership would obscure the fact that there is a considerable diversity of opinion on its essential nature. However, the same may be said of most concepts in the social sciences. Despite decades of intensive inquiry, theorists are well short of achieving a consensus in defining many of our important concepts (e.g., intelligence, creativity, motivation). Indeed, even the notion of *groups* that leaders are presumed to lead has proven difficult to define to everyone's satisfaction (Gibb, 1969; Shaw, 1976).

Gibb (1969) and Stogdill (1974) have reviewed the complexities involved in defining leadership and have offered numerous examples of the differing views of theorists. Four definitions that are but a sample of the major approaches to the topic are presented below. Hopefully, they will illustrate the range of viewpoints and some of the difficulties associated with attempts to reach anything more than a general agreement on the approximate nature of the leadership process.

> The function here figuratively defined may be called service, promotion of well-being, stimulation of progress. A general name, widely applied, is leadership. (Lehman, 1928, p. 8)

> To lead is to engage in an act which initiates a structure in the interaction of others as part of the process of solving a mutual problem. (Hemphill, cited in Gibb, 1969, pp. 214–215)

> Leadership, most broadly conceived, is a relation between leader and led in which the leader influences more than he is influenced: because of the leader, those who are led act or feel differently than they otherwise would. As a *power* [italics added] relation, leadership may be known to both leader and led, or unknown to either or both. (Gerth & Mills, 1953)

> The individual in the group given the task of directing and coordinating task-relevant group activities or who, in the absence of a designated leader, carries the primary responsibility for performing these functions in the group. (Fiedler, 1967, p. 8)

While leadership and even groups may be variously defined, there is general agreement that a leader's *effectiveness* or success in office, is reflected in the performance of her or his group. Any judgment or evaluation of the effectiveness of leaders, then, must be based on the group's progress toward meeting its objectives. This simple point is frequently lost in discussions swirling about the merits of individual leaders. In the words of one noted authority, "We must judge an orchestra conductor by how well his orchestra plays rather than by his ability as a musicologist or the elegance with which he waves his baton, or even the happiness and contentment of his musicians" (Fiedler, 1970, p. 2). Note that by a performance criterion, there is no requirement that the leader be liked or found to be exercising a style of leadership that is preferred by her or his subordinates. A group's performance, then, is the standard by which its leader is to be judged.

Leadership Versus Headship

In sports, when people speak of leadership at the time of a new appointment, they are usually referring to "headship." As in the military and the business world, sports leaders are chosen typically by owners, executive boards, and so on rather than by those they are expected to lead. With few exceptions, theorists hold that leadership involves a willing acceptance by subordinates of the leader's attempts to influence. Where that influence is unidirectional from leader to followers, and not voluntarily accepted, the relationship is more accurately termed headship. Of course, a sports team may function quite successfully under a head. Loyalty to the team and/or the fear of punishment for disobedience may be sufficient to ensure a motivated performance from team members.

Leadership and headship are not, however, mutually exclusive concepts. Consider the example of a coach newly appointed by the team owner. Shortly after taking office, he introduces a radical new training program that is followed by a string of league victories. As the coach gradually gains recognition from players for his contributions to their common cause, players adopt more favorable attitudes and soon come privately to accept his influence. Thus, although our coach began as an autocratic head, the success of his program in the eyes of his players brought with it their cooperation and eventual acceptance of his authority. At this point it can be said that he is functioning in a leadership capacity.

It would be an interesting and perhaps profitable exercise for those involved at the executive level of various sports to consider the extent to which "leadership" is present in their organization, particularly at the level of team captains. As noted, many major sports have adopted the headship model. Certainly, for teams chronically riddled with dissension and performing badly, experimenting with various forms of leadership can do little to harm their interests. Although the distinction between leadership and headship is often subtle (see Gibb, 1969, pp. 212–213), it is nonetheless important inasmuch as separate processes are thought to be involved, each with different implications for the performance of groups.

Three Approaches to Leadership

Trait Approach

> From the hour of their birth, some are intended to command, others to obey.
>
> Aristotle, *Politics*

> Herbert Spencer, who cannot be suspected of prejudice in this matter, divided the human race into a few clever individuals, many ordinary, some decidedly stupid.
>
> B.H. Lehman, *Carlyle's History of the Hero*

The idea that certain individuals are marked for leadership has long held a prominent position in the history of human thought. Sometimes referred to as the great man/great woman theory of leadership, a very small number of people—historically, nearly always men—are believed to possess a combination of traits that set them apart from others and predispose them to lead. This elitist view has been expressed by Aristotle and carried forward in the influential writings of Scotland's Thomas Carlyle (1840), who saw leadership as the proper role for those individuals who possess the stuff of which heroes are made. Indeed, as we look across the famous and infamous leaders of our time, they do seem generally to have certain traits in common. We might even agree on the contents of such a list. Might it not include a high energy level, intelligence, decisiveness, and a gift for verbal persuasion? Not surprisingly, early research efforts on the leadership process were guided by this compelling assumption, that is, that certain traits were a requisite for leadership and shared by those who exercise influence. It seemed a straightforward matter to simply identify those traits that distinguish leaders from followers. Leaders in a variety of fields could then be selected on the basis of that ideal combination of characteristics, thereby enhancing the effectiveness of those in society charged with the responsibilities of leadership. Unfortunately, efforts to identify the traits associated with the role of leadership have produced disappointing results overall.

Although a vast number of studies have sought to establish relationships between various personality/physical variables and leadership, no clear consistent pattern has emerged from those efforts (see reviews by, e.g., Gibb, 1969; Stogdill, 1974). At best, only a handful of variables show any degree of stability in their relationships with leadership across various settings, and even then the strength of those relationships is quite modest. Although the importance of particular traits varies greatly from situation to situation, leaders are generally more intelligent, of greater physical stature, better adjusted, more dominant/assertive, and more conservative in their attitudes (Gibb, 1969, pp. 216–224).

Perhaps the last word on the trait approach should be left to Lord, DeVader, and Alliger (1986), who emphasize a pivotal distinction. The question of who is chosen or otherwise *emerges* as a leader is separate from the question of how *effec-*

tive the leader is in his or her role. In the case of emergent leadership, three traits have been identified as centrally involved in the process. Based on a review of 27 studies, Lord et al. found that the emergence of leadership was strongly associated with stereotypical *masculinity* (e.g., aggression, decisiveness); *dominance;* and *intelligence.* However, in addressing the question of leadership effectiveness, a trait such as intelligence is not always an asset. As will be seen later in this chapter when cognitive resource theory is discussed, the relationship between the leader's IQ and performance is fairly complex.

It is important in considering questions of emergent leadership to keep the contributions of the trait approach in a balanced perspective. Singly, these traits have little predictive value; in combination, they *may* work to the advantage of the person seeking or being considered for a position of leadership.

A Situational Approach

An alternative and more recent approach to understanding leadership has been the situational view. Rather than emphasizing the leader's personal attributes, these theorists (e.g., Hollander & Julian, 1970) stress the importance of the situation for which leadership is required. Whoever is available and has the requisite skills/attributes called for by a situation is most likely to emerge as leader. Being in the right place at the right time with the needed qualifications will largely determine the choice of a leader. Change the situation and someone else may emerge as a leader. For example, the captain of the company's baseball team may clerk from 9:00 to 5:00 supervising nobody. Still other employees may lead the union in negotiations with management or plan the annual picnic. From a situational standpoint, those with task relevant abilities are most likely to be called upon to perform the various leadership functions in an organization. In short, being a recognized leader in one setting in no way guarantees the same recognition in different situations.

A Transactional Approach

A still more recent development in leadership theory—the transactional view—focuses on the *interaction* between the leader's attributes and those of the people he or she is attempting to lead. This transactional position (see, e.g., Beckhouse, Tanur, Weiler, & Weinstein, 1975; Hollander & Offerman, 1990) goes beyond the view that a leader unilaterally influences the attitudes and behaviors of subordinates or that the situation largely determines who leads. Rather, leadership is seen as a reciprocal process of influence between leaders and their subordinates. While followers are influenced by their leader, they in turn strongly influence the leader's behavior. It is this complex interplay of social influence between leader and followers that, from a transactional perspective, is at the heart of the leadership process. An example of the transactional view will be seen in Fiedler's contingency theory of leadership, to be discussed in the next section.

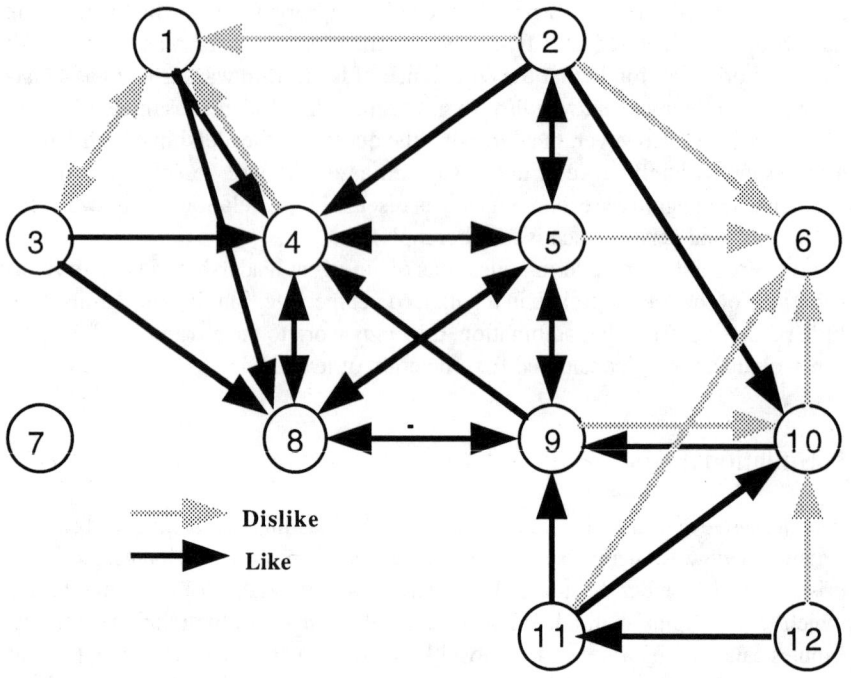

FIGURE 5.1 Team sociogram (adapted from Eberspächer, 1982).

Theories of Leadership

Sociometry

Although sociometry was originally developed as a means of aiding the rehabili-
tation of individuals in group therapy settings (Moreno, 1953), the technique has
also been used as a means of investigating leadership. In the process of assessing
the pattern of interpersonal relationships within a group, members are asked to
name, for example, the person whom they "go to for advice," the person whom
they "like the most," or the individual who "provides reassurance when things go
badly," and so on. Such questions then are intended to provide insights into the
dynamics of group interactions. However, it is also clear that certain of the questions might also identify the member(s) of a group or team who is (are) performing a leadership function. The pattern of responses to any single question emerges
when the members' nominations are combined pictorially in a *sociogram*. The
technique is well suited to analyses of the interactive patterns of smaller sports
teams. However, as the players increase in numbers, a point is soon reached
where an interpretation of the sociogram by a visual inspection becomes difficult.
(Computers will, however, ride to the rescue of those with unwieldy data sets.)

An application of the technique is seen in the work of Hans Eberspächer (1982), a physical educator from the University of Heidelberg. Figure 5.1 depicts a sociogram of a 12-man German handball team. The players were asked to indicate the teammate(s) with whom they like or do not like to play. The pattern of interpersonal relationships that emerged reveals a tightly knit clique (4, 5, 8, and 9), as well as an outcast (6). Number 4 appears as the narrow winner of the popularity contest and may play a leadership role on the team. On the other hand, 7 is socially isolated from the group.

Although the technique appears straightforward and directly applicable to sports teams, it is not without its shortcomings. For example, one would be mistaken if one simply equated "popularity" with leadership (Gibb, 1969). Also, slight changes in the wording of the question or the basis of choice can produce substantially different patterns of group structure (Bales, 1953; Criswell, 1961). As Gibb (1969) cautions, "sociocentrality is not necessarily leadership" (p. 211).

In an influential paper, Bales (1953) had group members first identify the "leader." He additionally asked members to identify those who were (1) "most liked," (2) "most disliked," (3) "contributing the best ideas," and (4) "guiding the discussion." A major finding of interest to the present discussion is that leadership was closely aligned with the contribution of ideas to the group and providing guidance to the members' discussions. On the other hand, leadership was only weakly related to "best liked."

The seemingly discouraging implications of Bales's (1953) evaluation of the sociometric approach to identifying leaders should not be taken as the final word. A negative conclusion would be premature. Recall, if you will, that the criterion for assessing leadership effectiveness is the *performance* of the group. The Bales study simply identified those individuals in various groups who were seen by the members to be their leader. Of the functions that those leaders might perform, only the contribution of ideas and guidance were related to their nomination. It was never intended that anything be revealed about how effective or ineffective those designated "leaders" might be in carrying out their responsibilities.

Fiedler's Contingency Model

The contingency model of leadership developed by Fred Fiedler (e.g., Fiedler, 1967, 1971, 1978; Fiedler & Garcia, 1987) perhaps offers us the most comprehensive account to date of the dynamics underlying successful leadership. Fiedler allows that most people can become effective leaders. However, the key to their success lies in being placed in the right situation, that is, a situation that is suited to their individual style in leading others. When the individual's leadership style is matched to the appropriate situation, effective leadership should result.

Sports organizations at all levels of competition and size differ in the challenge they pose for an incoming leader. For example, a team nearing the end of a disastrous season on the field and at the box office is advertising for a new coach. To make the position even less attractive, player conflicts abound and the club's management is riddled with dissension. In a more favorable scenario, the successful applicant may stand to inherit a well-managed, cohesive, and financially stable team with a winning record. Suffice it to say, regardless of whether an organization is in a state of complete disarray or enjoys a record of efficient and successful operations, both require effective leadership, to rebuild in the former case and to maintain the successful position in the latter.

A Matter of Style

One's style of leadership is assessed by means of the Least Preferred Co-worker (LPC) scale (Fiedler & Chemers, 1984), a measure that distinguishes between *relationship-motivated* and *task-motivated* leadership styles. The relationship-motivated leader can be characterized as one who prizes smooth and harmonious interactions among group members. The problems and challenges facing the group are also of concern but are secondary in importance. Conversely, the task-motivated leader has as the focus of his or her concern an interest in solving the problems at hand and moving the group toward its goals. This is not to say that the task-motivated leader is unconcerned about harmonious interpersonal relations. Rather, the leader is seen to be a necessary adjunct to the successful solution of problems. Although a concern of the task-motivated individual, being liked by subordinates is not a high priority in the leadership role.

What factors might be involved in the development of a particular style of leadership? Birth order appears a strong candidate. That is, firstborns tend to be more task-oriented in their interactions with subordinates; later-born leaders exhibit a more social orientation in their relationships (Chemers, 1970). Chemers accounts for the acquisition of different styles in terms of social development during the formative years, in which firstborns "are more completely socialized and develop as highly adult oriented and authority dependent persons. Later borns by contrast are more socially oriented being brought up in the company of older and stronger peers" (p. 243).

Situational Control

Before the leader's style can be matched to a situation in which it will be effective, it is first necessary to assess the situation itself. The model identifies the degree of *situational control* available to the leader as the key feature of the situation requiring a leader. What are the major elements that contribute to the leader's situational control?

Fiedler (1967) has identified three components: in order of importance, (1) *leader-member relations*, (2) *task structure*, and (3) *position power*. Briefly, leader- member relations is easily the most important factor and may be described as the extent to which goodwill is in the offing for an incoming leader. Task structure refers to considerations such as the clarity of the organization's goals and the means by which they might be achieved. For example, are the goals clearly understood or ambiguous? Is there one or several ways by which the goal can be reached? Finally, position power relates to the amount of power or authority vested in the office. For example, is the coach to be given a free hand in budgetary matters and in the hiring/firing, disciplining, and so on of his personnel, or must he seek prior approval for these actions from his superiors? Note that this aspect of the situation does not involve a consideration of the leader's qualifications (e.g., experience, training, or personal charm). Rather, it relates to how much power has been delegated to the leader while in office.

Scales have been developed to quantify each of the three components comprising the amount of situational control present in a leadership position (Fiedler & Chemers, 1984). This fact enables one to locate any given situation on a continuum of control ranging from very high to very low. That is, a position assessed as having good leader-member relations, structured tasks, and high position power represents a situation of high control. Where these components are all determined to be negative, the situation is one of low situational control. Situations moderate in control have a mix of positively and negatively assessed components.

The essential feature of the model is that of allowing for a *match* to be made between the leader's style and the situation in which he or she will be most effective. This can be seen in Figure 5.2. Note that over a large number of previous investigations, task-motivated leaders have been found to do especially well in sit-

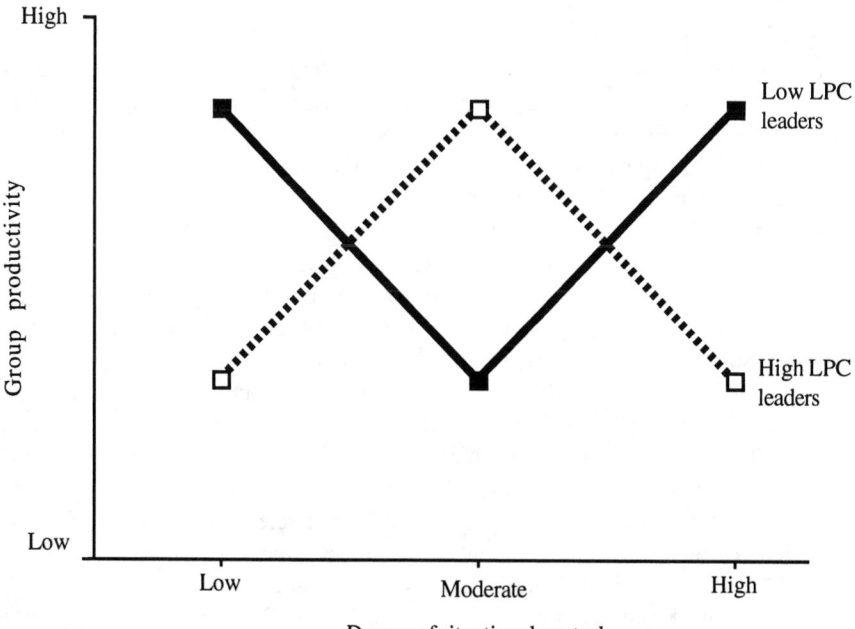

FIGURE 5.2 The contingency model (adapted from Fiedler, 1967).

uations that are either very high *or* very low in situational control. In the range of moderate control, relationship-motivated leaders excel in leading their groups to superior performances. Members in these circumstances respond better under a leader who shows concern for their personal views and well-being. On the other hand, groups that are in disastrous straits require strong, authoritative leadership to move them toward completion of their goals.

However, situations change. A leader who enjoys early and continued success is likely to improve the situation somewhat, perhaps to the point where his or her leadership style begins to interfere with the group's performance. The lack of a match dictates a change. Now, a different style is called for to restore the match between the leader and the situation in order to ensure a continuation of effective leadership.

Several interesting implications for the periodic restructuring of administrative positions arise from this aspect of Fiedler's (1967) model. As implied above, situations seldom remain static for long. Owners change, the group is given a new assignment, or the leader herself changes the situation through effective (or ineffective) leadership. One suggested means of meeting this difficulty is to provide for the rotation of leaders with differing styles. For example, a coach whose style of leadership is no longer suited to the situation could be moved to a management position and replaced by someone from the organization with the requisite style and comparable coaching credentials. The leadership skills of the displaced coach can be held "in reserve" and may again prove valuable to the organization as the situation undergoes further changes in the future.

A second means of ensuring a fit between the leader's style and the situation is to directly intervene and alter one or more components of the job until a closer match is achieved. For example, a board of directors might delegate more authority to a coach or manager, thereby increasing position power. Engaging in this sort of *job engineering* is generally regarded as the easiest and most preferable means of producing a closer fit between leadership style and situational control.

Finally, although one can successfully train the leader to adopt a different style and approach in her interactions with subordinates, such an undertaking is ill-advised on ethical if not practical grounds. While leadership effectiveness may be enhanced in the short run, the rather fundamental personality changes that accompany such training may have major disruptive consequences for the leader's ongoing social relationships beyond the organization.

The contingency model allows us to bring a more objective, empirically based approach to bear on the task of choosing leaders for sports organizations. The choice of a president, coach, or team captain need not be a totally subjective decision involving, as such choices often do, the individual biases, whims, and homespun theories of leadership held by the members of a selection committee. Rather, the chances of a successful appointment can be improved appreciably with a thoughtful application of Fiedler's model (see, e.g., Fiedler & Chemers, 1984).

Effective leadership obviously provides many benefits to an organization, not the least of which are the intrinsic satisfactions associated with improved performance. However, the contingency model can prove useful in yet another way.

An applicant for a position can herself make good use of the model by making an informal assessment of the control present in the situation in which she hopes to lead. The advantages of matching her style to the job are just as important to her interests as they are to those of the selection committee. Little is likely to be gained by attempting to lead in a situation that is unsuited to one's style. Rather, a different situation, one matching one's style of leadership, is more apt to yield success through effective leadership.

A Study

Researchers have chosen to test aspects of Fiedler's (1967) model in sports settings on only a handful of occasions. In one such investigation (Konar-Goldband, Rice, & Monkarsh, 1979) several predictions from the contingency model were tested using approximately 80 intramural university basketball teams. The leadership style of team captains, a measure of group atmosphere (an index of leader-member relations), and the performance of teams over their 9-week season provided the basic data of the study. The investigators found *stronger* relationships between group atmosphere and performance among low LPC leaders (task-motivated) than among captains scoring high on the LPC scale (relationship-motivated). Within this subgroup, then, the performance of teams playing under task-motivated captains is more readily predicted by a measure of leader-member relations than is the case with captains whose style of leadership is relationship-oriented. However, teams playing for high LPC captains were found to be more stable in their performance (i.e., from the first to second half of the season) than teams with low LPC leaders.

In an interesting sidelight, the authors note that, compared to the LPC scale norms, far more high LPC captains were identified than were low LPC leaders. Whether this imbalance is specific to the level of competition (intramural), the method of selecting team captains, or some other factor is an open question. Would intramural leagues in other sports similarly reveal a disproportionate number of relationship-motivated leaders? What is clearly needed in this area is a *series* of carefully designed investigations exploring, in particular, the role of sport-specific variables (e.g., skill level, type of sport) in affecting performance outcomes predicted by Fiedler's (1967) model.

A Caveat

Fiedler (1967) himself sounds a note of caution against generalizing the contingency model freely to all coacting groups. Many in positions of leadership are largely ineffectual in their role. In effect, the leader is a leader virtually in name only, with little influence over team members. Moreover, team sports played in a recreational vein tend not to create the anxieties of more intense competition, anxieties that a leader might be expected to actively dispel. Thus, where a leader is not sought out and/or has little control over the team, his style of leadership is unlikely to bear a relationship to performance. The results of two investigations in sports— bowling (DeZonia, 1958) and rifle shooting (Myers, 1962)—played in a recreational atmosphere dictate such a caution insofar as they yielded nonsignificant correlations between leadership style and team performance. As Fiedler (1967) concludes, "the leader's control over his team members may be simply too weak in these situations so that we cannot obtain meaningful relationships" (p. 225).

Both the contingency model and, ultimately, our understanding of leadership in sport stand to gain from studies conducted under the special circumstances afforded by sports. This is not to say that the model is without its critics (e.g., Graen, Alvares, Orris, & Martella, 1970) nor that all aspects of the model have received uniformly strong support. However, reviews of the theory (Peters, Hartke, & Pohlmann, 1985; Strube & Garcia, 1981) generally deem it to be valid in its major aspects. Leadership theory and sports psychology stand to be mutually enriched by its further application to sports.

Cognitive Resource Theory and Intelligence

As suggested earlier in regard to the trait approach, the strength of the relationship between the leader's intelligence and his effectiveness has been quite modest across studies despite a strong belief by most of us that highly intelligent leaders ought to be more effective in their roles than less intelligent leaders. A resolution of this perplexing question has been proposed by Fiedler and Garcia (1987) within the framework of cognitive resource theory. They suggest that two factors mediate or determine whether a strong association will be found between leaders' intelligence and the performance of their groups. The first of these factors is the *directiveness* of the leader. Unless the leader effectively communicates wishes, expectations, and commands to his followers, whatever intelligent plans he might want to implement are unlikely to take form. Among leaders who are able to communicate their plans to subordinates, intelligence would be predicted to have stronger links to performance.

The second proposed factor mediating the intelligence-performance relationship is *stress*. Evidence from a military study by Borden (cited in Fiedler, Potter, & McGuire, 1988) suggests that under highly stressful circumstances the relationship is virtually zero. In contrast, under nonstressful conditions the correlation between leaders' intellect and their groups' performance was an impressive .44.

In summary, intelligence is an important asset for those in positions of leadership. However, for intelligence to have a major influence it would seem that the leader must be directing in his interactions with subordinates and, ideally, be leading in nonstressful situations. Under these conditions, intelligence is likely to come to the fore as a predictor of group performance.

Other evidence (Fiedler, 1989) has considered additionally the role of the leader's job experience alongside IQ in relation to group performance. Again, stress is a critical determinant of the importance of intellectual ability in producing effective leadership. As mentioned previously, under low stress intelligence is used effectively by leaders to improve their group's performance; job-related experience makes a negligible contribution. However, under high stress leaders make little use of their intellect, instead drawing on their experience. In fact, in these conditions, less intelligent leaders tend to outperform leaders with higher intelligence. The effects of high stress seem to impair the leader's ability to assess problems facing the group and to make sound decisions.

Finally, a small-scale study of 20 high school basketball teams provided a bridge between the contingency model and cognitive resource theory (Richardson, cited in Fiedler, McGuire, & Richardson, 1989). The intelligence test scores and experience of team captains were examined in relation to their teams' win/loss records under conditions of either high or low situational control. It should be noted that the leader is under greater stress when situational control is low. It was under precisely these stressful conditions that the captains' years of playing experience were found to be strongly correlated with a successful season. Under conditions of high situational control, where stress is low, there was an indication that the intelligence of captains may instead contribute to effective leadership. Although these findings appear tentative, they do point to a number of important questions that might be addressed by sports researchers.[1]

To summarize, Fiedler's (1967) contingency model and cognitive resource theory cast considerable light on the often critical question of leadership in organized sports. It is surprising to the writer that there have not been more frequent tests of the models in sports settings, especially considering the relatively clearcut performance criteria that sports generally provide (e.g., win/loss, scores, times, etc.). Certainly, the wealth of results already obtained with the contingency model in diverse settings allows us to generalize with confidence to a variety of leadership situations. However, sports differ sharply from these other settings in several major respects. For example, is the model equally successful in predicting effective leadership across the full range of athletic motivation from recreational to that required of athletes training for an Olympic berth? To be sure, workers in military, organizational, and educational settings are rarely found to strive with anything approaching the zeal and dedication of a championship or Olympic-bound athletic team. Also, it is clear from Bird's (1977) study of collegiate volleyball that players' *preferred* leadership style may also interact with the levels of skill within a sport to differentially affect team performance. The role of these variables and their relationships to other aspects of the theory remain to be specified before Fiedler's model can be unreservedly applied to sports.

Leadership and Organizational Structure

Yet another approach to leadership has focused on the part played by the structure of an interactive situation in fostering the emergence of leaders from certain key

---

[1] For a review and evaluation of cognitive resource theory, see Vecchio (1990).

positions. Oscar Grusky (1963a, 1963b) has developed a theory of leadership specific to sports, one based on the formal structure of teams. Essentially, he proposed that one's advancement within an organization is largely a function of the position played by the athlete. More specifically, certain positions allow the development of the skills necessary for upward mobility within the organization.

Positions within the formal structure of an organization are seen to vary along three interdependent dimensions. These include (1) spatial location (central vs. peripheral), (2) nature of the task (independent vs. dependent), and (3) the frequency of personal interactions with those playing other positions. The combination of these factors allows one to identify two types of positions within an organization, those in which the occupant has a high "interaction potential" and those in which the individual is a low interactor. Those in positions calling for close and frequent interactions with others are presumed to be better liked, more socially skilled, and more strongly committed to the organization. In contrast, low interactors tend to be socially aloof and strive for individualistic rather than team values. The obvious prediction to be derived from the model is that high interactors will tend more often than lows to be recruited for executive or management positions.

The principal test of Grusky's organizational theory was conducted using the records of major league baseball (Grusky, 1963b). As specified by the model, infielders and catchers were classified as high interactors, outfielders and pitchers as low interactors. The results were entirely consistent with the model inasmuch as team managers have historically been drawn from high interactive positions. Catchers, in particular, were more likely than those playing any other position to later find employment as team managers. The original findings have also held up cross-culturally inasmuch as a similar pattern of advancement to managerial positions has been found in the records of Japanese professional baseball leagues (Loy, Curtis, & Hillen, 1987).

Loy and Sage (1970) conducted an interesting extension of Grusky's (1963b) study using high school baseball teams in Southern California. They predicted that high interactors (i.e., catchers and infielders) would (1) more likely be chosen as team captains and (2) be better liked than low interactors. It was further predicted (3) that those playing positions calling for the performance of highly independent and dependent tasks (i.e., pitchers and catchers) would be seen as more valuable to their club. All three predictions were borne out by their results (see also, Loy, Curtis, & Sage, 1978). Would similar results be found in other sports and cultures, as well as at different levels of skill? Two studies (Lee, Coburn, & Partridge, 1983; Massengale & Farrington, 1977) attempted to provide answers to these questions.

In the first of these, Massengale and Farrington (1977) tested the ability of the model to predict leadership in U.S. college football. Teams designated by the National Collegiate Athletic Association (NCAA) as Division I served as the focus for the study. Biographies of the head coaches, assistant head coaches (and coordinators), and assistant coaches were consulted to identify the principal positions these leaders had played during their college days. Playing positions classified as *central* included centers, guards, linebackers, quarterbacks, and several specialized positions (e.g., monster or rover); all other positions were regarded as *pe-*

ripheral. Two major findings emerged. Coaches tended to be drawn from among those who had played central positions in college. Also, as coaches moved upward through the ranks of management, centrality was increasingly evident in their backgrounds.

In a second study (Lee et al., 1983), British professional (First Division) and Schoolboy Association Football (soccer) records provided the data for an important test of the structural model of leadership. Players having the greatest amount of visibility/observability (*propinquity*) and interaction with teammates (*task dependence*) are found in the center-back and midfield positions. Among professional footballers, it was predicted that team captains would be likely to play these positions. However, because the soccer skills of schoolboys vary considerably, the authors predicted that (1) the best players would be appointed captains, and (2) coaches would assign them to play positions where their superior playing skills would be most effective (i.e., the midfield). The analyses revealed clear support for *all* of the predictions both at the professional and schoolboy levels. The results of this and the earlier Massengale and Farrington (1977) study considerably broaden the bases of support for a structural approach insofar as the model has successfully predicted leadership in different sports, cultures, and at two levels of skill.

Grusky (1963b) himself proposed several logical directions in which his research initiative might be extended. For example, "Is there a relationship between position played and managerial effectiveness? Is amount of experience as an infielder or number of different positions played a contributory factor affecting managerial recruitment?" (p. 351). These and other questions suggested by the structural model of organizational leadership remain to be answered. In the meantime, baseball, football, and soccer have provided settings for testing the merits of a theory of organizational leadership and at the same time advanced our understanding of the leadership process in sports.

Issues in Sports Leadership

This section is intended to acquaint the reader with several issues (among many) surrounding the question of leadership in sports. While some issues have been largely resolved, others wait on the results of research for clarification. Consideration of the issues to follow will hopefully provide a glimpse of the complexities involved in the leadership process, as well as implications for the design and conduct of research. The first issue concerns leadership that is largely ineffectual.

Leadership in Name Only

Formally designated leaders in many situations may be redundant. The principal functions traditionally ascribed to leaders (e.g., initiating task structure and fostering congenial interactions) may sometimes be performed by others or arise from the nature and structure of group activities. These "substitutes for leadership" may be present in some situations to such a degree that the formal leader is largely without influence. In short, the leader is superfluous and is seen as such by subordinates.

This view is expressed in an important though controversial paper by S. Kerr and Jermier (1978). These investigators allow that a group's need for a leader will diminish with the extent to which task structure and social support are provided to subordinates by other sources. They observe that historically there has been a widespread and deeply held conviction that leadership is always important, that "*some* leadership style will *always* be effective *regardless* of the situation" (p. 375). To clarify, consider how two sources of influence on group members, neither originating with the leader, might act to supplant the influence a leader might otherwise exert. If, for example, the task of a team member is intrinsically satisfying or if team members already possess an abundance of ability, experience, and knowledge, additional contributions on these matters from a leader are simply not needed.

Further, consider the diminished importance of the leader's role when team members develop a "professional" orientation. To paraphrase S. Kerr and Jermier (1978), such individuals characteristically establish horizontal rather than vertical relationships and tend to be guided by external referents. For example, academics frequently develop strong ties with colleagues at other institutions who share an interest in their specialty and are strongly influenced in their work by the opinions and encouragement they receive. Often, the department chair is not in the picture. Clearly, a formal leader can be largely without influence in such circumstances. In short, these and other factors sometimes operate as substitutes for leadership and as a consequence neutralize some or all the functions of hierarchical leadership.

Predicted relationships between various types of leadership and the performance of subordinates may fail to materialize for yet another reason. A study of leadership in 17 English First Division soccer teams will illustrate the point. Cooper and Payne (1967) administered the Orientation Inventory (Bass, 1962) to managers, coaches/trainers, and players alike. For present purposes, our interest is in the finding that the managers' styles of interacting with others was unrelated to the performance of their teams over the course of the season. That of the coaches and trainers, however, *was* related to the success of the teams in the case of those who adopted a task orientation with their players (a task orientation is similar to the style of Fiedler's task-motivated leader).

The result is, perhaps, not surprising. As Cooper and Payne (1967) point out, the club manager has only infrequent and relatively impersonal contact with his players. By contrast, coaches and trainers work closely with team members on a daily basis. Thus, a leader's style or orientation is largely irrelevant to the success of a team in the absence of frequent interactions with subordinates. As a consequence, predictions of leadership effectiveness are unlikely to be confirmed where the leader stays at arm's length from his followers. This failure to recognize that leaders of whatever stripe are not always influential may to some extent account for the lack of strong findings that has historically plagued much of the research on leadership.

Does a Leader Wear One or Several Hats?

It is often suggested that a leader can be all things to all men, in effect playing multiple roles. Yet the skills and efforts of some leaders appear to center almost exclusively on attempts to move their group toward its goals. The energies of other leaders seem to be directed toward maintaining a cohesive and harmonious following (i.e., group solidarity). This distinction between instrumental and expressive leadership, respectively, is at the heart of role differentiation theory (e.g., Bales & Slater, 1955). The question arises as to whether a leader can serve both instrumental and expressive functions, or whether these roles are mutually exclusive. The early view (Bales & Slater, 1955) was that instrumental leaders did not also function as expressive leaders, a position that has since been challenged.

A resolution of the issue was pursued by Roger Rees (Rees, 1983; Rees & Segal, 1984) within a sports setting. In the first of two studies, Rees and Segal had members of two U.S. college football teams nominate teammates who served (1) instrumental and (2) expressive leadership functions. The players also provided ratings of respect and liking for their choices. Analyses yielded a mix of results. Several of the players who were nominated as leaders displayed role integration; that is, they fulfilled both roles. However, other leaders performed purely instrumental functions, and still others played only an expressive role. Incidentally, all three types of leaders were liked and respected more than nonleaders.

In an attempt to shed further light on the issue, Rees (1983) followed a similar procedure using the members of 23 intramural basketball teams. A less ambiguous set of results led Rees to conclude that the important roles of instrumental and expressive leadership "are usually performed by the same people" (p. 24). Support was not forthcoming for the view that individuals play only a single leadership role.

It is noteworthy that both studies examined leadership in "interacting" groups where the smooth integration of members' skills is essential for team success. On the other hand, in coacting groups (e.g., golf and ski teams) little integration of skills is required, and consequently the expressive aspects of leadership are not as essential for group success. It thus seems likely that among coacting sports teams role differentiation may be more strongly in evidence. To conclude, leaders of teams competing in interacting sports tend to be generalists; those leading teams participating in coacting sports in all likelihood perform an instrumental function or a minor expressive function.

The Role of Coaches: Scapegoats for Failure?

How does a change in leadership affect performance? The reasoning behind most coaching changes is that fresh leadership will likely lead to an improvement in performance. This commonsense view might, however, be challenged by others who see instead the possibility of a worsened performance in the aftermath of the disruptions and tensions created by a leadership change. These two views are joined by a third that sees team performance being largely unaffected by a new face at the top (Gamson & Scotch, 1964).

Sports represent a special circumstance in which questions associated with managerial succession can be examined. Unlike organizations found elsewhere, sports organizations tend to be relatively homogeneous, that is, similar in terms of their size, goals, and organizational structures (Grusky, 1963b). This fact has made sports records from baseball, football, and basketball an attractive and valuable source of archival data for testing organizational hypotheses.

Grusky (1963a) concluded from his data that *frequent* managerial changes were dysfunctional to teams and led to a lowering of morale and poorer performance, a finding supported by Fabianic (1984) but only for long-established baseball franchises. For newer franchises, just the opposite is true! The greater the frequency of managerial changes, the greater a team's success on the field. Grusky's view has more recently been echoed by University of Calgary sociologist Robert Stebbins (1987), whose study of Canadian junior and professional football teams has highlighted the disruptive effects on morale and performance of frequent coaching changes. However, this view has not gone unchallenged (Eitzen & Yetman, 1972; Gamson & Scotch, 1964). Gamson and Scotch found that baseball teams generally fared no better or worse following changes in managers. A similar conclusion was reached by Eitzen and Yetman, who examined the relationship between the coaching changes of U.S. college basketball teams and their subsequent performance. After controlling for the record of the previous coach, there was no measurable impact on performance occurring as a result of a change in coaches.

Baseball provided the setting for a large-scale analysis of all major league teams over half a century from 1920 to 1973 (Allen, Panian, & Lotz, 1979). Using the "winning percentage" as the measure of team performance, these researchers found that the *frequency* of managerial changes is negatively related to teams' subsequent performances. While the overall effect of managerial changes on later performance is small, it does at the very least cast doubt on the common assumption that a change in leadership will necessarily lead to improved play. What seems a more consistent finding is that a record of declining team performance precedes a leadership change, a result found in several sports (Allen et al., 1979).

Other research has suggested that factors associated with the timing and type of managerial succession can also affect team performance. For example, performance deteriorates more when a change in leadership occurs *during* a football (Brown, 1982) or baseball (Allen et al., 1979) season rather than between. Thus, when the influence of teams' records in the prior season are controlled for "succession between seasons is more likely to improve team performance than succession during a season" (Allen et al., 1979, p. 178). Moreover, when teams find a replacement for their manager from outside the organization the effects prove somewhat more disruptive than when someone from within succeeds (Allen et al., 1979).

Among professional American football teams there is little evidence of an overall succession effect. Any improvement that might be seen to follow succession is not unlike that seen to follow a sharp decline in performance by teams that did not replace their coaches (Brown, 1982). Football played at the high school level may, however, be an exception (Penman, Hastad, & Cords, 1974).

In an interesting extension of this line of inquiry, Pfeffer and Davis-Blake (1986) examined succession effects occurring in the National Basketball Association (NBA) over five seasons. The results indicated that, overall, coaching changes had no effect on team performance, again controlling for prior performance. However, in taking their analysis one step further to consider the competence of the new coach, a succession effect was revealed. Coaches who had superior prior records, had NBA experience, and had previously led teams to improved performances were successful in improving the fortunes of their new teams.

It is further apparent that the outcomes of major team sports are to a considerable extent determined by the operation of random nonskill factors. Indeed, extraneous situational influences may be far more important in determining the outcome of contests than is generally recognized and may overshadow any influence associated with playing or coaching skills (J.H. Goldstein, 1979). In many instances, coaches are held responsible for events that are totally beyond their control.

A pervasive belief by the general public in a direct causal relationship between the exercise of leadership and performance extends even to situations where the leader could not possibly be responsible for the changing fortunes of his followers. R. Marshall (1927) beautifully illustrates this point with an analysis of rainfall and U.S. presidential election results for the century from 1824 to 1924, a period in which the U.S. economy was predominantly agricultural. The party in power was voted out of office in 11 out of 13 elections that were preceded by 4 years of below-average precipitation. However, the incumbent party remained in office in 11 of the 12 elections that followed 4 years of above-average rainfall! Generally speaking, then, the role of chance factors warrants much greater weight in the evaluation of a leader's performance.

Statistical Regression

Because leadership changes often follow on the heels of a poor season or an extended series of losses, it is important that the reader be alerted to regression effects. Coaches inheriting a team with a losing record in the previous season will generally appear to improve the team's performance; those taking over a team with a winning record will similarly appear to have led their team to a somewhat poorer showing. But these same trends also occur among teams that make no coaching changes whatsoever! In any season, previously weak teams can be expected to show improvement and formerly successful teams can be expected to experience a decline in performance, irrespective of any effects that might arise from a change in leadership. This tendency for unsuccessful and successful teams in any one year to drift toward the mean (or average) in the succeeding year is explained by regression effects. (For a detailed description of this statistical artifact see Campbell & Stanley, 1966.) Thus, the coach who inherits a team with a losing record may be credited with effecting a measure of improvement more accurately attributed to regression effects. A truly effective coach in the same situation will lead a team to an improved performance over and above that which can be credited to an expected upward regression toward the mean.

Regression effects occur as a result of the imperfect correlation between the final league standings in two succeeding seasons. The effect or movement toward the mean will be especially pronounced for those teams that in the previous year placed very high or very low in the standings (e.g., first or last place). Those teams finishing near the middle of the standings will show relatively little drift in the following year. But to return to the original question of the effect of periodic coaching changes, there is to this point no consistent evidence that a change in leadership per se influences the performance of a team. Why, then, are coaching changes so common?

The suggestion of Gamson and Scotch (1964) is that succession may represent a ritualized scapegoating. The removal from office of a truly inept leader can only benefit an organization and those it serves. However, the firing of a coach or manager merely to appease fans, alumni, or the media is a terribly shortsighted action. While short-term interests might be served, the organizational or personnel problems that often lie at the root of poor team showings are never addressed. So, while expressions of fan disenchantment may be temporarily silenced, the fundamental flaws in the organization itself remain.

Coaching Experience and Team Success

Do coaches, like fine wine, improve with age and experience? By the criterion of winning, the answer, with a few exceptions (e.g., Penman et al., 1974; Weiss & Friedrichs, 1986), appears to depend on the length of their tenure. Penman et al. (1974) compiled the win/loss percentages of head coaches in high school football and basketball. Winning was found to be unrelated to both the coaches' ages and years of coaching experience. However, Eitzen and Yetman (1972) compared the length of coaching tenure with team success in college basketball. Here the relationship was found to be significant but curvilinear. For approximately the first 13 years, teams show improved performance under their coaches' guidance. However, coaches who continued in their position beyond that point led their teams to steadily worsening records. Whether due to the ravages of age, complacency, or an impending retirement, the reduced effectiveness of "one-team" coaches who persist in the twilight of their careers seems well established.

I would hasten to add as a footnote that although leadership by senior coaches may in some cases deteriorate, it does not do so for reasons of declining intelligence. The occurrence of a disabling illness notwithstanding, the relationship between age and intelligence is a negatively accelerating function over most of the normal life span (Anastasi, 1988). Increments in intelligence (i.e., learned ability) continue to be realized by most people on up into their 60s, and beyond.

In contrast to sports, evidence of a relationship between years of leadership and the leader's effectiveness is not readily apparent in other types of organizational settings. Fiedler aptly summarizes the results of studies addressing this question in the title of his 1970 review article, "Leadership Experience and Leader Performance—Another Hypothesis Shot to Hell." The generally unquestioned assumption that experience in a leadership role is a prerequisite for advancement to higher positions of authority in an organization is rarely challenged. Yet the evidence for the assumption is sparse. After all, if experience simply means "time spent" in the lower ranks without opportunities to grow and hone leadership skills, then the lack of a relationship is not surprising. What, then, are we to make of the study of sports leadership noted above (Eitzen & Yetman, 1972) that tends to confirm this popular assumption?

Leadership in sports, specifically coaching roles, may provide the very conditions where leadership skills can be learned and refined over a number of seasons. Certainly, the actions of coaches are closely monitored by the owners, media, fans, and players alike, all of whom are only too willing to provide feedback on the wisdom of coaching decisions. So, too, does the win/loss column provide evidence, reinforcing or otherwise, of the success of a coach's efforts to improve the performance of players. It is only speculation on my part, but coaching may be an exception to the general pattern of negative findings on this question.

The Life Expectancy of a CEO?

It is generally recognized that coaches, managers, presidents, and so on of sports organizations—positions that contributors to the management science literature collectively refer to as chief executive officers (CEOs; e.g., Fredrickson, Hambrick, & Baumrin, 1988)—are frequently replaced after only a year or two in office. A model of CEO dismissal that has direct implications for the stability of sports leadership has been proposed by Fredrickson et al. One aspect of their model attempts to identify the factors that increase the CEO's chances of dismissal, especially during the early months in office when the CEO appears to be most vulnerable. In sports, as elsewhere, leaders appear to be quite insecure at the outset of their tenure. For example, coaches in the National Football League from 1970 to 1982 held their positions for an average of four years (Chakravarty, 1983). However, the number of modal years of service (i.e., the most common length of time spent as a coach) was one year! Our best advice to newly appointed coaches must be, *Rent, don't buy!* What, though, are the conditions that make the CEO vulnerable?

Fredrickson et al. (1988) propose that (1) attributes of the CEO and (2) factors associated with the departure of the previous CEO can hasten the dismissal of a new appointee. Two important characteristics of new CEOs that tend to be associated with early dismissal are whether their appointment was made from within or from outside the organization and whether they are excessively compensated or receive the "going rate" for their services. A board of directors is thought to have higher expectations for the performance of appointees from outside the organization and forms only weak allegiances to the new officeholder. The expectations for the performance of a "star" who has been lured away from a position in which they enjoyed outstanding success are similarly high, often unrealistically so. The first signs of failure on the part of the lavishly compensated star appear to bring disillusionment and an early end to his or her services. But characteristics of the new CEO's predecessor are also important, in particular the circumstances of his or her departure. Did the CEO leave for reasons of poor health, retire, or get fired? If the predecessor was dismissed, the board may be experiencing considerable turmoil and residual ill-will. This, and the likelihood that allegiances are slow to develop, does not augur well for the new CEO. At least for the early years, then, insecurity goes with the job.

Idiosyncrasy Credit

An awareness of the phenomenon of idiosyncrasy credit may allow a new appointee to avoid or at least forestall an early departure. Leaders of most groups require the support of their subordinates if they are to provide effective leadership. The support of subordinates is often tentative and conditional on the leader confirming their expectations regarding her behavior during her early days in office (i.e., providing a smooth transition from the previous officeholder). Yet leaders who truly "lead" often strike out in bold new directions. When should leaders innovate or alter their group's direction: at the outset or near the end of their term in office?

According to Hollander (1964), departures from previously established policies and practices are more likely to be accepted by group members when the introduction of an innovative program is carefully timed to follow a trial or honeymoon period. That is to say, followers expect their new leader to conform to the established standards, norms, or practices of the group, at least for a time. During these early days in office the leader by adhering to accepted practice amasses *idiosyncrasy credits*, credits that later allow her to introduce innovations and implement new programs, in effect to provide an important aspect of leadership. Attempts to implement major change immediately on assuming office are likely to create dissension and generate resistance from group members. By closely conforming to group norms for a period of time, the leader is permitted to deviate from established practice, that is, draw from her fund of accumulated credits in the interests of helping the group achieve its goals. For the newly appointed team manager anxious to introduce a new accounting procedure or the coach keen to try a radical new training regimen, the best advice must be to wait at least until the honeymoon is over.

When the Going Gets Tough, the *Complex* Get Going

Rather than risk embarrassment to anyone, I will avoid specific examples and assume that each of us can recall an occasion when a sports leader (e.g., captain, quarterback, coach, etc.) uncharacteristically performed badly in his or her play or

****

Speaking Tangentially 5.1: When to Pull the Goalie?
Your hockey team is one goal down, and time is running out in the third period. What is the optimum point at which the coach should pull the goalie in hopes of gaining a tie? The common practice is to wait until a minute or so remains in the game. Does a decision to pull the goalie at that point maximize the likelihood of tying the game?

To those with mathematical credentials, the answer is straightforward. Morrison and Wheat (1986) have determined that the goalie should be pulled with precisely 2:34 minutes left to play. Their general advice is to remove the goalie with 2 to 2:30 minutes left to play. However, all is not lost even when one's team is two goals down. In that case they recommend pulling the goalie with 2:30 to 3 minutes remaining. Actually, coaches have done reasonably well in simply following their intuition. Their suboptimal strategy of waiting until the final minute of play is still about 90% effective.

****

decision making under extreme stress. By any standards, the leader called the wrong series of plays or failed to use the clock and time-outs to the team's advantage in the dying minutes of a close championship game. Of course, a few of the decisions that are routinely taken under pressure have been mathematically predetermined so as to be maximally effective (see Speaking Tangentially 5.1). Is it common for leaders generally to perform less well under fire? Are some leaders perhaps better able than others to make judgments of superior quality under stress?

As you will recall from our discussion of cohesion (chap. 4), dissension within a group declines and members typically rally in support of their leader in the face of an external threat. But how does this same threat affect the leader himself? More specifically, how is the quality of decision making affected by high levels of stress? Here the evidence suggests that decision making suffers. That is to say, the typical leader under stress attends to fewer aspects of the situation, considers fewer options, and perhaps prematurely takes a decision that is resistant to change even in the face of changing circumstances (Schroder, Driver, & Streufert, 1967). However, a small number of leaders continue to process information effectively in stressful situations and make judgments that are qualitatively superior to those of other leaders. The leader who functions best under extreme stress is one who is cognitively or conceptually complex in contrast to his conceptually simple counterpart. (For details of the theory, see, e.g., Coates & Leong, 1988; Schroder et al., 1967.)

The conceptually simple decision maker may be briefly characterized as one who processes available information along fewer dimensions; tends to see matters as "either-or" (i.e., exhibits black-white thinking); has difficulty seeing an issue from another's perspective; seeks early closure on an issue; and displays a certain rigidity and inability to take new evidence into account once a decision has been made. An extended discussion of conceptual complexity is beyond the scope of this chapter, but Figure 5.3 will, hopefully, illustrate the effects of ex-

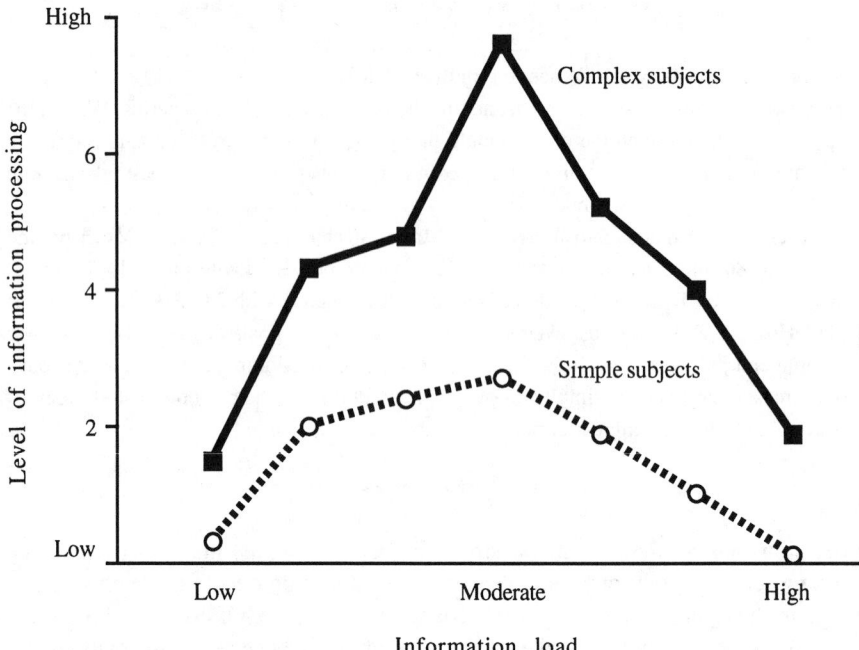

FIGURE 5.3 Performance under high and low stress (adapted from Schroder et al., 1967).

treme stress on two types of decision makers, the conceptually complex and the conceptually simple. In this study, the performance of groups comprised of either high or low complex individuals were compared in a tactical game situation (Schroder et al., 1967). Those in both types of groups were equally intelligent.

As stress increased from low to moderate levels, the number of pieces of information taken into account by both types of individuals steadily increased. However, as levels of stress moved upward into the high range, both conceptually simple and complex subjects processed the available information less and less effectively. Nevertheless, across all levels of stress, the complex decision maker demonstrates clearly superior information-processing skills.

The results of this early simulation have more recently been replicated in research by Peter Suedfeld at the University of British Columbia (Suedfeld, Corteen, & McCormick, 1986; Wallace & Suedfeld, 1988). Actual world leaders have shown similar patterns in their decision making through periods of international crises, exhibiting the same general tendency toward qualitatively inferior decision making under extreme stress. Incidentally, a remarkable exception to this tendency was the late Andrei Gromyko, the Soviet foreign minister. Throughout his long and distinguished career this conceptually complex diplomat exhibited dramatically superior decision-making skills during times of international tension. Still, one is entitled to ask if a leader's level of complexity can be shown to directly affect the outcome of a contest.

In the case of generals commanding troops in the American civil war, we see that their levels of integrative complexity were closely related to their success on the battlefield (Suedfeld et al., 1986). General Robert E. Lee as commander of the Confederate army consistently defeated superior forces led by Union generals with substantially lower levels of complexity. When Lee faced generals who were closer in complexity to him, his advantage was lost. Against General Ulysses S. Grant, whose complexity level was actually higher, the outcome as they say, is history.

It was noted earlier, in the context of cognitive resource theory (Fiedler & Garcia, 1987), that high IQ leaders are relatively ineffective under stress, tending to babble. While intelligence and conceptual complexity are themselves modestly related (Schroder et al., 1967), it would appear that it is the complex leader who should be at the helm in critical situations. Intelligence in a leader is advantageous in the general, nonstressful case. However, under conditions of extreme stress, it is the conceptually complex leader with above-average intelligence who is best able to guide his followers through perilous straits. Crucial moments are fairly commonplace in sports. At such times, conceptual complexity may be the single most decisive attribute in a leader that determines the team's success under fire. Intelligence is simply overshadowed in these circumstances. The critical variable mediating success under extreme pressure, then, is the ability to effectively process information.

And finally, do team members forgive a leader who folds under pressure? Is the leader retained following his best but unsuccessful efforts to lead his followers in times of crisis? At the conclusion of a shuffleboard game, teams for which Hamblin (1958) created crisis conditions quickly replaced their leader. Although they became increasingly accepting of and more strongly influenced by their leader as the crisis deepened, their leaders were nonetheless turfed out. Apparently, gratitude is not our strong suit (Chakravarty, 1983; R. Marshall, 1927)!

Leadership Preferences

Chelladurai has approached the leadership question from an interesting perspective (Chelladurai & Saleh, 1978). Basically, his program has involved efforts to determine what types of leadership are preferred by various athletes competing in a variety of sports. To this end, factor analytic procedures were used to identify the dimensions underlying preferences for "sport"-leader behaviors. (For a review of this innovative program, see Chelladurai, in press.)

Sex Differences

Chelladurai's analyses have revealed a number of major sex differences. Males prefer to be coached under an autocratic regimen, and females prefer instead a democratic style of leadership. On the other hand, in a nonsports setting, Kushell and Newton (1986) found that male and female speech communication students alike expressed greater satisfaction with a democratic form of leadership. Also, their satisfaction was unrelated to the gender of the leader.

Interestingly, the Chelladurai and Saleh (1978) study also found that males generally expressed a greater need than females for emotionally supportive coaching. This sex difference was especially pronounced in "closed" sports (e.g., golf, diving) in contrast to what the authors define as "open" sports (e.g., fencing, badminton). A closed sport refers to minimal variability in environmental changes with correspondingly less by way of a response required of the particular athlete. Athletes involved in team sports showed a greater preference for coaching that emphasized training than those participating in individual sports. Men and women did not differ in this regard.

Leadership Satisfaction

In subsequent studies, Chelladurai has turned to questions of the athlete's *satisfaction* with leadership (Chelladurai, 1984; Chelladurai & Carron, 1983). His measurement of satisfaction assesses the degree to which a preferred theme of leadership is discrepant with what the athlete perceives to be the case in his or her situation. For example, as athletes acquire increasing years of experience in sport there are corresponding increases in their preferences for social support and an authoritarian style of coaching (Chelladurai & Carron, 1983; Chelladurai & Saleh, 1978). To the extent that seasoned athletes perceive these to be lacking in their leaders, there will be dissatisfaction.

The preference of seasoned athletes for an authoritarian coaching style is likely founded on a belief that an authoritarian style of leadership will bring them success in their sport. Their confidence in the belief may be justified. Penman, Hastad, and Cords (1974) found that the more successful coaches of high school football and basketball teams adopt an authoritarian form of leadership.

Individual Satisfaction

A number of factors thought to be related to team and individual satisfaction have been tested in an investigation by Weiss and Friedrichs (1986). These researchers had the coaches and players of 23 college basketball teams complete a battery of questions and scales. Included among the scales were measures of institutional factors (e.g., size of school); coach's attributes (e.g., coaching experience); and the five dimensions of leader behaviors (i.e., training, democratic behavior, autocratic behavior, social support, and rewarding behavior) assessed by the Leadership Scale for Sports (Chelladurai & Saleh, 1980). Foremost among the results of extensive analyses was the finding that rewarding behavior on the part of coaches produced the greatest satisfaction among teams. Neither institutional variables nor attributes of the coaches were predictive of team satisfaction. Further analyses at the level of individual athletes revealed that greater satisfaction was expressed by athletes attending larger rather than smaller institutions and by those playing for coaches with better win/loss percentages. Interestingly, athletes playing under younger coaches with fewer years of playing experience expressed greater satisfaction than those playing for older and more personally experienced mentors. Of the five leader behavior variables, democratic behavior and social support were found to be modestly predictive of *individual* satisfaction.

Performance

Coaches' attributes and the set of institutional characteristics were found to be unrelated to team *performance* (i.e., win/loss records). Only one variable, that of social support provided a team by the coach, was related to performance. Whereas social support was associated with greater satisfaction among individual athletes, it was at the same time associated with *poorer* performance records (Weiss & Freidrichs, 1986). Thus, while satisfaction is a worthy topic of investigation in its own right, it would be naive to conclude that satisfaction necessarily leads directly to improved team performance. Certainly, Fiedler's (1978) contingency model allows for "satisfied" but unproductive workers in situations that are unsuited to the leader's style. As Chelladurai (1984) has acknowledged, the relationship between the satisfaction of athletic team members and their actual performance remains to be clarified.

Summary

In the foregoing, I have attempted to provide an overview of leadership, a topic whose importance to athletic performance is greater than is generally recognized. In so doing, several theoretical views of leadership, among many, were emphasized along with a number of practical issues having implications for selection practices and organizational structure in a variety of contemporary sports. However, my sense is that unlike other organizations, there has generally been a reluctance to abandon traditional means of filling leadership positions in sports. Yet at the same time, these organizations go to extraordinary lengths and expense to recruit athletes with just the right combination of skills to complement and enhance the overall performance of their team. Surely, if leadership has an impact on team performance, just as much time and care should be given to the selection of leaders, be they coaches, managers, or team captains. Otherwise, the most painstaking search for talented players goes for naught if they are unable to function effectively because of an inept or mismatched leader.

Suggested Readings

Hunt, J.G. (1991). *Leadership: A new synthesis.* Newbury Park, CA: Sage. The current views of this noted authority on leadership processes are presented in a well-organized volume.

6

Sports Heroes:
An Extension of Leadership

Virtually every field of human endeavor has produced its share of heroes, both for the benefit of those aspiring to success and for those who merely wish to admire or relive their heroes' past glories. The sports world in particular has historically demonstrated an ability to create heroes instantly and/or keep alive the exploits of those from an earlier era. Given the fleeting nature of fame, it is not surprising that institutions have been established in most sports designed solely to perpetuate and keep before the public the flickering memories of past achievements.

Lewis and Redmond (1974) observe that halls of fame are peculiarly an American phenomenon and have multiplied at an astonishing rate since World War II. In addition to serving as quasi-religious shrines to honor the past, halls of fame fulfill other important social functions. Frequently, they provide a boost to tourism and serve as a repository for archival information. Perhaps equally important, they provide a setting that allows visitors to experience collective and individual nostalgia (Snyder, 1991).

However, it is not only sports officialdom that shows an interest in preserving the memories of great achievements. Many outstanding athletes are themselves mindful of their opportunities for a place in sports history. As a consequence, some will persist, often in the twilight of their careers, in pursuit of even more records simply to ensure that their mark in a sport will not be lost to future generations. Their interest in the *postself*, that is, "the concern of a person with the presentation of his or her self in history" (Schmitt & Leonard, 1986, p. 1088) manifests itself in the athlete's striving to surpass past performances with a view to extending her or his name into the future. A question to be asked once an individual is established as a contemporary hero or enshrined in a hall of fame is the extent and quality of their influence on those who elevated them to their position of social prominence.

The Impact of Heroes

As noted in the previous chapter, nearly all definitions of leadership include a notion of influence. The case in support of the common assumption that heroes similarly influence their admirers in significant ways is best illustrated by Wolfenstein and Kliman's (1965) comprehensive assessment of children's reactions to the assassination of President John F. Kennedy. For many of these children (and their parents) the president was a personal hero. Kennedy's widespread popularity is seen in the results of a 1961 Gallup poll in which 41% of respondents with a grade school education and 17% of those with a college education chose him as the person they most admired (cited in Hyman, 1975, p. 282). Among the diverse reactions observed in the aftermath of his death, perhaps the most important was a loss of the children's motivation to achieve. The effects were far from transitory. Wolfenstein and Kliman collected their data several months after the tragedy. One can only speculate on the longevity of this and other residual influences, both positive and negative, arising from the loss.

Certainly, there is a wealth of testimonial and anecdotal evidence suggesting that deceased and living heroes are frequently credited with serving as an inspiration to others who strive for life goals. Be that as it may, the important and basic point to be established here is that heroes have the *capacity* to influence their admirers in fundamental and profound ways. The extent and quality of the influence exerted by prominent sports figures is a central theme of this chapter.

I would stress at this point that the act of choosing an exemplar is considerably more than a lighthearted exercise having few real-life consequences. Rather, a serious choice may reveal a great deal about a person. One possibility is that the values, traits, or behaviors that an individual sees displayed by a heroine/hero may be the very ones to which that person aspires and that motivate and guide his or her behavior. While the crash course on correlation (chap. 7) reminds us that we cannot infer causality, let alone any direction of influence, still links have been established between exemplar choices and attributes of their admirers. These relationships will be highlighted later in this chapter. In the meantime, let me underscore the central role of exemplar choices by reference to behaviors that often have serious, far-reaching social consequences. An example from the literature on wife battering will hopefully illustrate the point. Don Dutton (1988) has developed a comprehensive theory of spousal violence that profiles men who batter their female partners. A central component of the model that is predictive of assaultive behavior is "exposure to violent role models" (p. 68). Notwithstanding the question of whether all such models serve as personal heroes for batterers, the models' violence is presumed to legitimize and provide scripts for men to enact similar tactics in their own relationships with women.

The importance of exemplar quality is also suggested by an early study that compared U.S. high school graduates to dropouts (Cervantes, 1965). The study revealed that both graduates and dropouts cited parents (followed by relatives) as the principal influences in their lives. A critical difference between the groups was seen in the nomination of peers. Almost twice as many dropouts (15%) as graduates (8%) indicated that peers were the most influential people in their lives. The percentage differences arose from the dropouts' nomination of peers who did not meet with the approval of their parents.

Fortunately, the availability of prosocial heroes/heroines for children is not a matter that need be left entirely to chance. During the formative years in particular, parents, teachers, and others can actively expose youngsters to a wider circle of quality choices both on informal occasions and through the educational process. Perhaps of greater importance is the example that they themselves set.

A sidelight to the Cervantes (1965) study that should be of more than passing interest to those of us in the teaching profession was the almost total absence of teachers in the youngsters' nominations. As Cervantes concludes, "the central figure on the academic stage—the teacher—is all but a nonentity when viewed through youths' brutal binoculars" (p. 117). In further expanding on the lack of evidence in his data for a student-teacher link he observes that "educators seem to be suffering from delusions of grandeur when they infer that a great number of students are 'identified' with the teacher" (p. 113). The same result was found in a Canadian study (Russell & McClusky, 1985). Among a sample of several hundred high school students, only one nomination was for a teacher. For most of us, a deflating result! Perhaps we would do better on a second or third ballot.

Heroes as Leaders

Unsought Leadership

The idea of unilateral influence (i.e., from the hero or heroine to the admirer) consistently emerges from a consideration of the hero's role in society. On this basis alone, it is appropriate to regard sports heroes as leaders, albeit of a special type. For the most part, sports heroes fit the category of *unsought* leadership (Gibb, 1969) inasmuch as their outstanding achievements rather automatically thrust them into the spotlight of public acclaim. In their new role, they are called upon to assume many of the responsibilities of leadership. Additionally, they are accorded the status of "expert" on the topic of their sport by virtue of their record setting or championship performance. Such authority is bestowed on the hero despite the fact that other lesser lights are often equally or even more knowledgeable regarding the fundamentals and intricacies of their sport.

Impact Champions

A subcategory of media figures who have been ascribed hero/heroine status should also be recognized. Among those athletes popularized by the media, a few can be classified as *impact champions*, a term coined by sportswriter Frank Deford (1969). While an excess of talent is a necessary condition for media superstar status, it is not always a sufficient condition. Beyond possessing outstanding abilities, some athletes are able to "establish a notoriety and an impact that can be turned into box office" (p. 33). The extracurricular activities of such former notables as tennis player Ille Nastase, hockey's Derek Sanderson, and Broadway Joe Namath placed them squarely in the mold of impact champions.

Celebrities

Barney (1985) makes a similar distinction between *heroes* and *celebrities* in noting that "the celebrity is always contemporary, and is destroyed by this passage of time. Eventually, the media, the agency which made the surrogate hero, is the agency of destruction of that image. A celebrity is really a personality."

The value of hero status has not been lost on political (Petrie, 1975), religious (Deford, 1976; G.J. Smith, 1976), and commercial interests. The potential gains to be realized through association with successful athletes have not escaped the attention of politicians. In recent years, White House staff members have made arrangements for the U.S. president to phone the winners of various national championships immediately after their victory, that is, in the dressing room while the network cameras are still rolling. This is followed by a White House reception a week or so later, again a media event.

The most blatant exploitation of the hero's lofty standing with the public is probably seen in the promotions of Madison Avenue that feature popular athletes endorsing everything from breakfast cereals to feminine hygiene products. It matters little that the sportsperson's area of competence has nothing whatsoever to do with the products with which he or she is associated. A long-standing tradition of research on attitude change, however, recognizes that the sheer prestige and/or attractiveness of a communicator, irrespective of any product-relevant knowledge he or she might possess, is often sufficient to effectively persuade some of us to purchase what he or she recommends (e.g., see Rosnow & Robinson, 1967, Part I; Zimbardo & Leippe, 1991).

However, one's admiration for a subgroup of these commercially minded athletes is sorely tested when they lend their name to the promotion of deadly alcohol and tobacco products. It is refreshing from time to time to see a celebrity-athlete take a stand against the attempts of these industries to reach their markets through association with the images of health and fun portrayed by sports (Zimbardo & Leippe, 1991, p. 26). Canada's outstanding downhill skier Steve Podborski once refused to accept the Export "A" Cup for winning the Canadian downhill championship sponsored by the RJR Macdonald Tobacco Company ("Podborski Turns," 1984). In a similar gesture of protest, England's two-time Olympic decathlon champion Daley Thompson competed through the first five events with the name of the Commonwealth Games sponsor scratched from his vest. The International Guiness Brewing company was reported to be "very unhappy" about the incident (*USA Today,* July 28, 1986). Such personal statements by athletes are all too rare.

Heroic Types

Just as there are different categories of leaders, so too are there types of heroes. The writer of a letter to the editor of a national magazine (*Maclean's,* March 8, 1982) intuitively recognized this point in declaring the following:

> Your editorial statement about Wayne Gretzky is wrong, wrong, wrong! Gretzky is a magnificent hockey player and by all accounts a fine young man. He is *not* a hero. Terry Fox was a hero.
>
> Roger Wellman
> Richmond, B.C.

Stephen Fonyo and the late Terry Fox clearly fit the mold of classical hero in their valiant efforts to run across a continent despite having each lost a leg to cancer. Millions of North Americans were moved to tears and altruism by their example of self-sacrifice. But to take slight issue with Roger Wellman (above), Wayne Gretzky is also a hero, although of a distinctly different type. The reader interested in pursuing questions of definition and the classification of heroes may wish to start with Barney (1985), Klapp (1962, 1969), and Lehman (1928) for historical background to the topic. In this regard, Klapp has developed an extensive taxonomy of heroes, an outline of which is presented in Table 6.1.

Of immediate interest is the fact of sports heroes having been relegated en masse to the subcategory of "heroes of play." It should be noted that although classificatory schemes are often useful in bringing order to a welter of seemingly unrelated elements within some particular realm, they are seldom without deficiencies. Often, certain individuals do not fit comfortably into existing categories, suggesting that further refinements are required in the system. Moreover, other

Table 6.1. A classification of heroes.

Category	Theme
I. Winners	
(a) Strong man	Getting what you want,
(b) The brain	beating everyone, being
(c) The smart operator	a champ.
(d) The great lover	
II. Splendid Performers	
(a) Showmen	Shining before an audience.
(b) Heroes of play	
(c) Playboy	
III. Heroes of Social Acceptability	
(a) The pin-up	Being liked, attractive,
(b) The charmer	good.
(c) The good fellow	
(d) Conforming heroes	
IV. Independent Spirits	
(a) Bohemian	Standing alone, making
(b) Jester	one's way by oneself.
(c) Angry commentator	
V. Group Servants	
(a) Defenders	Helping people, cooperation,
(b) Martyrs	self-sacrifice, group
(c) Benefactors	service and solidarity.

heroes may appear equally suited to two or more of the available categories. For example, the late-night social activities of England's former soccer great George Best and football's Joe Namath qualify them for membership in both the "playboy" and "heroes of play" categories.

Finally, bear in mind that taxonomies are merely a starting point in our attempts to understand the "whys" of human behavior; by themselves, they provide few answers. Moreover, some taxonomies are more useful than others. Fortunately, guidelines have been developed solely to evaluate the adequacy of classification systems. Altman (1968) proposes that six key questions be addressed by the developers and users of taxonomies. For example, one question asks, "Can variables, relationships, and phenomena be reliably located in the classification space?" (p. 63). By this criterion, users must be in agreement as to where in the system an item is to be found. In the absence of a consensus, there is likely to be chaos. Another question asks, "Can new facts be incorporated into the classification system?" (p. 64). If new items can be fitted in only with difficulty, then modifications and refinements in the system are obviously needed. Altman notes that in these and other respects the standards for judging a taxonomy are much like those used in evaluating the merits of a theory.

The Functions of Exemplars

Just as heroes are not all of the same stripe, neither do they perform the same functions in society. Assuming for the moment that heroes have the capacity to influence their admirers, we turn to the question of how their influence might affect their social constituency. That is to say, how is society led or misled by its heroes? Janet Harris (1986) has identified three major functions of heroes as (1) displaying idealized versions of social order, (2) compensation, and (3) providing opportunities for social interaction.

Idealized Social Order

In the first of the three major functions of hereos, admirers are inspired to strive toward idealized societal forms. The particular forms displayed can, of course, range from "things as they are" to the stretching of existing behavioral norms, to the creation of new modes of normative behavior (Klapp, 1969). More specifically, Klapp labels one who represents the status quo and who sets directions within the existing social order as the "reinforcing hero." The goals and values pursued by the admirers of the reinforcing hero are those of which society has traditionally approved. The "seductive hero" tempts us instead to violate social norms. Secret agent James Bond, with his penchant for an excessive life-style featuring fast cars and faster women, illustrates the second direction in which heroes lead. Finally, Klapp's category of "transcending hero" includes those prominent figures who urge us to step outside of the existing structure to create a new, fresh approach to social order. Utopians and the present crop of various and sundry gurus perhaps best represent this category.

Compensatory Function

To return to the second function of Harris's (1986) model, heroes sometimes play a compensatory role in rekindling the salience of valued traits that seem all but lost in modern society but that people would nonetheless like to see restored. The epic journey of Sir Francis Chichester, the 65-year-old English adventurer whose solo voyage around the world in his 54-foot boat, *Gypsy Moth IV*, stirred Britishers to relive the glorious days of empire when heroic deeds seemed far more commonplace.

In an epilogue (Chichester, 1967), Anderson has attempted to capture the essential Chichester achievement:

> He has succeeded in making dreams come true, his own private dreams, and the dreams that most men have from time to time as they fare on that long fool's errand to the grave. (p. 224)

But more than that:

> He was the nation's hero, but to me he seemed to epitomize not scarlet and lace, but that incredible endurance that the people of England have shown when it was needed of them, the endurance of the men who sailed with Drake, Anson, Cook and Nelson, for England. (p. 226)

Interpersonal Involvement

Third, heroes provide opportunities for involvement with others. Of course, when the exemplar is in the *personal* domain of his or her admirer (e.g., parents, acquaintances), involvement is the rule rather than the exception. However, in the case of heroes in the *public* domain, personal interactions with their following are unlikely except as interactions may be fantasized by their admirers. Even so, social relationships may be strengthened among individuals who find they share in their admiration of exemplars in the public domain. A prime example are those caught up in the mania of collecting and trading sports cards. They are in regular contact with other enthusiasts, as additionally are members of fan clubs that allow for even more formal social bonds to be established.

Expanding this notion to an international scale, it has been suggested (Goodhart & Chataway, 1968, pp. 152–154) that nations that share in their admiration of a common hero are, as a result, drawn closer together. Support for these ideas has been forthcoming from the social laboratory. Subjects led to believe that they hold similar attitudes subsequently express greater liking for each other than subjects told they have few attitudes in common (e.g., Berscheid & Walster, 1969).

The industrialization and technological advances of today's modern societies are frequently held responsible for alienating people from one another. This sense of isolation and/or loss of identity can have tragic personal and social consequences for some individuals. It has been suggested that the effects of alienation can be greatly offset through an identification with a hero in which the individual vicariously shares in the exploits of the hero (Klapp, 1969). Evidence that hero worship may serve this function has been provided by G.J. Smith (1976). Respondents choosing a sports hero were found to be more socially integrated than those not choosing someone; that is, they held a greater number of memberships in organizations. Similarly, there was less alienation among those choosing a *reinforcing* sports hero than among those without a sports hero. Smith also found an interesting sex difference. Females choosing sports heroes were less well socially integrated than their male counterparts. An interest in sports seemingly distances females from the mainstream interests of other women.

Fitness Motivation

A further function confined to sports heroes has been cryptically described by Averill (1950). Assuming that the idealization of the sports figure is not spent solely "in mere mouth honor and vociferous oral adulation" but instead leads to participation in physical activities, he concludes that "this shift from an ideational to a muscular motif may prove to be a not unfortunate one" (p. 52). Support for the proposition that heroes can actually motivate their admirers to participate in sports activities has been forthcoming from in-depth interviews with deeply committed fans (G.J. Smith, Patterson, Williams, & Hogg, 1981).

Economic Function

Finally, an economic function is often served by the sports celebrity. Modern-day entrepreneurs are certainly not the first to recognize the financial rewards to be reaped from the appearance of a hero in the lineup. Sandiford (1982) documents the financial impact of British cricketer Dr. W.G. Grace during the Victorian era. Grace is described as "perhaps the most dynamic sports hero in British history" (p. 6) and "lionized all across the Kingdom" (p. 9). His scheduled appearance in a match consistently drew enormous crowds. Some cricket clubs even took the unusual step of doubling the admission prices for matches in which he played.

But we are entitled to ask whether the "excessive" salaries paid hero-celebrities are justified. Noll (1974) has determined that the drawing power of "star" baseball and basketball players contributes substantially more to team revenues than they individually receive in salaries. This is true even discounting their contribution to the win/loss record of their team, a factor that, in turn, is recognized as additionally affecting attendance (e.g., Russell, 1986; Schollaert & Smith, 1987). While Noll concludes that stars are not overpaid (i.e., by the standard of pre-1974 salary schedules) in terms of the financial benefits they provide their organizations, his analysis leaves unanswered the question of "whether they are overpaid in relation to their value to the sport at large" (p. 135) and, I might add, their value to society. The question that springs to mind for all of us, I'm sure, is whether Noll's conclusion would still hold with an analysis based on the lavish contract settlements being reached in 1992.

Trends and Category Importance

Early Trends

Writers have referred to heroes by a variety of terms that are far from synonymous (e.g., exemplars, ideals, reference idols, role models or significant others, etc.). Even so, I will use the terms somewhat interchangeably in keeping with the preferences of authors I cite.

Research on heroes enjoys a long history dating back to the 19th century (e.g., Darrah, 1898). Until recent decades, most of this research took the form of a single poll-type question being asked of large samples of schoolchildren. Unfortunately, the wording of the question varied considerably from study to study, often restricting the children's favorite or most admired persons to those who were well-known public figures or in some sense famous. We know more recently that friends, relatives, and the not-so-famous frequently serve as models (e.g., Harris, 1986; Russell & McClusky, 1985).

Those who have examined trends in these early studies (e.g., Averill, 1950; Greenstein, 1964; G.J. Smith, 1973) note a major shift in exemplar categories beginning in the 1930s. That is to say, earlier categories such as national historical characters, religious figures, and representatives of the "serious arts" were largely supplanted by sports stars and personalities from radio; the silver screen; and, more recently, television. Thus, entertainment figures and sports heroes have emerged as visible categories providing models for North American youngsters. The shift in choices speaks to the powerful and pervasive impact of communications technology. With the introduction of each new innovation in communications, media figures have been thrust into our presence in increasingly personalized ways. More immediate sources, then, are drawn upon at the expense of traditional sources, now overshadowed and in many ways relatively less accessible.

An even more recent trend also warrants comment. Whereas a "Relatives & Acquaintances" category remained unchanged at 10% from Darrah's (1898) study to that of Averill in 1950, its importance since appears to have sharply increased. More recently, over 50% of the exemplar choices of teenagers have included friends and relatives (Russell & McClusky, 1985). In all likelihood, the restrictive phrasing of earlier questions produced the smaller category. However, this particular category is also sensitive to regional differences. U.S. national poll data (Hyman, 1975, p. 270) shows that among white Southerners, family members or local individuals are chosen twice as often as they are among non-Southerners.

A Comment

Several methodological comments are perhaps in order at this point. Asking respondents to name someone they "most admire," "their greatest hero," or someone "they would most like to be like" appears to yield roughly similar results (Harris, 1985, cited in Harris, 1986). Moreover, these particular wordings do not restrict choices to the *public* domain but rather also allow for choices from the *personal* realm (i.e., friends, relatives). There is, then, some latitude available in the framing of questions. However, sampling differences and other issues aside, the standardization of questions would nevertheless go a long way toward increasing the validity of comparisons across studies.

A second point concerns the fact that studies in this tradition have typically asked youngsters for a single exemplar choice when in fact a majority of respondents would prefer to name several individuals who possess attributes they find attractive. Interestingly, when multiple exemplars are sought, a youngster's choices reflect somewhat different sets of attributes (Harris, 1986). In a sense, many people maintain a "composite ideal."[1] This being the case, a more complete mapping of the modeling influence process through an exemplar choice approach can best be achieved by allowing for multiple nominations.

The Importance of Sport Heroes

Before attempting to provide answers to questions of the *bases* of hero selection in sports, the extent of their influence, and the lessons they teach their admirers, we might first pause to ask how large the sports exemplar category is. A study conducted in Medicine Hat, Alberta, provides some preliminary answers to these and other questions (Russell & McClusky, 1985). As Rosenberg (1973) observes, the identification of exemplars must necessarily begin with the individual: "significance is in the eye of the beholder; ultimately, he alone can determine whether a particular other is significant to him" (p. 831). Guided by this perspective, virtually all Grade 10 students ($N = 280$) in the public school system were asked to "indicate the person, past or present, from any walk of life, whom you admire the most." With the question worded in this nondirective, open-ended form, four major identifiable exemplar categories emerged.

---

[1] A Methodist church school asked its students which individual in the history of the world they most admired. Bart Starr (quarterback of the Green Bay Packers) and Jesus tied for first. Jesus was on the ballot; Starr's votes were write-ins (G.C. Roberts, personal communication, June 19, 1991).

Table 6.2. Relative size of boys and girls exemplar categories.

	Sports	Entertainment	Friends	Relations	Miscellaneous
Boys	16.1%	23.8%	21.0%	19.6%	19.5%
Girls	5.7%	20.7%	36.4%	26.4%	10.8%

As can be seen in Table 6.2, sports figures represent the smallest category over-all. Strikingly similar results were obtained with a U.S. national sample ($N = 2,258$) of 7- to 11-year-old children (Foundation for Child Development, 1977) using a question worded so as to preclude the nomination of friends and relatives. Asked the question "Can you tell me the name of a *famous* person you want to be like?" [italics added], 28% mentioned a popular entertainer and 13% nominated athletes. Averill (1950) replicated a study of children's ideals conducted by Darrah (1898) half a century earlier. Whereas a category of sports figures was virtually nonexistent among 12- to 14-year-old Americans at the turn of the century, the category accounted for fully 23% of the choices by midcentury.

A survey conducted in Brazzaville, Congo (Didillon & Vandewiele, 1985), re-vealed that sports are a relatively minor source of exemplars in West Africa. The classification of children's responses to the question "Who would you like to resem-ble the most?" shows athletes *and* entertainers sharing a very minor category. Final-ly, it is instructive to note that even with the use of a question directly asking Cali-fornia youngsters to name their favorite *sports* figure (Bredemeier, Weiss, Shields, & Cooper, 1986), fully 37% of the boys and 57% of the girls left the item blank.

The Gallup poll has, since 1947, almost annually asked Americans to nominate a living man and woman from any part of the world whom they most admire. The wording of the question has changed slightly from year to year, and further has di-rected respondents to consider individuals "they had heard or read about." Al-though this wording favors those in the public domain, sport heroes have nonetheless remained a negligible category (i.e., less than 1%) over the past 37 years (Tom Smith, 1986). Adult Americans have consistently looked beyond the sports world for their most admired man or woman. It is evident from the forego-ing and the earlier examination of historical trends that sports, by and large, do not represent a major source of personal heroes for the general population. With 73% of adult Americans participating in keep-fit activities and/or sports and 71% describing themselves as sports fans (R.M. Thomas, 1986), it might seem surpris-ing that more sports figures are not chosen as personal heroes. It must be said that their appeal as individuals to be emulated is fairly limited.

Summary

To summarize, it would appear that sports have only recently emerged as a stable, al-beit minor, category from which principally youngsters and young adults choose indi-viduals whom they admire. Furthermore, the size of the category can be expected to vary considerably with the age and sex of respondents as well as across cultures. This is not to say, however, that sports are any the less important in the lives of young people. For many youngsters, sports play a variety of important roles. For example, sports may provide entertainment, promote the development of motor and social skills, or serve as a common topic of conversation with peers. However, youngsters do not at the same time appear to draw their exemplars from this category in large numbers.

A Question of Quality

A Statement of the Problem

Expressions of concern regarding the quality of our heroes accompanied the shift noted in exemplar choices through the middle decades of this century. In summarizing this concern, Klapp (1969) states,

> not only is there *doubt* that celebrities of today are better than the people who admire them, but there is an uncomfortable possibility that the proportion of reinforcing ("good") to seducing ("bad") and transcending models has shifted to a critical point of imbalance—that more "heroes" are tearing down consensus than building it up. (p. 253)

Similar concerns regarding the suitability of heroes in particular sports have surfaced with some regularity throughout this century. The emergence of Babe Ruth as a cultural hero and the relative obscurity of his equally talented teammate Lou Gehrig perhaps best epitomize this concern. Although both were gifted ballplayers, Ruth's character was seriously flawed whereas Gehrig displayed the finest of personal qualities. As Zeigler (1987) states, "it is high time that we give the highest acclaim and pay the most reverence to those who demonstrate through sport *both* a high degree of athletic ability *and* the finest of personality and character traits" (p. 328). As for those athletically outstanding but personally deficient sport champions, he suggests that we should "not revere them for faults that are often glossed over and desirable traits they never possessed" (p. 328).

The True Hero

Throughout this discussion, I have cast a wide net in considering a variety of individuals who, although they may be perceived as role models, significant others, heroes, and so on by their admirers, often come up short by other standards, standards involving more than a singular achievement or performance. To be sure, even record-setting performances are not all equal. Occasionally, one record rises above all others (see Speaking Tangentially 6.1).

What then, are the general criteria that might be applied to determine whether an individual is a true hero or someone whose memory should be allowed to quietly

****

Speaking Tangentially 6.1: Against All Odds

Historically speaking, the practice of recording exceptional performances in sports is a fairly recent invention (Mandell, 1976). Records are, however, the stuff of which heroes in the modern era are made. The longest throw, the fastest time, the most points, the first to do whatever, appended to an athlete's name is an important prerequisite if one is to achieve hero status. Of course, ties notwithstanding, someone will own every record. Considering the staggering number of sports records that are kept, often dozens of categories in a single sport, innumerable athletes can lay claim to some form of special recognition.

Record performances are achieved through a combination of superior abilities and a generous measure of luck. But how are we to distinguish between those records that are "merely" outstanding and those that defy the laws of probability? Are there any? In the view of Stephen Gould (1991), baseball owns only one such record, that belonging to Joe Dimaggio, who in 1941 hit successfully in 56 consecutive games. The second longest streak is 44 games held jointly by Wee Willie Keeler and Pete Rose. Gould's conclusion is based on statistical analyses of baseball records by Nobel laureate Ed Purcell, whose work Gould describes (pp. 463–472). Simply put, the record of 56 games is off the curve, that is, so many standard deviations from the historical mean of such streaks that neither your grandchildren nor their grandchildren can expect to see Dimaggio's feat eclipsed. Otherwise, "nothing ever happened in baseball above and beyond the frequency predicted from coin-tossing models" (p. 466). Dimaggio's mark is a record among records.

****

fade? Historically, a number of writers have attempted the task of specifying the criteria by which one can distinguish between the truly great and the "great but really not *that* great." I think that Robert Barney (1985), in extending the work of earlier theorists, has proposed a useful model. Essentially, he suggests that a bona fide sports hero should excel in each of four categories. Within each category, he identifies *ideal* standards, criteria that most hero/heroine candidates only approach.

1. The individual must exemplify *physical excellence* in terms of health, vigor, fitness, and skill as an athlete. Too often, contemporary sportspeople are judged solely on the criterion of this more public and publicized category. However, would-be heroes must also be shown to be outstanding in three other realms before they can be accorded true hero status.

2. The hero must also exhibit *moral excellence*. In all areas of his or her life, the hero should display those moral values that have stood the test of time, such as honesty, humility, generosity, sportsmanship, self-control, and courage.

3. On a *social* level, Barney's model additionally requires candidates to unselfishly direct their energies and talents toward helping others in their social groups. Their commitment may be to family, community, or even beyond to assist mankind in general. Their efforts may be made on behalf of the poor, in the fight against disease and injustice, or in government service. In all such endeavors they must use their lofty position to improve the plight of others less fortunate than themselves.

****

Speaking Tangentially 6.2: Rose 1, Sabin 0
September 11, 1985, marked the day that Pete Rose got his 4,192nd hit, surpassing the long-standing major league baseball record of Ty Cobb. The following day, Cincinnati's city council sought to honor his achievement by changing the name of the street that runs past Riverfront Stadium to Pete Rose Way. The council's action aroused the ire of the medical community, who since 1982 had been lobbying the committee on names to dedicate a public area to Dr. Albert E. Sabin, the medical researcher who discovered the oral polio vaccine in the 1950s. The controversy may yet be resolved by the Committee on Names, who continue to debate the merits of Dr. Sabin's candidacy (*New York Times*, September 29, 1985, p. 28).

Rose 1, Sabin 1
All is well in Cincinnati. The city council has voted unanimously to name its convention center after the famed medical researcher. The city now boasts an Albert E. Sabin Convention and Exposition Center *and* Pete Rose Way (*New York Times*, November 17, 1985, p. 18).
(Recent indications are that one of the decisions may have been taken prematurely!)

****

4. The fourth area in which the true hero must excel is the *intellectual* realm. Barney allows for two types of intellectual development. First, what he calls *theoretical wisdom* is that education acquired through formal channels (i.e., completing a high school diploma, college, and so forth). Second, he cites *practical wisdom* as a standard toward which the hero must strive. Practical knowledge is seen in the manner in which the individual deals with the problems and decisions that confront most people in life (e.g., money management, choices on alcohol, drugs, gambling).

An additional overriding factor to be applied before elevating a candidate to hero status is the sheer passage of *time*. The application of this criterion requires us to resist the rush to enshrine people as heroes in their lifetime. The judgments of future generations are seen as necessary to provide an objective and balanced view of the candidate's success in approximating the fourfold qualifications proposed in Barney's model. Speaking Tangentially 6.2 offers a case in point.

When Heroes Fall, as They Sometimes Do

It is for good reason that Barney (1985) and other writers allow for the sheer passage of time before bestowing true hero status on an athlete. Among the vast array of modern-day hero candidates, more than a handful have fallen or at least stumbled in the years following the performances that brought them acclaim.

The reputations of current sports figures such as baseball's Pete Rose and sprinter Ben Johnson have also suffered irreparable damage. In both cases, the injuries were self-inflicted while the athletes were at the heights of their careers. However, few events in sports history have produced greater shock and distress among admirers than the fall of Canadian Ben Johnson during the 1988 Olympics in Seoul, South Korea. Having tested positive for anabolic steroid use, Ben was stripped of his gold medal, and his world record 100-meter time was disallowed.

Canadians sought answers to this rare and unexpected turn of events in the aftermath of the Seoul announcement. A question for sociologists Ungar and Sev'er (1989) concerned which of the explanations that surfaced in public and media discussions of the event were ultimately adopted by Canadians. More specifically, did Ben's countrymen attribute the fall of their hero to external, situational causes or to dispositional causes? Also, where did the responsibility lie for what happened, with Ben or with his handlers? In the days immediately following the disclosure of steroid use, four plausible explanations emerged. The first of these suggested that the test results were in error, and the second that Ben was the victim of sabotage. The remaining explanations were that Ben had either knowingly or unknowingly been taking steroids.

Following from the discussion in chapter 3 on the *fundamental attribution error*, the results of this study should have been straightforward. That is, observers in ordinary situations tend to assign more weight to dispositional factors than to situational factors in accounting for an event. However, this was far from an ordinary event. As Ungar and Sev'er (1989) point out, Canadians had formed a close *unit relationship* (Heider, 1958) with their national hero such that the unexpected announcement that threatened Ben's future was also personally threatening to everyday Canadians. These factors suggested that a different pattern of attributions might be made.

Unlike the almost reflexive top-of-the-head judgments that form the basis of the vast majority of our attributions, the unexpected and threatening announcement in Seoul could instead lead to *biased hypothesis testing* (Pyszczynski & Greenberg, 1987). From the perspective of this attributional model, the resulting attributions would be predicted to reflect a *defensive* interpretation of events, that is, an interpretation in which more responsibility is assigned to situational than to dispositional factors. This was indeed what happened.

Students ($N = 338$) at the University of Toronto completed a questionnaire within eight days of the announcement that Ben had tested positive. Two sets of questions addressed, first, the causal locus for the alleged steroid use and, second, whether responsibility for the incident lay with Ben or with his handlers. The mean ratings of causal locus appear in Figure 6.1.

It is clear that very few respondents thought it likely that the Olympic tests were in error. Evidence of this sort is virtually irrefutable. However, consistent with the authors' predictions, subjects believed that it was more likely that Ben had been using steroids unknowingly than knowingly. Thus, under the special circumstances surrounding the affair (i.e., an unexpected and personally threatening outcome), the response of observers was just the opposite to that predicted by the fundamental attribution error. In this instance, situational factors were judged as more likely to have caused Ben's downfall than dispositional factors. Incidentally, the explanation that Ben was the victim of sabotage was judged to be at least as likely as the suggestion that he knowingly took steroids. The second part of the

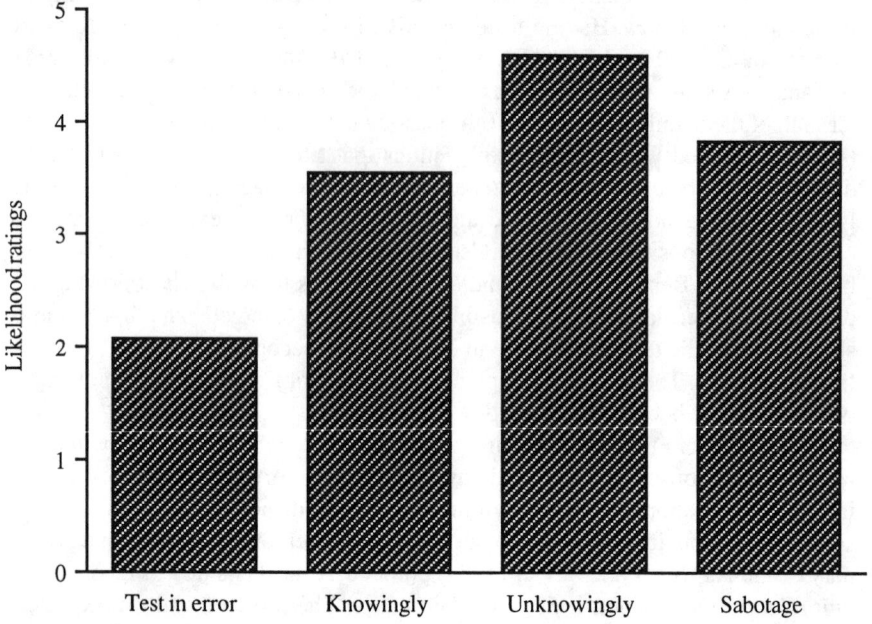

FIGURE 6.1 Attributions for the Ben Johnson affair (adapted from Ungar & Sev'er, 1989).

analysis attempted to determine where subjects placed responsibility for the incident, with Ben or with his handlers. By a wide margin, subjects assigned more responsibility to Ben's handlers than to Ben himself.

In summary, then, a rare set of circumstances in sports has provided a successful test of theory (Pyszczynski & Greenberg, 1987) under real-life conditions. At the same time, these and similar results tend to limit predictions from the perspective of the fundamental attribution error to those off-the-cuff judgments that we all make every day. In sports, as elsewhere, when the event is unexpected or novel and self-threatening, observers seemingly engage in biased hypothesis testing. This active hypothesis testing mode is further facilitated when observers have formed a unit relationship with the actor. Almost certainly this was the case for Canadians who at the time were basking in the reflected glory (Cialdini et al., 1976) of Ben's Olympic achievement. From a sad day in sports history, we move on to consider the related question of the influence we derive from those whom we choose as our personal heroes.

The Influence Process: For Better or for Worse

How does a hero influence an admirer? After all, the hero is usually far removed from the would-be learner and makes no direct effort to teach anything about his or her skills, attitudes, values, or life-style. While we tend to think that most learning results from direct experience in which the learner proceeds in a trial-and-error fashion, the fact is that a vast amount of learning also occurs through observing the behavior of others. At the same time, however, the observer additionally takes note of the consequences for the model of their actions, that is, whether they are rewarded or punished for their behavior. This observational learning view, in which learning is acquired vicariously, has been summarized by Stanford psychologist Albert Bandura in several sources (e.g., Bandura, 1969, 1973, 1986).

Under what conditions does observational learning occur? Basically, four interdependent processes govern observational learning. First, the learner must actively attend to the model's behavior. Next, the particular behavior must be symbolically represented in images and/or words. This subprocess of memory representation provides a continuing guide to behavior and allows a later transformation of the symbolic representations into actions when motor production processes are engaged. Finally, should circumstances arise that prompt the observer to put into practice what he or she has learned, such responses will be regulated by incentive and motivational processes.

It is important at this juncture to emphasize a distinction between the acquisition of learning and the performance of what has been learned. Social learning theory allows that a great deal of what we learn through observation may never be put into practice either because it serves no particular function for the individual or because its expression would invite disapproval from others. As a consequence, the hero's influence likely extends much further than can be inferred solely from observing the overt behavior of her or his admirers.

Considerable importance attaches to the question of the *quality* of heroes inasmuch as they are presumed to influence the attitudes, values, and behaviors of their admirers. Whether the influence of a particular hero is "good" or "bad" is very much a value judgment that can be expected to vary from one person to another. That is to say, the same hero may be regarded as a good model by one person and as an inferior model by another. Despite the highly subjective nature of "quality," Butt (1987) has ventured this observation: "To the extent the athlete serves as a constructive cultural force, combining competence at sport with strong character, he contributes a healthy model to the young" (p. 256).

In the case of celebrated sports heroes, they might in general be presumed to exert a near maximum level of influence. As Bandura (1973) notes, those models most highly attended to in society are those who "possess high status in prestige, power, and competence hierarchies." This is in contrast to those paid little heed "who are socially, occupationally and intellectually inept" (p. 70). The superstars of the sports world—adored by the media, skilled, and lavishly compensated for their efforts—signal "success" to legions of followers who cherish and strive for similar goals in their own lives. By any standard, their potential for influence assumes impressive proportions.

In the case of malevolent influence, sports stars have the same capacity to shape the behavior of their admirers. The modeling of antisocial behaviors would, however, have its greatest influence under slightly different circumstances. For instance, in the matter of aggression, "the combination of prestigious aggressive modeling with positive reinforcement of fighting and other manifestations of toughness creates the most effective condition for cultivating aggressiveness" (Bandura, 1973, p. 98).

Of course, the behavior of sports heroes is generally subject to public scrutiny both on and off the field of play. Those who flaunt the norms of society or run afoul of the law, although they may be euphemistically described as "colorful" or "controversial" by their followers and the media, nonetheless teach aspiring youngsters lessons that can only retard their development into mature and socially responsible adults. The wider responsibility of athletes to provide their admirers with a positive model both on *and* off the field of play has also been noted by Butt (1987). She aptly observes, "The athlete contributes more to the audience than an enactment of competence and competition. He also contributes his way of life. Whatever the admired athlete does, the crowd, particularly the young, tend to emulate" (p. 257).

Correlates of Hero Selection

Personality

A sample of the research conducted beyond the realm of sports will serve to illustrate the linkages between heroes and our attitudes/behavior in everyday life. One of the classic undertakings in the area of personality has been that of Adorno, Frenkel-Brunswik, Levinson, and Sanford, whose efforts to understand the psychological roots of fascism led to the publication of *The Authoritarian Personality* in 1950. One aspect of this massive work sought to establish a relationship between authoritarianism and the type of person we admire by means of the question "What great people do you admire most?" (p. 559). Briefly, these investigators found that highly authoritarian individuals admired those in the categories of (1) power and control (e.g., Churchill, Carnegie); (2) conservative Americans (e.g., Washington, J. Edgar Hoover); and (3) parents and relatives. Those most admired by subjects who scored low on measures of authoritarianism tended to fall in the categories of (1) the arts and philosophy (e.g., Shakespeare, Bertrand Russell); (2) physical and biological sciences (e.g., Madame Curie); and (3) social scientists and liberal radical political figures (e.g., Benjamin Franklin, Karl Marx). Additionally, the admiration of nonauthoritarians is more diffuse, lows often expressing the opinion that "no one person stands out" (p. 560).

Building on this previous work, H.P. Smith and Rosen (1958) sought to determine if the "ego-ideals" of individuals whose outlook could be described as "worldmindedness" differ from those displaying more nationalistic sentiments. Worldmindedness was measured by means of the W-scale, a typical item being "All national governments ought to be abolished and replaced by one central world government." Subjects scoring high on worldmindedness chose ego-ideals predominantly from an "artistic-intellectual-humanitarian" category; those scoring low on the W-scale tended instead to choose ego-ideals from a "political-military" category. From the examples provided, it would appear that the categories of Smith and Rosen have their counterpart in the *power and control* and the *arts and philosophy* categories of Adorno et al. (1950). Finally, as you might have guessed, those scoring low on the W-scale tend also to exhibit attributes of the authoritarian personality.

Media

Several points dealing with the media's role in influencing the hero selection process bear mention. First, the media report first and foremost on their own culture, giving greater coverage and emphasis to nationals at the expense of foreign athletes. For example, in the study of Finnish heroes (described below) it is hard to imagine that any of the top choices of the Finnish children would even be mentioned by North American youngsters (e.g., Pentti Nikula, Field Marshal Mannerheim, Paavo Nurmi, and Curt Lincoln). Second, the media selectively filter candidates for stardom, choosing those from sports that have a wide following among the general public. For example, Laurie Skreslet, the first Canadian to climb Mount Everest; Susan Nattrass, world champion trapshooter; and Vicky Keith, long-distance swimmer, were given only sporadic coverage by the national media and today are scarcely known beyond their sport. Far better known are the American stars of Canadian baseball and football in addition to a crop of homegrown hockey players.

Finally, the media make little pretense of selecting for quality, focusing instead on the "newsworthiness" of the athlete and his or her performance. If the star is personally flawed and an inferior model for others to emulate, his or her shortcomings are minimized or glossed over. Thus, the distinction between media popularity and the hero's personal merits are frequently blurred. Boorstin (1968) succinctly summarizes this point in noting that while the media "can so quickly and so effectively give a man fame, we have willingly been misled into believing that fame—well knowness—is still a hallmark of greatness" (p. 327).

Cultural Influence

The powerful role played by one's culture in determining the choice of heroes is clearly seen in a Finnish study (Toukomaa, 1969). Boys ($N = 846$) aged 10 to 18 were asked to rate their admiration for each individual on a list of eminent people. Sportsmen dominated the choices of the youngsters. By far the most admired figure was Pentti Nikula, the then world record holder in the pole vault, followed by the legendary distance runner, Paavo Nurmi. Field Marshal Mannerheim placed third, with another sports figure, race-car driver Curt Lincoln in fourth place. Non-Finns such as Albert Schweitzer, Albert Einstein, Elvis Presley, and Robin

Hood drew little admiration by comparison. A culture, interpreted by its media, thrusts its own nationals into the spotlight, which in the Finnish case reveals choices that honor their strong tradition of sporting excellence.

Sex Differences

A number of sex-linked differences are apparent in people's selections of exemplars. Foremost among these differences is the consistent finding that considerably more males are chosen *overall* as exemplars (Balswick & Ingoldsby, 1982; see a review by Harris, 1986), a finding that extends to the singular sports category (Cooper, Livingood, & Kurz 1981; The Miller Lite Report, 1983; Russell & McClusky, 1985; Vander Velden, 1986). Moreover, sportspeople are nominated more often by males than females, a result Bredemeier et al. (1986) attribute to the relatively lower rates of participation in sports by young females. The suggestion draws support from the results of a national survey of 1,460 Canadians (Bibby, 1991). Among those who indicated that they follow the four major professional sports "very closely" or "fairly closely," men outnumber women by a ratio of more than 2:1.

There is some additional evidence to suggest that individuals make same-sex exemplar choices (Cooper et al., 1981; McElroy & Kirkendall, 1980; G.J. Smith, 1976). Cooper et al. found that whereas girls chose both male and female sports figures, the boys chose *only* male heroes. However, in an exception to this trend, Balswick and Ingoldsby (1982) failed to find any greater tendency for males to nominate male exemplars than females over all exemplar categories.

Among Canadian respondents, G.J. Smith (1976) found sex to be strongly related to the nationality of the sports hero. Males were far more likely than females to choose American athletes. Smith suggests that Canada at that time had produced few male sports heroes beyond hockey, whereas Canadian women had earned international reputations in several sports. Sex differences also emerged in an interesting sidelight to Smith's study. Sports heroes were found to be far less often the topic of conversation among women, a result supported by Bibby's (1991) finding that sports occupy a more central position in the day-to-day lives of men.[2]

Racial Differences

The tendency for individuals to select exemplars with whom they have personal attributes in common extends also to race (e.g., Vander Velden, 1986). Among a college sample of black athletes, not a single white sports idol was nominated (Castine & Roberts, 1974). This clear preference for same-race sports heroes was

----

[2] Sports themselves differ considerably in the size of their Canadian following: hockey (NHL) 36%; baseball (AL) 23%, (NL) 23%; football (CFL) 16%; (NFL) 11%; basketball (NBA) 5%.

also expressed by young boys in a study by Cooper et al. (1981). The relationship was not found, however, among the girls in their sample. In yet another study (Balswick & Ingoldsby, 1982), the race of the subjects was unrelated to their preferences for "heroes" versus "heroines."

Age Differences

As Harris (1986) notes in her review of athletic heroes, evidence on the role of age as a variable in the exemplar selection process is fragmentary at best. However, within the range from adolescence to older adults it is clear that with increasing age people are less likely to acknowledge having a sports hero (G.J. Smith, 1976). After piecing together a number of scattered findings, Harris (1986) reaffirms earlier suggestions of a *curvilinear* relationship between age and the frequency with which people nominate exemplars (i.e., an inverted-U function). That is to say, whereas young children have relatively few exemplars, adolescents nominate considerably more, followed by a decline in nominations that continues through the adult years. A further interesting, but as yet unanswered, question concerns the relationship between the ages of respondents and the ages of their exemplars.

Other attributes likely form a common basis for exemplar selection. For example, among aspiring tennis players, do the left-handers disproportionately select John McEnroe and Jimmy Conners as their same-sport idols? Do disabled athletes also tend to choose other handicapped athletes (e.g., gymnast Kathy Johnson and wheelchair marathoner Rick Hansen) as their exemplars?

It also appears that shared interests and/or team roles form the basis of exemplar choices for some individuals. For example, 59% of children who named a sports hero chose an athlete who was outstanding in the child's favorite sport (Cooper et al., 1981). An even more specific basis for selection is seen in the tendency for young hopefuls to nominate athletes playing the same position as they. Among black college athletes participating in baseball, football, and basketball, 56% played the same positions as their high school idols (Castine & Roberts, 1974). Also, junior hockey players consistently choose as models those from the professional ranks who play their position (Russell, 1979).

The reasons aspirants choose a star athlete who plays their sport or position is still pretty much an open question. In addition to their unqualified admiration, two possibilities seem likely: to learn playing skills or, in some sports, aggressive tactics. Interestingly, if a youngster's choice of hero is based on an expectation that his own playing skills will benefit by the association, such hopes may be most cruelly dashed. As Bandura (1969) notes, mere observation of a model's performance may be a relatively ineffective means of learning a complex and coordinated set of skills. Internal responses certainly are beyond the view of the would-be learner. When observing excellence in performance, it may not be possible for even the most vigilant observer to detect the subtle differences in motoric responses between say a star and a teammate warming the bench. Moreover, the aspiring youngster may simply not possess the where-withal (i.e., speed, agility, strength) to reproduce the model's superior per-formance. In the case of aggression, fighting prowess, or perhaps simply a will-ingness to fight, may seemingly be enhanced through observational learning (M.D. Smith, 1974, 1983). Such evidence as we have on the lessons learned by admirers has been deferred to a later section in this chapter.

The Response of Admirers

Admiration

The Medicine Hat study (Russell & McClusky, 1985) also sought students' rat-ings of how strongly they admired their choices. Fairly high but *equal* levels of admiration were revealed across the four exemplar categories of sports, entertain-ment, friends, and relatives. However, it must be acknowledged that among the general public there is considerable variability in expressions of admiration. Ex-cessive outpourings of admiration are not uncommon in individual circumstances and on particular occasions. *Certain* teams and athletes have at various times en-gendered such passionate loyalties among their followers that "admiration" seems wholly inadequate to describe the surge of affection fans extend to their he-roes. As Dervin (1985) has observed, "fans often behave as fanatics, and their de-votion to their cherished stars is just shy of idolatry" (p. 280).

Influence

In addition to admiration, the students were also asked to provide self-reports of the extent to which they felt they are actually influenced by their exemplar. En-tertainment personalities were the least influential. Sports figures were some-what more influential, followed by friends and relations, the most influential. Admiration and influence, of course, are matters of degree. In other words, *"not all significant others are equally significant"* (Rosenberg, 1973, p. 830). It might further be assumed that "those who are more significant should have greater in-fluence on our self-concepts" (p. 830). While we can assess the degree of influ-ence that respondents believe their heroes exert on their behavior in the manner above, the particular *form* that influence takes remains an open question. Does the exemplar merely draw our appreciation, or are lives affected in more pro-found ways?

G.J. Smith (1976) approached the question of influence somewhat differently by asking subjects if there were a particular sports figure that they would like to be like. More than half responded in the vein of "I like the way I am now" or "I would rather be myself" (p. 266). Smith concludes that the bonds between heroes and their admirers may not be especially intense or personal but rather represent "a detached form of admiration. It is the difference between appreciation and emulation; respondents like what they see the athlete doing but they would not necessarily want to trade places" (p. 266).

McEvoy and Erickson (1981) conducted in-depth interviews with college students as a preliminary step in their efforts to more thoroughly understand the nature of the influence process. They made an initial distinction in their data between two types of public reference idols, "heroes" and "villains." Both types of idols elicit a range of responses from admiration (heroes) and disdain (villains) to extreme personal sacrifice either in support of heroes or in opposition to villainous figures. Their scales of influence include five descriptive levels of increasing influence exerted by public idols on individuals who attend to them. It would be an interesting extension to sports hero literature to identify the specific ways that admirers are influenced by their idols beyond aspects of same-sport performance.

Efforts to Emulate

A question arising from the above concerns the capacity of heroes to generally motivate their admirers to emulate aspects of their behavior. The question was approached by asking the Medicine Hat sample to rate the strength of their *efforts* to be the kind of person their choice represents (Russell & McClusky, 1985). As can be seen in Figure 6.2, the analysis yielded a fairly complex result (i.e., an interac-

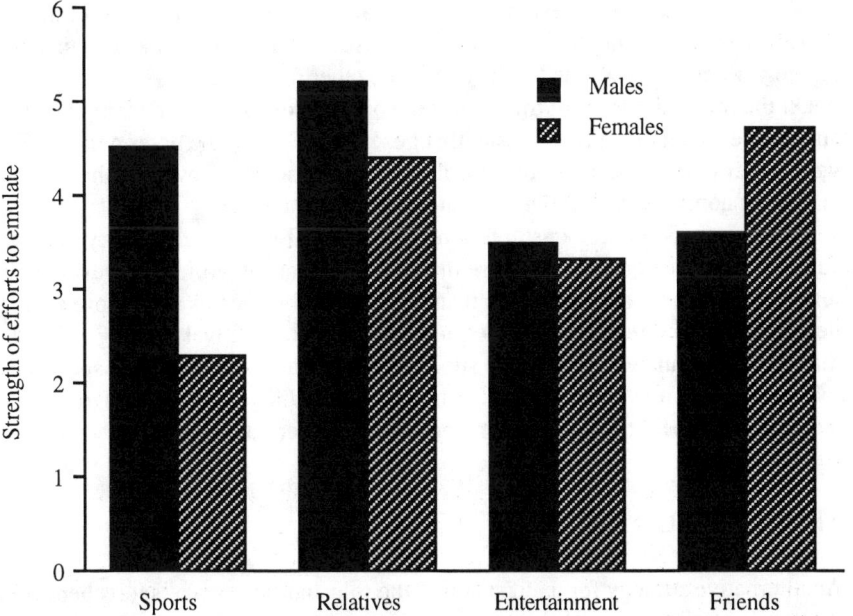

FIGURE 6.2 Efforts to emulate exemplars (adapted from Russell & McClusky, 1985).

tion). Although males and females expended equal efforts to emulate their exemplars overall, males made greater efforts to emulate their choices in the sports and relatives categories whereas females made the greatest efforts on behalf of their nominees from among friends. However, questions of whether or not the admirer's efforts to emulate the exemplar are successful or indeed, what specific aspects of their hero's behavior they strive to emulate, remains a matter for conjecture.

Again, the Question of Quality

To return to the critical question of the *quality* of sports heroes relative to those in other categories, students in the Medicine Hat study (Russell & McClusky, 1985) were also asked to select five traits that best described their exemplar. The particular list of traits used offered the advantage of having previously been rated with respect to the *desirability* of each of the trait adjectives (Anderson, 1968). These norms provide a quantitative basis for determining the quality of the nominee's traits, as seen from the particular perspective of his or her admirer. For instance, tennis professional John McEnroe may be perceived and described in quite different terms by two admirers. One might describe him as "sincere," "skillful," and "intelligent," a very desirable and plausible set of traits. Another admirer might attend to other behaviors and consequently describe his hero in completely different terms. This alternative view might characterize Mr. McEnroe as "loud-mouthed," "immature," and "petulant." Two admirers, two views. The more important point, however, is that we typically *act* on the basis of our perceptions quite apart from any objective reality in the external world we are perceiving. Thus, Mr. McEnroe's two fans, each attending to different characteristics, stand to be influenced in qualitatively different ways, one for the better, the other for worse.

On the important issue of the quality of sports heroes and other exemplars, the analysis revealed that girls consistently chose exemplars on the bases of traits that were superior to those that boys ascribed to their choices. However, the overall quality of nominees across the four categories did not differ.

In sum, sports heroes constitute a relatively small exemplar category and are admired no more nor less than those in other exemplar categories. However, their relative influence is seen to be less than that exerted by choices from those classified as friends or relatives. Furthermore, boys make relatively stronger efforts than girls to emulate their favorite sports figure. Finally, the quality of sports heroes is equivalent overall to that of nominees from other exemplar categories, although girls appear to choose exemplars with superior qualities.

The Lessons Learned

An alternative strategy for understanding the role and function of sports heroes is through a consideration of the *basis* for their selection in the first instance. Are heroes chosen because of their skill, physical attractiveness, sportsmanship, aggression, or their charitable deeds on behalf of those less fortunate in society? Several studies have addressed aspects of this question. Garry Smith (1976) conducted interviews with a large number of Edmonton residents. His subjects indicated overwhelmingly that the basis for the selection of their hero(ine) was the athlete's outstanding *ability* in their sport. In the case of National Hockey League *player* popularity, those receiving the most nominations from Canada Winter Games competitors were also those with the best NHL performance records, that is, goals, assists (Russell, 1979). The preeminence of ability as a basis of exemplar choice has since been confirmed by *The Miller Lite Report on American Attitudes Toward Sports* (1983) and by the work of Vander Velden (1986).

Other investigations within a single sport have provided evidence that the hero's aggression may also form a basis of attraction for aspiring athletes. Michael Smith (1974; 1979; 1983, pp. 114–116) used an interview method in asking young hockey players to name their favorite NHL player and to estimate how "aggressive" their choice was in league play. His analysis resulted in a positive correlation between the heroes' aggression and that exhibited by their young admirers in their own junior league competition. There is also an indication that the relationship may be *causal* insofar as the youthful respondents admitted learning dirty tactics from their heroes and attempting to put them into practice in their own games (e.g., M.D. Smith, 1978).

In an attempt to avoid reliance on the "perceptual" estimate of hero aggression used by Michael Smith, Russell (1979) used the actual records of aggressive play (i.e., aggressive penalties) in assessing the bases for hero selection by teams representing their provinces at the Canada Winter Games. Perhaps because of the limited number of games played by each team in the competition (6 to 10), the previous association between hero aggression and that of their admirers reported by Smith was not replicated. There is a likelihood that a somewhat greater number of games may be required in order to achieve a valid ordering of players in terms of their characteristic levels of aggressive play. Further regarding aggression, the individual popularity ratings of these same stars bore no relationship to their NHL penalty records.

Mugno and Feltz (1985) have provided support for the proposition that specific acts of aggression may be learned and practiced by youngsters through observation. Teenage football players were asked to identify any illegal tactics they learned from players in the college and professional ranks and also, to indicate whether they put these tactics into practice in their own games. Players admitted to learning the intricacies of numerous illegal acts including spearing, facemasking, late hits, and stepping on a downed opponent while getting back on their feet. Overall, the findings revealed a strong relationship between the learning of aggressive tactics and players' use of these specific acts in their own play. Bredemeier et al. (1986) confirmed the previous findings that young boys choosing athletes from high-contact sports tended to be more aggressive in their own sports play. However, she additionally established the very important point that they were also more aggressive in other settings outside of sports (see also Olweus, 1979). The malevolent influence of a favorite athlete, then, is not restricted to the playing field.

Aggression has also been found to be an important basis for the selection of favorite sports *teams* or what might be termed reference groups (Hyman, 1975). The popularity of NHL teams with junior hockey players at the Winter Games was significantly related to the teams' records of scoring and on-ice aggression (Russell, 1979). That is to say, the higher the ratings of NHL team popularity, the better their scoring performance *and* the greater the number of aggressive penalties they incurred.

The specific means by which Pee Wee hockey players (11 to 13 years) learn to emulate aggressive aspects of the professional player model have been described in detail by Nash and Lerner (1981) in a study that used the method of participant observation. Over and above learning "the time, place, and the form for aggression" (p. 242), the youngsters learn to distinguish among four types of peers (i.e., "enforcers," "stickers," "tempermentals," and "passives"), who differ in the nature of their aggressive acts and their proclivity for aggression. Stickers, for example, take responsibility for disrupting the play of the opposing team and are known to fight in self-defense, although not in defense of teammates. That role is assumed by the team's enforcer. It is further known that while stickers are not unwilling to threaten others with their sticks, they are only occasionally "chippy" in their own play. Such knowledge is acquired in impressive detail in the course of participating in youth hockey, always though, with an eye to the professionals' way of doing violence.

Hero selection is associated with yet another important aspect of a youngster's personal development: the acquisition of standards of morality. To the extent that the boys' favorite athletes are involved in contact sports, the youngsters are less mature in regard to their own level of moral reasoning (Bredemeier et al., 1986). Moreover, children who actively *participate* in high-contact sports were similarly found to have attained a lower level of moral maturity.

Several supplemental factors also appear to be important to an understanding of the hero selection process. Regional loyalties may also influence choices. In the study of Winter Games competitors (Russell, 1979), teams from provinces with NHL franchises tended to nominate Canadian teams more frequently than those without NHL representation in their province. However, perhaps because the NHL rosters are comprised largely of Canadians, the Winter Games competitors chose favorite players equally from Canadian and American based teams. An explanation for regional loyalties is to be found in the intense coverage given a local team by the media. Inasmuch as familiarity generally breeds liking (e.g., Zajonc, 1968), repeated exposure to individual team members and their exploits not surprisingly serves to increase their stature among members of an admiring public.

Summary

In summary, sports figures—a minor exemplar category—often achieve a slice of immortality and in so doing likely exercise a leadership role for as long as they are remembered. Perhaps the most important question centering on their role is the quality of whatever influence they have. Any assessment of the quality of their influence is only relative to that exerted in other exemplar categories. It would appear that the interests of boys, at least, would be better served by sports heroes who embody traits that are more likely to stand them and society in good stead during their adult years. Finally, the powerful role of the media in cultivating and interpreting the values and behaviors of "selected" heroes is an awesome responsibility having far-reaching social consequences. It is at this interface, between the media and hero selection, that future research might profitably be focused. The last word in this regard should perhaps be left to K. Young (1946), who nearly half a century ago observed, "The problem is not to try to prevent heroics and myths and legends but to control them within a moral framework which will prevent their abuse in the hands of unscrupulous men" (p. 221).

Suggested Readings

Bredemeier, B.J., & Shields, L. (in press). Moral psychology in the context of sport. In R. Singer, M. Murphy, & L.K. Tennant (Eds.), *Handbook on research in sport psychology*. New York: Macmillan.
    A thorough review that summarizes empirical findings and sets the agenda for future research on this important topic.

7

Personality

Entering university freshmen, indeed the general public, share a belief that psychology is mostly about one's personality. The possibility of finding out what makes ourselves and others "tick" would appear to be a major reason for taking one or more psychology courses. It often comes as something of a surprise for students to discover that the study of personality is only one of a number of emphases within the discipline that attempt to understand behavior. Within departments of psychology, however, personality is firmly entrenched as a core course in the curriculum. For those interested in gaining a fuller understanding of the behavior of athletes and others involved in the sports process, the topic of personality is essential and of fundamental importance.

A general fascination with personality has spawned a vast amount of vigorous research activity resulting in an abundance of findings. Unfortunately, much of this literature is of inferior quality. Seemingly, many of those attracted to the topic are, for whatever reasons, enthusiastic but ill-prepared to design and carry out investigations that meet acceptable scientific standards. The result is that findings are frequently contradictory, confusing, and difficult to interpret. Thus, despite the investment of enormous amounts of energy, time, and money in researching personality in sports settings, the return on that investment has been meager. We know relatively little as a result. Those who have formally reviewed the topic (e.g., Eysenck, Nias & Cox, 1982; Martens, 1976) have made similar observations. Eysenck and his colleagues expand on this theme in making the following observation:

> There has been an alarming failure to consider the complexities of the topic, to allow for the weaknesses and deficiencies of many existing personality questionnaires, or to make distinctions which are absolutely crucial in this field, e.g., between outstanding and average practitioners of a given sport, or between different types of sports, such as individual versus group sports. Last but not least, there has been little effort to consider the relationship between sport and personality in theoretical terms, i.e., to try to elucidate the possible relationships in terms of causal factors that might be mediated by differences in personality. (p. 1)

Rainer Martens (1976) has presented a more detailed description of the methodological problems and interpretive errors associated with this body of research findings. Among the flaws common to many investigations are the use of inadequate sampling procedures and statistical analyses that are ill-suited to the data. Such results as are sound are often generalized to situations and persons well beyond what is justified by the findings. Finally, Martens notes the prevalence of the sophomoric error of inferring causality from the fact of two variables being significantly correlated, a point that will be discussed shortly in an upcoming section.

The focus of those interested in personality is on individual differences, an emphasis that recognizes the unique makeup of each of us. Some within this tradition of inquiry have chosen to adopt an *idiographic* approach to questions regarding human behavior, whereas others have used a *nomothethic* research strategy. The idiographic approach seeks to understand the laws or rules governing the actions of a single individual(s). The following would be an idiographic statement: "Lydia consistently steps up her training following a disappointing performance." A nomothetic strategy is concerned with identifying the rules governing the behavior of aggregates, for example, "Low-skill players attribute their failures to external conditions (e.g., luck), whereas highly skilled players attribute their failures to internal causes (e.g., their lack of preparation)." Such a conclusion represents a nomothetic statement, summarizing as it does the difference in response to failure of two groups of athletes that differ in ability.

A Matter of Definition

As with most concepts in the social sciences, theorists seldom agree on matters of definition. The concept of personality is no exception. The diversity of opinion is reflected in the sample of definitions that follow:

> Personality is the dynamic organization within the individual of those psychophysical systems that determine his characteristic behavior and thought. (Allport, 1965, p. 28)

> Personality represents those structural and dynamic properties of an individual or individuals as they reflect themselves in characteristic responses to situations. (Pervin, 1970, p. 2)

> Personality is a stable set of characteristics and tendencies that determine those commonalities and differences in the psychological behavior (thoughts, feelings, and actions) of people that have continuity in time and that may or may not be easily understood in terms of the social and biological pressures of the immediate situation alone. (Maddi, 1968, p. 10)

Among other things, definitions of personality generally share in a recognition that personality is to an important degree shaped by influences within the socialization process, that is, those influences arising during the formative years from our interactions with others in the home, community, institutions, and elsewhere. Moreover, one's personality is presumed to be relatively stable and enduring over time, although from some perspectives the situation in which we find ourselves may effectively determine how we behave. This latter point is at the heart of an ongoing debate, namely, the trait-state controversy.

Is It a Trait, a State, or Even Something Else?

People are seen to exhibit certain regularities in their behavior, their values, and attitudes in their day-to-day interactions with others. Even over extended periods of time, we recognize a considerable degree of consistency in the behavior of others to the point that those we know well are largely predictable. We expect and have learned over the years that our friend, known to be scrupulously honest in her golf play, is also honest in all of her other dealings. It would come as a terrible shock to learn that she had recently been convicted of shoplifting. Seldom are our predictions about those we know disconfirmed. Expressions of underlying values and behaviors that show such evidence of stability are generally ascribed *trait* status.

An alternative perspective would instead propose that the behaviors we display on any particular occasion are largely determined by the circumstances in which we find ourselves. This *state* view of personality sees any stability in one's behavior as arising from similarities across situations rather than as a result of a relatively permanent feature of one's psychological makeup. There is additionally an *interactionist* view that strikes a middle ground.

One of the earliest studies of moral development provides a good example of the evidence supporting the situation-specific position. Hartshorne and May (1928) had children mark their own true/false examination questions and also participate in an athletic competition along with several other activities. In all settings the youngsters were provided with ample opportunities to cheat. And cheat they did! Interestingly, the children showed no particular consistency in dishonesty from one situation to another. While some cheated in one situation, others refrained. In another situation some of those who had earlier refrained were now found to have cheated. However, in all fairness to the trait view, it must be acknowledged that Burton (1963) reanalyzed the data from this classic study and found some modest evidence of cross-situational consistency in honesty. Nevertheless, honesty is generally regarded as a behavior more strongly influenced by state-specific factors than a fundamental personality trait.

While numerous studies exist to support both extreme positions in the "person-situation" controversy, a more current position takes the view that our behavior is influenced by both sources. This interactionist perspective recognizes contributions from the features of a situation and the personality traits of the actors in that situation. In general, however, it is a matter of explanatory or predictive emphasis. Neither the person nor the situation is dismissed as an inconsequential source of influence. Perhaps the staunchest proponent of the situationist position, Mischel (1977) has modified his view to take person variables into account: "To understand the interaction of person and environment we must consider *person variables* as well as environmental variables" (p. 251). To some, the interactionist position represents a satisfactory resolution.

To recap, some behaviors may be best understood as traits; other behaviors can be better accounted for in terms of situational constraints. Narrow traits (e.g., aggression) provide somewhat stronger predictions of human behavior (Olweus, 1979). On the other hand, more diffuse, less focused traits (e.g., outgoingness) generally predict less well (McGowan & Gormly, 1976). Certain individuals come to be recognized by all who know them as being aggressive irrespective of the sport or workaday activities in which they are observed. In the case of a broader trait such as extroversion, there is less agreement among observers that a particular individual consistently displays this characteristic.[1]

An individual differences variable on which people are usually in full agreement is whether others are left- or right-handed. Speaking Tangentially 7.1 highlights the important part played by sports records in allowing for a test of a major hypothesis associated with handedness.

****

Speaking Tangentially 7.1: The Dark Side of Left-Handedness
Sports have provided basic data for the investigation of a fascinating line of research into handedness. Incidentally, if you are a lefty, you'll find yourself in good company with the likes of da Vinci, Picasso, Chaplin, Queen Victoria, and four recent U.S. presidents—Carter, Ford, Reagan, and Bush. However, there is a downside to being left-handed. In addition to being required to function in a world designed by and for right-handers, early evidence suggested that lefties also have a shorter life expectancy. It was this question for which Diane Halpern and Stanley Coren (1988) sought answers in the records of major league baseball.

Halpern and Coren first identified two groups of ball players, strong left-handers and strong right-handers. That is, players were included in the analysis only if they both batted and threw from the same side. Their refined samples included 1,472 right-handers and 236 left-handers.

The two groups were found to have differed significantly in their survival rates. Whereas 2.5% of the right-handers survived to age 90, only .5% of the southpaws celebrated their 90th birthdays. The oldest surviving left-handed ball player was 91; the oldest surviving right-hander was 109. A number of explanations have been offered, ranging from a less effective immune system to greater involvement in accidents over a lifetime of trying to navigate in an environment designed for right-handers.

****

Measurement of Personality

Despite the extensive and often bewildering array of tests that are available, a number of important guideposts exist that can help in the selection of the appropriate and best test for a particular purpose. An understanding of the criteria for

---

[1] A classification of personality traits as they emerge in infancy through adulthood has been proposed by Buss and Finn (1987). See also a special issue of *Journal of Personality* (June, 1992) devoted to the Big 5 dimensions of personality.

judging the merits of tests is vital to both the fledgling researcher and consumers of research. That is to say, vast numbers of people read the published accounts or popularized summaries of research findings, findings that are frequently absorbed as part of common knowledge. As a consequence, many individuals are prompted to alter their behaviors and still others may be affected by policy or program changes implemented by those in authority. If the measure used in a study is seriously flawed, then clearly, any conclusions and subsequent changes in programs are indefensible on grounds of the study's findings. Most of us, then, have a vested interest in acquiring at least a smattering of psychometric theory. After all, of what use are the results of a study purporting to show that participation in an exercise program reduces depression if the measure used is known to assess something other than depression? It is to this critical question of the *validity* of a test that we will shortly turn. First, however, a major statistic used in this and nearby chapters will be briefly reviewed.

Correlation: A Crash Course

It would seem timely at this point to refresh the reader's memory regarding several aspects of the correlation coefficient. A correlation simply provides an indication of the strength of the relationship between two variables. A variable is an attribute of the real world, hopefully one that can be quantified. (Angels pose particular difficulties in this regard.) A correlation can range in value from +1.00 down and through 0 to -1.00. Whether the correlation is positive or negative merely reflects the fact that the values associated with the two variables tend to rise and fall together (a positive correlation) or that as values associated with one of the variables rise those associated with the other variable fall (a negative correlation).

Consider the variables of height *and* weight. Intuitively at least, one senses that these physical attributes are to a considerable extent related to each other. That is, with some exceptions, tall people tend to be heavier, whereas shorter individuals generally tend to weigh less. In fact, were we to actually record the height and weight of all students attending a large first-year class and then compute the correlation between these two variables, a correlation in the range of +.60 to +.80 would not be unexpected. That is, as the heights of people increase, there is a corresponding increase in the weights of these same individuals.

Consider now the variables of golf scores *and* earnings on the tournament trail. Again, we intuitively recognize that earnings are directly tied to golf scores (i.e., lower scores/higher earnings; higher scores/lower earnings). The values representing the two variables, scores and earnings, are in a sense moving in opposite directions. Those in the field of players who have shot high rounds stand to earn very little. In contrast, golfers shooting low rounds will be more generously rewarded for their performance. An actual calculation of this relationship would likely yield a correlation coefficient in the range of -.75 to -.95. Thus, positive and negative correlations are equally important, the sign (+ or -) merely indicates to the reader the direction of increases in the values on one variable relative to those on the second variable.

The actual magnitude necessary for a correlation coefficient to be statistically "significant" (i.e., other than due to chance) depends on the size of the sample. In general, a correlation calculated on the basis of a *small* sample must be quite large to be significant. In contrast, a relatively smaller correlation based on a *large* sample may also be significant. Tables that enable one to determine whether a particular correlation is significant, taking sample size into account, can be found at the back of most textbooks on statistics.

Many variables, of course, are unrelated to each other. Nonsignificant correlations of zero or near zero indicate a lack of association between two variables. For example, one does not anticipate nor would one be likely to find any relationship between eye color and measures of performance in baseball (e.g., batting average, stolen bases, or home runs). It might interest you to know that these eye-color hypotheses have recently been tested (Beer & Beer, 1989). It is not too surprising that the relationships were found to be nonsignificant.

A final point that continues to elude many personality researchers as well as their students (Martens, 1976) should be noted in regard to correlation coefficients. Simply stated, one cannot infer *causality* from the fact that two variables are significantly related. One might, for example, find a significant correlation between the financial worth of junior tennis players' parents and the youngsters' regional rankings. That is, the children of wealthier parents are generally ranked higher than children whose parents have more modest incomes.

Obviously, money per se does not produce excellence in the sport. Instead, it is the coaching expertise that money can buy that improves tennis skills. Money merely mediates or underlies the relationship between the amount of expert instruction and the caliber of a player's game but does not itself produce improved play. The fact of a significant correlation, then, does not allow one to infer that changes in the values associated with one variable are producing or causing changes in the values associated with the second variable. You may strongly suspect that they are, but support for your suspicions will have to wait on evidence from other sources (e.g., a controlled experiment).

Validity

When we ask about the validity of a measure we simply want some indication that the test measures what it claims to measure. Thus, while the title of a test may describe it as a "Test of Gymnastic Aptitude" and give every appearance (i.e., *face* validity) of tapping the relevant and requisite skills/attitudes for attaining some level of competence in the sport, we still want hard evidence to substantiate the claim that an aptitude for gymnastics is in fact being assessed.

Although the question of test validity can be approached and assessed in a number of different ways (see, e.g., Anastasi, 1988, chapters 6 and 7), the present sketch of the topic will deal with three of the more important types of validity.

1. Predictive Validity

To stay with our hypothetical test of gymnastics aptitude, one would anticipate that if the test indeed measures what it purports to measure, then the scores obtained by students at the start of a physical education class in gymnastics should be related to their final grades or standing in the class some months later. That is, assuming both that all students tested complete the course and that the instructors remain unaware of the students' initial scores, a significant correlation between the original test scores and final grades should result. Evidence of such a relationship would support a contention that the test is valid.

While such a validity coefficient may be statistically significant, it may not be especially large in absolute terms. But then again, a number of factors can intervene between the original administration of the test and the awarding of grades some months later (e.g., illness, injuries, loss of interest, etc.). For these and other reasons, a relatively low-order validity coefficient in the range of +.20 to +.40 is to be expected.

Forecasts of how teams in various sports will fare in upcoming league play are a popular feature of many magazines. As with other measures, these preseason forecasts can readily be evaluated in terms of their predictive validity. Blumenfeld (1985), for example, assessed the validity of preseason predictions by *Sports Illustrated* for football teams competing in 10 U.S. college conferences. Preseason rankings were significantly correlated with final standings at the end of the season for only 4 of the 10 conferences. Blumenfeld's findings certainly raise doubts about the ability of those at *Sports Illustrated* to predict the outcomes of conference play any better than their readers.

2. Concurrent Validity

Essentially the same procedures are followed in establishing the concurrent validity of a measure except that the criterion is available at the *same* time as the test is administered. It is not necessary to wait on the eventual emergence of a criterion. To return again to the example of our gymnastics aptitude test, it might be administered to all members of a university team. If our test truly measures aptitude, then those currently among the top-ranked members of the team should obtain generally higher scores, whereas those with lower rankings should obtain generally lower scores on the test. A claim that our test measures an aptitude for gymnastics is substantiated to the extent that test scores and gymnastic ratings are significantly correlated.

The two types of validity, predictive and concurrent, differ mainly in terms of time, the former being validated against a criterion that has yet to mature, the latter against a criterion presently available. But now, yet another type of validity deserves mention.

3. Content Validity

A further means of establishing the validity of a measure is seen in the *known groups method*. Let us imagine that we are in the process of developing a scale that we believe will assess the degree of concern on the part of the public for protecting our wilderness areas from encroachments by land developers. With a final set of cohesive and refined items in hand, we identify a group whose members, by the very nature of their ongoing activities, would be expected to get high scores on our test: the Sierra Club. The case for our test being valid is strengthened considerably if a sample of Sierra Club members scores substantially higher than, for example, members of the chamber of commerce. Few would challenge the a priori assumption that the protection of our environment is a higher priority for the Sierra Club than for members of the business community. Thus, results showing that members of the Sierra Club score very high on our test and the chamber of commerce members substantially lower gives us cause for optimism that our test measures environmental attitudes (indeed, has content validity).

Reliability

A second important psychometric property of a test is reliability. Here the concern is with the consistency of measurement. Is there stability over time (e.g., test-retest reliability) or agreement between two or more trained observers/judges (e.g., interjudge reliability)? Is there a degree of consistency in responses to the test items themselves (e.g., split-half reliability)? Again, a correlation coefficient is used to represent the strength of the relationships.

1. Test-Retest Reliability

One expects considerable stability in a measure from one test occasion to the next. To be acceptable, a test administered to a group of individuals today should yield a roughly similar pattern of individual scores when the same people take the test again 3 weeks from now. With few exceptions, those scoring high on our test today would tend to again score high on the readministration; those who score low today would be expected to get generally lower scores in 3 weeks. Because of the nature of the question asked of our test (i.e., evidence that it yields similar results on two test occasions involving the same people), we demand a relatively high correlation to satisfy the requirement of a stable, consistent measure. By convention, correlation coefficients in excess of +.80 are generally regarded as providing sufficient evidence of reliability.

2. Interjudge Reliability

When individuals in their capacity as trained observers or judges provide measures of athletic performance, we require some assurance that they are largely in agreement on their ratings. It would obviously be folly to base a prizefight decision solely on the judgment of the referee and to ignore the opinions of the judges at ringside. *Independent* ratings by two or more trained observers clearly provide a superior means of assessment. Although the same performance is rated from different vantage points, one should nevertheless expect a high level of agreement or interjudge reliability, again in the region of +.80 or above. As straightforward as this judgmental task might appear to be, especially for highly trained and experienced judges, they often fail at their task.

By any standard, a world boxing championship title fight ranks among the top events on any sports calendar. Prestige and millions of dollars are riding on the outcome. Barring a knockout, ring officials assigned to the match declare a winner based on round-by-round judgments of boxing skill. How *reliable* are their judgments?

In a 1971 title fight, Joe Frazier was declared the winner in a controversial decision over Muhammad Ali. An estimate of the interjudge reliability (i.e., the referee and two judges at ringside) was calculated on a round-by-round basis by Stallings and Gillmore (1972). The reliability coefficient was a dismal +.57. Little wonder that boxing seems to have more than its share of controversial decisions. You might well ask, Just how reliable is the judging of performance at other major sports events such as ski jumping, diving, figure skating, synchronized swimming, body building, bronc riding, and so forth?

Other studies, however, give us greater cause for optimism. For example, Showalter (1985) calculated the extent of agreement between the United Press International (UP) and Associated Press International (AP) football polls. The UP poll is the result of weekly rankings of U.S. college teams by a panel of coaches, whereas the AP poll is derived from rankings provided by the nation's writers and sportscasters. Despite the different perspectives from which team performances are judged, the two polls are substantially in agreement on the national rankings. Reliability coefficients ranged from +.73 to +.94.

3. Split-Half Reliability

Yet another aspect of the reliability question deals with the internal consistency of test items. One common means of determining the reliability of a test is to simply correlate the first half of the test with the second half. Occasionally, however, the items in a measure are arranged in order of increasing difficulty (an aptitude test might take this form). In that case the *odd-even* method of calculating reliability is used. The biasing effect of increasing item difficulty is virtually eliminated by correlating the odd-numbered items in the test with the even-numbered items. However, having split the measure in two halves, we are in one sense calculating the reliability of a test that is now just half its former length. Inasmuch as shortening a test lowers its reliability, a correction is required to provide an estimate of the reliability of the full, undivided test that will ultimately be used in practice. The Spearman-Brown formula (e.g., Anastasi, 1988, p. 121) provides just such a correction of the original Pearson r that we calculated for the two halves of the test.

An example is seen in an analysis of the records of a youth soccer team (Schuh, 1986). During the first half of the schedule ($N = 25$ games), 11 performance measures from the first half of their games were correlated with those from the second period of play. Reliabilities were again calculated in the same way for the remaining 24 games played during the second part of the season. Although the reliability of all 11 measures was assessed and adjusted by the Spearman-Brown formula, only 2 were shown to be reliable. These were *goals* (+.90), but only during the first part of the season, and *win-loss* (+.87) during the latter half of the season. Schuh's results suggest that most indices of soccer activity may fall short of acceptable levels of reliability by the criterion of internal consistency.

An Aside

With few exceptions, the Pearson product-moment correlation is suited to calculating reliability coefficients. However, a word of caution: The formula for computing a Pearson r (see, e.g., Anastasi, 1988, pp. 110–115; Rosenthal & Rosnow, 1984, chap. 17) assumes a linear, or straight-line, relationship between the two variables. One is always well advised to first draw a scatter plot—or have the computer do so—to see if there is visual evidence of curvilinearity in the data. If there is, a measure of association that takes curvilinearity in the data into account is appropriate and will provide a more accurate estimate of the strength of the relationship (see Rosenthal & Rosnow, 1984, pp. 222–224).

Norms

Yet another important criterion by which one can judge the usefulness of a test is the extent to which norms have been established. Norms are developed by initially administering a test to a very large number of people with identifiable characteristics, such as all Grade 10 students in the city of Montreal or 5,000 members of the Sierra Club. Thereafter, the score of an individual taking the test can be compared to the previously established norms. The individual's raw score can be meaningfully interpreted as, for example, falling slightly below the mean or, more precisely in another case, at a point 1.5 standard deviations above the mean of the normative group. Of course, to provide a meaningful comparison the test taker should share a common cultural background and personal attributes (e.g., sex, age) with the normative sample. For example, it would be patently unfair to compare the

"Test of Baseball Knowledge" score of a 10th grader from London, England, with the norms developed with 10th graders in Indianapolis, Indiana. By the standard of norms developed in Indianapolis, the London student's knowledge will appear scant, yet a comparison with other 10th graders in the London school system may reveal instead that the same youngster is reasonably well informed on the topic.

It should be noted that the test features sketched above are ordered in terms of their importance. If a test is not valid, it serves no useful purpose even though there may be some evidence of its reliability. Acceptable reliability in no way ensures that a test is valid. The relationship between the psychometric properties of validity and reliability are brought into perspective in the following summary: If a test is valid then it must be at least somewhat reliable; however, if a test is reliable, it may or may not be valid. Validity, then, is the prime consideration in the evaluation or selection of a test.

Finally, a note of caution on the choice of a test: A major pitfall for the unwary lies with the use of measures that have *ipsative* properties. Such a measure "yields scores such that each score for an individual is dependent on his own scores on other variables, but is independent of, and not comparable with, the scores of other individuals" (Hicks, 1970, p. 167). As an example, a hypothetical scale using a forced-choice format purports to measure one's preference for recreational activities involving same-sex, coeducational, or solitary pursuits. Each question requires respondents to choose between two items describing either a solitary or coed activity, a solitary or same-sex activity, a coed or same-sex activity, and so on. It might be hastily concluded from the results of a survey that a group of graduate students in astronomy is less interested than the rest of the student body in coeducational activities. Astonomy majors' very low scores on the coed scale seems to point to such a conclusion. However, by some other (absolute) measure, our astronomy majors may instead be found to have an equal or even stronger preference for coeducational recreation than other students. (After all, those long, lonely all-night sessions in the observatory can play havoc with one's social life.) The point to note is that given the forced-choice item format, low *coed* scores might be the result of high *solitary* scores. Consistently choosing the solitary item in solitary–coed pairs must inevitably result in a depressed score on the coed scale. It follows that comparisons between individuals or between groups using purely ipsative measures are at best spurious.

Tests and measurement procedures vary in the degree to which they are ipsative. Hicks (1970) provides a review of the topic and identifies a number of measures having ipsative properties, measures that appear in the sport psychology literature from time to time. In this regard, particular note should be taken of the Edwards Personal Preference Schedule (Edwards, 1954), the Strong Vocational Interest Blank (Strong, 1951), and Sheldon's (1940) typology of body types. The choice of a test, then, is far from a casual undertaking.

Means to Evaluate

A number of major reference sources are available and provide a means by which most published tests can be evaluated. A general source covering the full range of tests is the *Mental Measurements Yearbook* (*MMY*), edited by O.K. Buros (1978). Tests are critically evaluated by qualified psychometricians in regard to the considerations noted above. The *MMY* is regularly updated and additionally available through an on-line computer service (see Anastasi, 1988, pp. 19–22). One is further aided in a choice by a number of other reference sources for attitude and personality measures (Robinson, Shaver, & Wrightsman, 1991; Shaw & Wright, 1967), a classified listing of tests (Anastasi, 1988, Appendix D) and a sports-specific compendium of test summaries by Ostrow (1990).

Tests

The following sections are intended to acquaint the reader with some of the more popular tests appearing in the sports literature. Although passing reference will be made to the psychometric properties of some of the measures, this section is not an adequate substitute for the detailed descriptions and evaluations offered in the sources cited above.

Projective Measures

Advocates of the diverse class of projective measures share an underlying assumption: that as the test materials are increasingly unstructured, vague, or ambiguous, respondents are better able to reveal more of their innermost selves. For example, presenting the client with single stimulus words (e.g., *mother*) in a word association test administered in the accepting atmosphere of the clinician's office may elicit a wealth of previously repressed experiences important to an understanding of the individual's current state. As in diagnostic or therapeutic settings, it is important that those using these procedures in sports research have graduate training in advanced testing. Courses and supervised practica specifically on the Rorschach and/or Thematic Apperception Test (TAT), which are described below, generally form part of the core curriculum in clinical psychology.

The Rorschach Test

Perhaps the test most closely associated in the public mind with clinical diagnosis, the Rorschach involves a set of 10 cards of inkblots presented individually by the clinician. The client provides an interpretation with only slight prompting from the therapist. A complex scoring procedure (e.g., Exner, 1986) designed to identify areas of conflict is applied to the protocols and interpreted against the background of the clinician's experience and theoretical perspective.

Thematic Apperception Test (TAT)

The TAT (Murray et al., 1938) is similarly intended for use as a clinical diagnostic tool. Clients are asked to tell a story in response to each in a series of 19 cards depicting an ill-defined, ambiguous scene. In addition to their interpretation, they are asked to suggest what preceded and followed the scene as well as what the characters are feeling and thinking at the time. Again, a detailed procedure for scoring the protocols accompanies the test and dictates that users of the test be suitably qualified.

With regard to the psychometric properties of the Rorschach and the TAT, it must be said that despite many decades of research on these instruments acceptable validity has yet to be clearly demonstrated. Reliability fares only somewhat better (e.g., Anastasi, 1988, pp. 612–622).

Notwithstanding these major limitations, Davis (1990) has apparently used projective measures with considerable success in addressing an important issue, namely, the role of imaging in performance. Both the TAT and Rorschach were administered to members of the Calgary Flames Hockey Club. Measures of achievement imagery and action imagery were derived from the test protocols in an independent context that did not draw upon the athletes' sport experiences. The results of this study are impressive. Seemingly, the ability of players to develop imagery in a nonsports context is predictive of their on-ice performance in the National Hockey League. That is, those players able to produce greater amounts of achievement and action imagery were also those who led their club in goals and assists.

Objective Measures

Minnesota Multiphasic Personality Inventory (MMPI)[2]

The MMPI is easily our leading clinical diagnostic tool. It is a self-report inventory comprised of 550 items tapping areas ranging from psychosomatic symptoms, to sexual and religious attitudes, to obsessive/compulsive states. Ten basic scales are derived from the test items (e.g., depression, "D"; paranoia, "P"; social introversion, "Si") in addition to several validity scales. For example, a high K, or correction, score denotes defensiveness in answering items or "faking good." It should be noted that a number of the scales have inadequate reliability (Anastasi, 1988, p. 532). Moreover, the original norms are based on the responses of a small sample of approximately 700 Minneapolis adults. As with the Rorschach and the TAT noted above, the MMPI is intended for use with *clinical* populations.

---

[2] A revision, the MMPI-2, is currently available for use (Hathaway & McKinley, 1989).

California Personality Inventory (CPI)

The CPI is adapted for use with "normals" and consists of 462 true/false items, approximately half of which were drawn from the MMPI. It has acceptable reliability and includes 3 validity scales in addition to 17 basic scales (e.g., self-control, femininity, etc.). The norms are based on a sample of 6,000 males and 7,000 females. It is suited to the assessment of people age 13 and up. Thus far, it appears to be a good predictor of such criteria as high school grades and delinquency.

Sixteen Personality Factor Questionnaire (16PF)

Cattell's 16PF is a personality inventory (Cattell, Eber, & Tatsuoka, 1970) developed by means of factor analyses of large numbers of trait ratings. The approach taken was one of trying to identify the primary source traits that underlie personality as causal factors. Sixteen scores on independent traits can be calculated providing measures of, for example, shy versus venturesome and reserved versus outgoing. The 16PF has proven to be an especially popular measure among sport researchers seeking to identify differences in the psychological profiles of those engaged in different sports and at different levels of skill within the same sport. At the same time, a distressing feature of this literature is the considerable number of published reports using the 16PF in which the authors apparently ignore or are oblivious to criticisms of the inventory. As Mischel (1986) has noted, "Some fourteen or fifteen source traits have been reported...but only six have been found repeatedly" (p. 126). When there are major concerns associated with a test—and the 16PF is certainly not alone in this regard—they should be acknowledged or addressed rather than leaving the nonspecialist reader to incorrectly infer that there is a consensus that a test meets acceptable standards of measurement in all respects.

The clinical tests noted in this section are but a few of the more popular and better known instruments that have served to test hypotheses in sport psychology. It bears repeating that the measuring instrument or procedure chosen should be psychometrically sound and in the hands of qualified persons for use with those populations and purposes for which the test was intended.

Mood Measures

Another important class of measures is concerned with providing self-reports of one's current affective mood states. Several carefully developed instruments are available for this purpose.

Profile of Mood States (POMS)

This popular and easy to administer scale (McNair, Lorr, & Droppleman, 1971) provides measures of the following dimensions of mood: *tension, depression, anger, vigor, fatigue,* and *confusion.* Among the many applications to research derived from the POMS, perhaps the best known is Morgan's (1980) investigation of elite athletes. Morgan found a common *iceberg profile* to underlie the mood states of topflight competitors in several sports. For example, wrestlers successful in making their Olympic team scored generally lower on all mood measures than did those not making the team, the single exception being *vigor.* On the measure of vigor, the Olympians peaked dramatically higher than their unsuccessful rivals, hence the iceberg analogy. This program represents a significant contribution to the efforts of those attempting to distinguish the very best performers from those who are just off the pace.[3]

Mood Adjective Check List (MACL)

The development of the MACL was based on extensive factor analyses of adjectives that are descriptive of a full range of mood states (Nowlis, 1965). Its short form provides an attractive alternative to the POMS. Eleven clusters of adjectives or independent (uncorrelated) factors were found to underlie the domain of moods. In its application, subjects are instructed to attend to how they feel at the moment with respect to a particular state (e.g., *affectionate)* and to indicate the degree to which *affectionate* describes the way they presently feel. Of course, *affectionate* is only one of several adjectives that best represent a dimension of *social affection*; others include *kindly* and *warmhearted.* In sum, both the MACL and POMS are psychometrically sound, with good evidence of their validity and reliability.

An Ethical Comment

The researcher using a test of individual differences bears a heavy responsibility to ensure that the highest standards of ethical conduct are observed. Inasmuch as test items frequently probe personally sensitive matters, the tester must among other things assume responsibility for the confidentiality of results, limit access to test data and seek information only on matters that are relevant to the investigation at hand. In short, considerable care should be exercised to protect those who volunteer to help us with our research from later being dealt a disservice as a result of their participation. Research is a joint undertaking that can succeed only as long as our subjects feel that their interests are protected and their participation makes an important contribution to our understanding of human behavior.

A second area of ethical concern centers on the qualifications of test users. Although the level of training necessary is, to a certain extent, dependent on the particular test being considered, training in psychometric and test theory, in addition

[3] A useful sports bibliography of the measure has been provided by LeUnes, Hayward, and Daiss (1988).

to supervised practica in the case of specific tests, is a prerequisite to engaging in the administration of most tests. Usually this entails course work at the master's and doctoral levels. It is inappropriate, indeed unethical, for unsupervised individuals whose only qualification is an enthusiasm for research to be administering and interpreting test results.

The above digression is intended to alert the reader to the fact that a host of various ethical concerns surrounds psychological testing. Note should be taken of the *Ethical Principles of Psychologists* appearing in Volume 36 of the *American Psychologist* (pp. 633–638). Whereas the statement addresses ethical issues on a variety of professional topics, Principle 8 specifically deals with matters of assessment. More detailed discussion of the ethics involved in testing is available in other sources (e.g., Anastasi, 1988, chap. 3).

Social Personality Models

In this section, five models of personality with especial relevance to sports will be outlined. Each such outline will be followed by a sample of studies that provide tests of the theory in sports settings. The set of personality models chosen for discussion includes those that social psychologists interested in individual differences have traditionally found useful in their research. For the most part, the results of these investigations will be shown to have implications for athletic performance, coaching practice, or the structure of some sports.

1. The Macho Personality

Machismo, or variants of the original Spanish concept, is a pervasive theme found in many contemporary sports. A dominant and culturally prized trait in Hispanic cultures, machismo has been a growing influence in recent years throughout North American sports and leisure-time activities. Examples of machismo are close at hand. Turnbull and Brown (1977) felt compelled to comment on the "super males" of Western Canada in observing that, "there seems to be a sense of pride involved in living under adverse weather conditions, manifested by the often grossly inappropriate (under)dress for those conditions worn by Saskatchewan males" (p. 77). The authors see such expressions as an outgrowth of the "pioneer/farmer tradition," a tradition that incidentally elevates contact sports to an exalted status.

Far from being an anomalous theme of the North American culture, the counterpart of the macho man can also be found on other continents. Everett (1988) describes the stereotype of the Australian *ocker* as "the pot-bellied, singlet-clad, can-in-hand Australian male" (p. 138). The origins of the ocker and the part he plays in society have been skillfully portrayed in G. Lewis's (1983) book *Real Men Like Violence*. Because of its considerable potential for mediating antisocial behaviors, such as rape and family violence (Everett, 1988; Mosher, 1991, in press), machismo and its variants are deserving of more than passing interest by sports researchers.

Seldom have machismo themes found greater cultural expression than in the German dueling practice, or *Mensur*, that flourished at universities during the latter half of the 19th century and into the early years of this century. Swordsmanship and the accompanying ritual were rehearsed by young boys in the gymnasium and even by children at play in the nursery. The duel itself was believed to develop the traits of coolness and courage in German youth, although at least one witness to the Mensur (Jerome, 1900) saw it instead as a brutalizing experience. At the risk of offending your sensibilities, what follows are excerpts from a particularly lurid eyewitness account provided by the British playwright and journalist Jerome K. Jerome.

The setting:
> The room is bare and sordid; its walls splashed with mixed stains of beer, blood, and candle-grease; its ceiling, smokey; its floor, sawdust covered.

The combatants:
> Quaint and rigid, with their goggle-covered eyes, their necks tied up in comforters, their bodies smothered in what looks like dirty bed quilts, their padded arms stretched straight above their heads, they might be a pair of ungainly clock-work figures.

The duel:
> The whole interest is centered in watching the wounds. They come always in one of two places—on the top of the head or the left side of the face. Sometimes a portion of hairy scalp or section of cheek flies up into the air, to be carefully preserved in an envelope by its proud possessor, and shown round on convivial evenings; and from every wound, of course, flows a plentiful stream of blood. It splashes doctors, seconds, and spectators; it sprinkles ceiling and walls; it saturates the fighters, and makes pools for itself in the sawdust.

"Doctors" (actually medical students) rush in and make deliberately clumsy efforts to repair the wounds. The duel continues:
> Now and then you see a man's teeth laid bare almost to the ear, so that for the rest of the duel he appears to be grinning at one half of the spectators, his other side remaining serious; and sometimes a man's nose get slit, which gives to him as he fights a singularly supercilious air.

Who emerges as the victor? Paradoxically, the fighter with the most extensive and severe wounds. The wish of the mutilated victor is that his scars will last a lifetime, a wish almost certain to be granted thanks to the inept efforts of those attending his wounds. For the victor there is the assurance of becoming "the envy of German youth" and of drawing "the admiration of the German maiden. He who obtains only a few unimportant wounds retires sulky and disappointed" (pp. 153–154). The value of a gaping wound can also be calculated in purely monetary terms. As Jerome noted, "such a wound, judiciously mauled and interfered with during the week afterwards, can generally be reckoned on to secure its fortunate possessor a wife with a dowry of five figures at the least" (p. 154).

The starting point for any scientific examination of the role of the macho individual in sport is a ground-breaking article by Mosher and Sirkin (1984). These authors developed a theoretical model of the macho personality constellation. They specify three basic components that characterize the hypermasculine personality. First, macho males exhibit calloused sex attitudes toward women whereby "sexual intercourse with women establishes masculine power and female submission, and is to be achieved without empathic concern for the female's subjective experience" (p. 152). Second, they share a belief that verbal and physical aggression is manly and serves as a preferred means of expressing one's dominance over other men. Finally, danger is seen as exciting and parallels an attitude that their masculinity is reaffirmed or enhanced with demonstrations of survival in a dangerous environment. Among other things, the macho man tends to be impulsive, reckless, fearless, and adventurous in the sense of seeking out new, often risky, experiences that allow him to tempt fate.

At other times, expressions of machismo can be enjoyed vicariously as a spectator at combatant sports. The response of hypermasculine men observing violent events is predictably one of heightened aggression; by contrast, nonmacho males show no appreciable increase in their aggression (Russell, in press).

Future research on the role of a macho personality in sports has been aided by the development of a 30-item scale based on the three components of the constellation noted above. Early indications are that the Hypermasculinity inventory has construct validity and external validity insofar as predictions of drug use, aggression, dangerous driving after alcohol consumption, and an earlier record of delinquent behaviors were confirmed among a population of university males (Mosher & Sirkin, 1984).

In recent decades we have witnessed the promotion of alcohol, tobacco, sportswear, colognes, and so on by the advertising industry using macho themes as a vehicle. The ads are slick and undoubtedly profitable for advertisers. The entertainment media have similarly enjoyed notable success in marketing programs and films that cast actors in macho, often violent, roles. One of the subtle consequences is that many have uncritically come to adopt the macho man as an *ideal* whose behaviors parents and their male children strive to emulate. However, there is a darker, a much darker, side to the macho man. Mosher and Sirkin's profile of the macho personality (above) might already have alerted you to the downside of the macho male's behavior.

The major concern, I believe, should lie with the macho man's proclivity for violence, in particular, the threat he poses to women on a day-to-day basis. Macho men are more willing than other men to use coercive tactics to obtain sex with females. Threats and even physical force are willingly used in their conquest of women. It comes as no surprise, then, that they are also more tolerant of rape (Mosher, 1991; Mosher & Anderson, 1986) and less sympathetic to the plight of female victims of physical assault (Russell, 1992a) than their nonmacho counterparts.

The expression of macho tendencies in real-world violence is likely seen results of a *Philadelphia Daily News* survey of 350 U.S. colleges. The resul gested that football and basketball players are overrepresented in campus statistics, especially in the category of sexual assault. A report of the survey (Kirshenbaum, 1989) indicated that compared to male students in the general campus population, those playing football and basketball were 38% more likely to be involved in assaults on women. Society clearly is not well served by the promotion and glamorizing of the macho male.

While the origins of hypermasculinity lie in the early parental socialization experiences (Mosher, 1991; Mosher & Tomkins, 1988), later involvement in sports and other peer group activities (e.g., delinquency) can serve to reinforce and further influence the adolescent boy in specific ways toward a macho ideal. Certainly, there is no shortage of all-male sports containing elements of physical danger in which the lessons of machismo can be effectively learned. Marc Fasteau's (1975) *The Male Machine* provides a detailed portrayal of the idealized and pervasive image of masculinity toward which most American men strive. Of even greater relevance for the present discussion is his description of the various forces operating specifically within sports that foster and sustain the development of stereotypical male behavior. Sports, then, may provide a superior investigative context for those interested in understanding the etiology of the hypermasculine personality.

The next section provides a discussion of the Type A personality. Before introducing the topic, however, I should point out that Type A's are closely related to the macho personality. So close is the resemblance that Virginia Price (1982) has been prompted to conclude that "Type A behavior and 'macho,' or masculine behavior are in many respects indistinguishable" (p. 72). Price recounts an anecdote involving the behavior of two Type A men, behavior that would equally typify the macho male. In separate incidents, two men known to be Type A were accosted by armed attackers on the streets of San Francisco. Both chose to challenge their attackers; both were killed (p. 73). Where others might be reflective, Type A's are not. Where most of us display fear in situations that are dangerous, macho and Type A individuals appear fearless. The next section, then, examines this close relative of the macho personality.

2. Type A and Type B Behavior Patterns

The Type A behavior pattern is perhaps best known for its widely publicized association with coronary heart disease (Glass, 1977; Houston & Snyder, 1988; Price, 1982). The greater susceptibility of Type A's presumably derives from their hard-driving, competitive style in pursuit of "success." These individuals exhibit impatience and hostility in pursuing their goals and work with an overriding sense of urgency; that is, time is short, there are deadlines to be met, there is never enough time. Although some might judge that too big a price is paid, it should be noted that the achievement strivings of Type A's often meet with success (Matthews, Helmreich, Beane, & Lucker, 1980).

Of particular interest is the prediction that Type A's readily react with hostility to any thwarting of their feverish activities. Support for this assumption was provided in an experiment by Carver and Glass (1978). Type A's and Type B's were individually provoked by an experimental accomplice who was both insulting and interfered with their attempts to solve a puzzle. Given an opportunity to later shock the confederate, Type A's administered substantially higher levels of shock than did Type B's. However, under normal circumstances (i.e., in the absence of frustrations), Type A's and B's do not differ in their aggressiveness.

Type A's are further characterized by nonaggressive dominance in competitive situations. For present purposes, dominance will be taken to mean behavior intended to achieve "control of situations or individuals" (Straub, Grunberg, Street, & Singer, 1990, p. 1052). Within competitions, two forms of behavior in particular appear to express dominance. First, dominance is expressed through the amount of *resistance* one offers in response to pressures to concede or submit. It is also seen in the *persistence* shown by an individual when faced with an unrelenting opponent. A modified version of the classic Deutsch and Krauss (1960) trucking game provided a setting in which Type A's could be assessed with regard to these forms of dominance. Both male and female Type A's persisted longer in their efforts to control the situation than did Type B's. Type A women additionally showed a greater resistance than B's to caving in to pressures to back down when their route was blocked by the rival trucking company. However, Type A and Type B males did not differ in their resistance; both stood their ground for an equal length of time.

Straub et al. (1990) went on to propose "that women may be more apt to display and use nonaggressive dominance than men" (p. 1060). The suggestion remains speculative at this point. However, the hypothesis certainly warrants investigation in other competitive settings and would make an important contribution to the expanding literature on sex differences.

There are, of course, occasions when the ultracompetitive Type A fails. Their reactions are interesting. Musante, MacDougall, and Dembroski (1984) had Type A and Type B subject pairs compete in games of video "Pong." Unlike Type B's, Type A's attributed their failures to internal factors (i.e., their own lack of ability or skill) rather than to external causes such as luck. Further evidence (K.V. Jones, 1985) collected in the context of a competitive reaction time task suggests that having experienced failure, Type A's quickly lose interest in the competition. Jones explains the tendency of Type A's to quit when success eludes them as an elective strategy whereby they husband their resources. These reserves can later be applied to other competitive situations where they feel they stand a better chance of winning.

A Word to Coaches

Coaches concerned with the physical well-being of their charges should be especially mindful of the behaviors of Type A athletes in a competitive environment. It has been shown that Type A's will complain less about hard work (Weidner &

Matthews, 1978), report less fatigue than Type B's following training sessions (Carver, Coleman, & Glass, 1976), and play with injuries (Carver, DeGregorio, & Gillis, 1981). However, once injured, Type A's are rated by their physicians as making worse than expected progress through the course of their treatment. These noncompliant Type A's (i.e., those who make a poor recovery) also attribute responsibility for their injury to themselves, see it as a condition to be fought, and express more anger than other injured athletes (Rhodewalt & Strube, 1985).

Assessment Procedures

The most widely used means of assessing the Type A behavioral pattern is the Jenkins Activity Survey (JAS; Jenkins, Zyzanski, & Rosenman, 1979). This 52-item, self-report test is presented in a multiple-choice format. Respondents are asked to report on their typical behavior in a variety of day-to-day situations, such as how rapidly they eat, patterns of sleep, how often they take work home.

The Structured Interview (SI; e.g., Price, 1982, 1988) in some ways represents a superior means of assessing Type A behavior. The measure is derived from an interview in which the interviewee's motor behaviors are seen to be more important indicators of a Type A personality than the actual content of their verbal responses. A sense of time urgency is seen in knee jiggling or rapid finger tapping; a clenched fist indicates hostility. Its weaknesses are those associated with any interview technique. Differences in the age, sex, and attitudes of the subject vis-à-vis those of the interviewer, as well as the subjectivity of the scoring system, leave the procedure open to several sources of bias. For diagnostic purposes, then, the SI has much to recommend it; for predictive purposes, the JAS may be better suited to the needs of most researchers.

Even a superficial overview of the JAS items makes it apparent that Type A athletes and others have the potential to restructure their style of behavior and increase their life expectancy as well as enhance the quality of their interpersonal relationships (e.g., peer relations, family life, etc.). If this seems an attractive goal, Type A individuals, aided by a qualified clinician, can effectively approximate the easygoing, more affable Type B's.

The further fact that two independent (uncorrelated) dimensions, *Achievement Striving* and *Impatience-Irritability*, underlie the JAS items opens the possibility of a further option that might combine the best of both worlds. It is generally recognized that the hostility component is responsible for the life-shortening consequences of Type A behavior. Programs designed to reduce what is called the AHA syndrome (i.e., anger-hostility-aggression) in Type A's could conceivably reduce the health risks and at the same time leave the drive to excel untouched.

Not to downplay the health risks, there is much to recommend Type A behavior. For example, Type A researchers in social psychology outperform their Type B colleagues both quantitatively (number of publications) and qualitatively (number of times their works are cited). Additionally, Type A students outperform their Type B classmates. Generally speaking, Type A's earn higher grade point averages (Spence, Pred, & Helmreich, 1989). All in all, then, there is some good news and some not-so-good news associated with Type A behavior.

3. Internal-External Locus of Control (I-E)

A further construct that has given us numerous insights into the behaviors of sportspeople is Rotter's (1966) distinction between an internal and an external locus of control. This popular social psychological model and scale assesses the extent to which individuals believe they can exert a degree of control over the course of day-to-day events. Some feel they can influence events; others believe that the course of events is virtually beyond their control. More specifically, some people see outcomes in their day-to-day lives as being partly contingent on their own actions; others see no connections between their behaviors and subsequent outcomes. In effect, the latter group, those with an external orientation, see events largely occurring as a result of external forces (e.g., luck, fate).[4]

There are several important implications for athletic performance arising from the distinction between those with an internal versus an external locus of control. When a task calls for cooperation, internals and externals perform equally well. However, if the structure of the task is instead competitive, internals generally excel (Nowicki, 1982). This point is seen in a study of women competing on the Ladies Professional Golf Association (LPGA) tour. A battery of physiological and personality measures was administered to a sample of players just prior to a tournament. Locus of control emerged as an important predictor of scoring average (Crews, Shirreffs, Thomas, Krahenbuhl, & Helfrich, 1986). Those golfers with an internal orientation (i.e., those who believed that the quality of their play was largely the result of their own actions) fared better in competition than their externally oriented rivals.

On the other hand, the execution of other athletic skills may instead favor those with an external orientation. Ice hockey players with an external locus of control are credited with more assists than their internally oriented teammates. While locus of control does not differ across playing position, players with an external orientation are involved in more on-ice altercations (Russell, 1974). In regard to frustration-induced aggression, internals make a greater effort, and see it as within their power, to bring about outcomes other than a fight. In a nutshell, internals respond more constructively to frustration. As Brissett and Nowicki (1973) suggest, "externals regard obstacles as 'insurmountable' in comparison to internals who regard them as 'surmountable'" (p. 41). As a consequence, externals may just let the "inevitable" happen, believing there is little or nothing they can do to alter the course of a developing confrontation.

The role of situational factors in shaping one's orientation is seen in a study of football players. Members of a university team have been found to score higher

---

[4] Type A's typically have an internal orientation, $r(273) = -.17, p < .01$ (Glass, 1977, p. 185).

on a "powerful others" dimension of externality than students not involved in the program (LeUnes & Nation, 1982). Additionally, black players were found to be more externally oriented than their white teammates (Nation & LeUnes, 1983a). As LeUnes and Nation are quick to point out, a university football program is a social situation where one's outcomes or eventual success as a player is largely in the hands of significant others (i.e., coaches and scouts). Their advice, approval, and influence may have a considerably greater impact than anything the individual athlete can do to further his career. Participation in football, or any sport with a similar social structure, might understandably foster a belief that the important outcomes in one's life are determined by external forces. By contrast, nonathletic students can more easily credit their academic success to their own efforts, and for many, an internal orientation is acquired or maintained.

4. The Machiavellian Personality

The historical figure most closely associated in the public mind with guile, deceit, and the manipulation of others is Niccolo Machiavelli (1469–1527), the 16th-century advisor to the princes of Italy's feuding states. Indeed, his recommended tactics for gaining and holding power—described in *The Discourses* and *The Prince*—have served the unscrupulous well over the centuries. For psychologists Richard Christie and Florence Geis (1970), the question was whether Machiavellians are still among us today, that is, those who share the same beliefs and employ the same tactics. In developing a scale of Machiavellian tendencies, these researchers drew many of their items directly from the writings of Machiavelli. The scale itself has undergone a number of revisions with the Mach IV perhaps enjoying the greatest use. It is comprised of 20 true/false items, whereas its successor, the Mach V scale, employs a different scoring procedure that requires respondents to select their answers from triads of alternatives.

The psychological profile of high Mach individuals recognizes four major features of their personality. First, Machiavellians exhibit a lack of affect or emotional involvement in their interpersonal relations. Were they not aloof and devoid of empathy, their deceptions and manipulation of others would be made that much more difficult. Second, their breaches of moral standards are not in any way troubling to them. Again, abiding by the normative code of morality that governs the actions of most people would limit their ability to lie, cheat, and bend the rules to suit their purpose. The third noteworthy aspect of high Machs is their lack of any serious commitment to the ideology or goals of those groups in which they are members. As a consequence, they can readily sacrifice idealistic group goals in favor of attaining immediate, personally advantageous ends. Finally, it should be recognized that the high Mach individual is neither out of touch with reality nor has a distorted view of the surrounding world. Quite the opposite! Such individuals have a very clear view of social situations, in particular, where the power lies and how it might be used to their advantage. These characteristics, then, allow high Machs to engage in a range of unethical, immoral, and sometimes illegal activities without suffering the pangs of conscience or remorse that most of us would experience in such circumstances.

High Mach individuals are, of course, to be found in sports as elsewhere. Sports that feature social interactions afford the Machiavellian superior opportunities for the manipulation of individuals. Evidence of the success of Machiavellian tactics is seen in the results of a study by Paulhus, Molin, and Schuchts (1979). The Mach scores of football and tennis players were found to be positively correlated with their proficiency ratings. The authors propose that high Mach football players gain an edge by a willingness to push "every rule to the limit" (p. 204) and by exploiting their relationships with the coaches to get more playing time. Similarly, high Mach tennis players would not hesitate to resort to a variety of shabby tactics intended to "psych out" or otherwise unnerve an opponent.

However, the success of Machiavellian tactics does not appear to extend to ice hockey. Neither goal scoring nor assists has been found to be associated with a Machiavellian outlook. High Machs are, however, more likely to be penalized for acts of on-ice aggression and to be found playing on defense (Russell, 1974). It may be that high Machs are attracted to the defensive position on a team where their superior interpersonal skills (e.g., reading cues, inferring intentions) can be put to good use.

Christie and Geis (1970) have themselves expressed a qualified respect for the cunning of the high Mach in commenting that "we found ourselves having a perverse admiration for the high Mach's ability to outdo others in experimental situations" (p. 339). There is, then, a seductive appeal and general fascination with Machiavellian skills, first because they are often seen to "work" and, second, because such tactics are generally condoned and even applauded in the media.

The Machiavellian personality is put squarely into perspective in a monograph by Robert Smith (1978). He undertook a comprehensive review of the psychopathic personality that included a comparison with Machiavellians. He concluded, "There seems hardly a single serious contradiction between the two profiles emerging from theory and research" (p. 92). The Machiavellian, as with his fraternal if not his identical twin the psychopath, is a disconcerting presence in sport. It is unfortunate that some athletes have adopted Machiavellian values and tactics. Even so, they may be doing little more than reflecting the dominant values of their culture. As Robert Smith observes with reference to the psychopath:

> Because of "encouragement from without," i.e., the market place, it may be argued that psychopathy can be much more fruitfully looked at as the logical extreme, or the fantastic exaggeration perhaps, of what our Western societies not only tolerate, but virtually demand of us if we want to win fame and fortune. (p. x)

The erosion of the principles of sportsmanship and fair play is a disheartening step back from the ideals of sport. But hopefully not all of the horses have left the barn. Any further retreat should be resisted.

5. The Aggressive Personality

A clinical profile of the aggressive personality type has been provided by Millon (1969). Millon has offered an extended account of the aggressive personality in describing an active-dependent pattern of behavior characteristic of such individuals. In sketching the aggressive personality, he notes their irritability and the ease with which these persons are given to outbursts of anger (see also, Josephson, 1987; Wilkins, Scharff, & Schlottmann, 1974). They also tend to use projection as a defense mechanism and in so doing attribute their own malevolent motives to others. Millon further characterizes the aggressive individual as possessing an assertive self-image, a pride in her or his energy, realism, and "hard-nosed" style. At an interpersonal level, the aggressive person is described as vindictive, intimidating, and punitive. To make their hostile behavior appear acceptable, aggressive individuals routinely cloak their actions in rationalizations. To quote Millon: "He espouses such philosophical balderdash as: 'Might is right,' 'This is a dog-eat-dog world,'. . . 'It's better to get these kids used to tough handling now before it's too late,' and 'You've got to be a realist in this world, and most people are either foolish idealists, appeasers, commies or atheists'" (p. 247). By putting a thin veneer of respectability on their behavior, the chronic aggressor can make their actions seem justified and even to be operating in the best interests of society.

The aggressor's interpersonal relations are in many ways blunted, lacking in genuine feelings of affection, sentimentality, and empathy for others. These qualities are instead deprecated. Note that the profile of the Machiavellian, also aggressive, overlaps with that of the chronic aggressor in regard to the lack of emotional empathy. Suspicious by nature, the aggressive individual frequently seeks out an adversary whom he provokes to the point of conflict. Such encounters may be reinforcing and even enjoyable for the aggressor and further allow for a test of his strength and aggressive prowess.

A similar characterization of chronic aggressors has been provided by Susan Butt. In the course of developing her empirically based motivational theory of sport participation (Butt, 1976, 1987), she has succinctly described the aggressive athlete as especially energetic and one who as a consequence "appears to be eager, active, and impulsive. If frustrated the aggressive athlete is quick to find fault with others and may verbally or physically attack them" (Butt, 1987, pp. 4–5). Millon (1969) also draws attention to the provocative actions of the aggressive individual. "He carries a 'chip on his shoulder,' seems to be spoiling for a fight and appears to enjoy tangling with others to prove his strength and to test his competencies and powers" (p. 275).

The above is not to say that aggressors are all of the same stripe. Rather, just as there are different types of aggression, so too there are different types of aggressors. Those identified as chronic aggressors can be expected to differ considerably in terms of personality factors, the tactics they employ and the situations that favor their aggressive outbursts. The next section describes an attempt to develop a system of classification for violent prison inmates. The system is one that can be readily generalized to noninmate populations (including sports) to account for the underlying personality dynamics of aggressive individuals.

A Typology of Violent Males

Hans Toch is a social psychologist who has provided a particularly useful means of classifying and understanding the psychological dynamics of aggressors. A highly readable account of his analysis of those who repeatedly become involved in interpersonal aggression is provided in *Violent Men* (Toch, 1984). The subjects who offered detailed information on their violent encounters were prison inmates and parolees who had a history of assaultive crimes. In a departure from the traditional means of conducting interviews, Toch used a peer-interview technique. Carefully trained prisoners and recent parolees conducted the interviews and subsequently contributed in a major way to the interpretation and analyses of interview content. The technique, of course, capitalized on the insights of those sharing similar values, backgrounds, and subtleties of language with those being interviewed. Also, a chronic problem with traditional interviewing techniques— that of the interviewees being reluctant to discuss personal matters with interviewers who differ substantially in status, education, and so on—was bypassed. Seemingly, those interviewed were less guarded and more forthcoming in their discussion with peers. From all accounts of the interviews and the role of peers in interpreting the data, it is clear that the quality of the resulting system of classifying violent individuals was greatly enriched by their contributions.

The interviews produced data from which Toch (1984) and his colleagues developed a classification system that recognized 10 distinct types of aggressors. The resulting typology described the nature and antecedents of the aggressive act for each category as well as the motives and personality dispositions that underlie the behavior of each of the types of aggressive individuals.

Several of the categories of community violence clearly have their counterpart among the aggressive elements in sports. In some instances the types are consistent with research findings involving athletes; in others, devotees of a sport will recognize the existence of one or more of the types among participants in their favorite sport. The five categories I have chosen as illustrations are those I would judge are most likely to be found among sports aggressors or, alternatively, those that the reader is most likely to recognize from his own involvement and personal analysis of sports. The size of each category—expressed as a percentage of the total sample—is based on the inmate sample interviewed in Toch's (1984) investigation and may or may not correspond to a sample of violent sportsmen.

1. Self-Image Promoters

Toch's (1984) largest category (28% of the interviews conducted) describes individuals who engage in interpersonal aggression for reasons of self-image compensating by way of either (a) promoting or (b) defending their self-image. The first type, *self-image promoters*, actively seek out or contrive situations that can only lead to violence. Hoping to convince others of their toughness and courage, they at the same time derive feelings of worth from having assaulted someone. As you might suspect, this person feels that he is actually of little worth and insignificant in comparison with others. Through his violent actions, then, he attempts to overcome or compensate for a negative view of himself. The typical sequence of events initiated by the self-image promoter as a means of reducing his sense of inadequacy is illustrated in one case study. In the exchange, verbal aggression is minimized in favor of physical assault; indeed, he has never fared particularly well in verbal debate. In his words, "'somebody says something to offend me, I provide the person the opportunity to challenge me to a duel, and then I make mincemeat out of him'" (Toch, 1984, p. 141). Thus, the target is first maneuvered into a confrontation from which he can scarcely withdraw and is then savagely attacked. The aggressor feels no remorse, seeing the situation he has contrived as one in which violence is both justifiable and necessary. The intensity of his assaults generally go well beyond what might be seen by his peers as equitable to redress a real or imagined insult. Toch observes, "he just doesn't teach people a lesson—he puts them out of commission. He doesn't just vindicate himself—he destroys people" (p. 140).

2. Self-Image Defenders

As with the "promoters," those who engage in *self-image defending* (13%) do so from a background of insecurity and low self-esteem. Their focus is on the words and actions of others that might in some way detract from the positive view of themselves they would like others to adopt. Always on the alert for slights or challenges—even anticipating or arranging a confrontation—these individuals privately suspect that derogatory remarks directed at them may in fact be true. Aspersions on his self-image often elicit a swift reaction, one so sudden and exaggerated that his victim is caught by surprise.

3. Rep Defenders

Yet another distinct category of aggressor is the *rep defender* (15%), whose presence on football and hockey teams many will recognize. This person has assumed a social role on a team that calls for his involvement in violent exchanges. Toch (1984) describes this role as follows:

> He knows he must champion his people, execute the guilty, and put on a good show. He may not derive much joy from this special awareness; some gang leaders, for instance, may try hard to negotiate, and some muscular "gorillas" may discourage aspiring youngsters who feel im-

pelled to challenge them. But the assumed obligation pursues such persons relentlessly and hard. (p. 149)

4. Self-Indulgers

A small but interesting type of aggressor has been given the label *self-indulger* (4%). These people have chronologically reached adulthood but have somehow managed to retain a preschooler's view of the world, that is, that others have been placed on Earth solely for the purpose of catering to their every need. Toch (1984) characterizes them as follows: "They view the world from the vantage point of infants, and toddle about their way expecting to find a crib or breast around every corner" (pp. 165–166). The failure of others to fulfill their needs, and others do eventually tire of this, is regarded as treachery. Indignantly, and with no insight into the needs of his providers, he unleashes a tantrum-like attack.

5. Bully-Sadists

Perhaps the most reprehensible category is the bully-sadist (6%), who has come to derive pleasure from the pain and suffering he brings to his victims. Toch (1984) suggests that an intense fear underlies the bully's behavior. His encounters are on his own terms, never on even grounds, and the violence itself "unfair, unmerciful, and inhumane" (p. 160).

The work of Olweus (1978) on *school* bullies provides a somewhat different picture of the bully's psychological makeup. School bullies are marked by self-confidence and low levels of anxiety. They are further characterized by "a low tolerance for frustration, coupled with strong aggressive inclinations, a generally hostile attitude, and a positive view of violence" (p. 152). Considering the bully's carefully orchestrated "successes" in vanquishing weaker opponents, his acts of violence and/or the pain of his victims can gradually acquire reinforcing properties. The work of Berkowitz (1970) and, incidentally, Olweus (1978, pp. 144–145) would additionally emphasize the role of learning in accounting for the reinforcement value that violence and acts of cruelty hold for some people. Of course, whether one can equate prison, school, and sports bullies is at this juncture a matter for future research. For example, do youngsters identified as bullies at school extend their reign of terror to the locker rooms of community sports facilities? Are their hapless victims or "whipping boys" (Olweus, 1978) at school similarly victimized in other settings?

Clearly, an important task for future research is a cross-validation of Toch's (1984) typology using athlete-subjects. Such an undertaking would provide a stronger basis for generalizing the framework to sports and other settings, as well as providing evidence of category size in a noninmate population. Here again, the peer interview technique seems suited to the research question and could be expected to yield superior data. From considering aggression as a personality trait, the focus widens in the remaining chapters to examine a range of factors that facilitate aggression, the merits of a cathartic hypothesis, and collective violence.

Suggested Readings

Dervin, D. (1985). A psychoanalysis of sports. *Psychoanalytic Review, 72,* 277–299.
> Have you ever wondered why sports teams are named after animals or symbols of authority? Why do the John McEnroes of the world carry on as they do? Is a ball something more than a ball? I doubt that many of us have spent sleepless nights pondering these questions, but to our colleagues in the psychoanalytic community they may be profoundly significant. Dervin's intriguing and thoughtful essay seems to me to convey the full richness of the psychoanalytic view. Besides, you will find answers to the questions I asked above.

Gavin, J. (1988). *Body moves: The psychology of exercise.* Harrisburg, PA: Stackpole.
> This engaging book represents an attempt to establish details of the relationship between exercise/movement and personality.

Stanovich, K.E. (1992). *How to think straight about psychology* (3rd ed.). New York: Harper Collins.
> If I had my druthers, I would make this paperback required reading for all students entering psychology, or the social sciences for that matter. It is above all entertaining and cuts through the mystery surrounding scientific investigations. The reader is also provided with the intellectual tools to debunk the misleading claims of pseudoscience practitioners.

Strube, M.J. (Ed.). (1991). *Type A behavior.* Newbury Park, CA: Sage.
> An advanced book that features contributions from experts describing recent developments in Type A theory and measurement. Current issues are also discussed, as are applications of Type A findings to a number of real-life settings.

8

Sports Aggression

In this chapter I intend to present an overview of the research and theoretical speculations of those who have sought answers to questions of human aggression. A single chapter allows little more than the opportunity to present an outline of several theoretical positions and to focus on some of the basic data of aggression in areas that have direct implications for sports. As one of several underlying themes in this book, aggression is also highlighted in the upcoming chapters on catharsis and spectatorship. Specific discussions covering the broad range of issues surrounding sports aggression can be found in books by J.H. Goldstein (1983) and M.D. Smith (1983). Other major texts that provide a general treatment of the topic of aggression are those of Bandura (1973), R.A. Baron (1977), Geen (1990), and Zillmann (1979).

Outside of wartime, sports is perhaps the only setting in which acts of interpersonal aggression are not only tolerated but enthusiastically applauded by large segments of society. It is interesting to consider that if the mayhem of the ring or gridiron were to erupt in a shopping mall, criminal charges would inevitably follow. However, under the umbrella of "sport," social norms and the laws specifying what constitutes acceptable conduct in society are temporarily suspended. In their stead is a new order of authority, namely the official rules of the sport. These dictate the forms of aggression that are illegal (e.g., a low blow) and the conditions under which aggression is unacceptable (e.g., a late hit).

This double standard was brought to light in the aftermath of a widely publicized criminal case in which an on-ice hockey fight with racial overtones was later resumed in the parking lot. A young midget player died after choking on his own vomit. Writing in the *New York Times*, Runfola (1974) noted that had the fatal attack taken place during the game, the accused "would have been liable for a five-minute major penalty. Off the ice he was liable to a term in prison" (p. S2).

The responsibility for enforcing the rules and the punishment of transgressors rests with the governing body of a sport. Their powers to punish flagrant violations are, however, generally restricted to fines and the suspension of playing privileges. Unlike convictions in the public domain, the only "record" one acquires is that contained in the league files or in newspaper accounts of the incident. Only on rare occasions has the legal system seen fit to involve itself in cases of excessive player violence, and that with mixed results (Barnes, 1983).

It is worth pointing out that the conduct of spectators and athletes is governed by different legal systems during a contest. Physical violence among spectators is summarily dealt with by the police and thereafter by the courts, whereas a few feet away the same violence by players is adjudicated by referees or umpires under the de facto authority of the "rules of play." Thus, players in most combatant sports risk considerably weaker punishments for illegal aggression than do their fans. In general, the threat of punishment acts to deter would-be aggressors under conditions where it is swift, certain, and severe (R.A. Baron, 1977, pp. 228–239). The relatively mild punishments meted out to athletes in some sports ensure that current levels of interpersonal aggression are likely to continue unabated. In contrast, the greater certainty and severity of sanctions against violence in the public domain have generally proven effective in deterring aggressive outbursts, at least among North American audiences.

Historical Trends

The North American public has expressed a continuing concern with levels of violence in society. Pollsters periodically ask national samples to indicate the issues that most concern them. With great regularity, respondents mention law and order as a major issue alongside the economy and environmental concerns. While social violence is troubling to many people, it has at the same time been accompanied by a belief that violence has been rising steadily in recent decades. Certainly, the annual *Uniform Crime Report* (*UCR*) of the U.S. Federal Bureau of Investigation would support such a belief. Although the report is not without its shortcomings (Skogan, 1979), the *UCR* has shown fairly dramatic increases in the major categories of violent crime through the middle decades of this century to the present. While rates of violent crime in Canada are only a fraction of those in the U.S., they show the same upward trend over the same period. Against this background, is it conceivable that sports have somehow been insulated from the social forces that have driven levels of violent crime steadily higher through the latter half of this century?

Evidence on trends in sports violence is scarce and largely anecdotal. Soccer authorities have expressed alarm over rising levels of hooliganism during much of the post–World War II era. Even cricket, that most staid of sporting institutions, has witnessed riotous behavior in recent years. An international match played in Barbados between England and West India saw fans hurling bottles at the English side. The riot squad was called out and used tear gas to quell the melee. Then again, in a sport such as ice hockey, oldtimers will often dismiss suggestions of escalating violence by asserting that hockey has always been a violent sport. Why, they remember when. . ., and so on.

In the case of hockey, the public record can speak for itself. Game summaries have routinely been published in major newspapers since the inception of the National Hockey League (NHL). Russell (1991) tallied the aggressive penalties awarded in *all* games played in the NHL during the 1930–1931 season. The procedure was repeated thereafter at five-year intervals to the present. (Recent seasons were randomly sampled.) The record of interpersonal aggression spanning over half a century of play is depicted in Figure 8.1. Following the 1930–1931 season, aggression gradually declined through the years of World War II until shortly after 1945. Thereafter, aggression rose steeply, easily surpassing levels seen in 1930 and reaching levels four times that of the immediate postwar years. There is no indication that the upward trend is leveling off. It is an interesting ex-

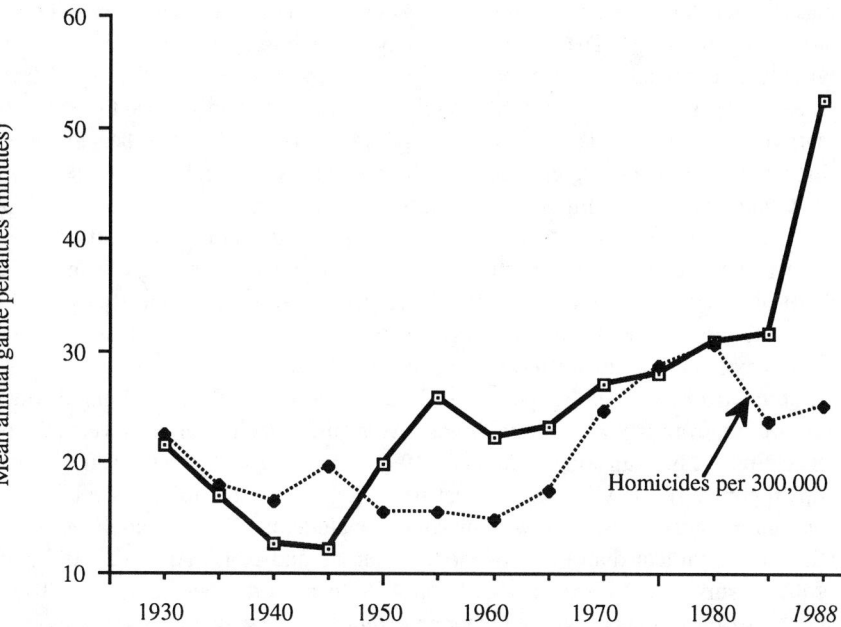

FIGURE 8.1 NHL aggression 1930–1988 (adapted from Russell, 1991).

ercise to speculate on the specific historical factors that might have influenced the course of aggression in hockey since 1930, such as the depression, World War II, and the formation of the rival World Hockey Association. However, an equally interesting question is the relationship between levels of hockey aggression and a measure of societal violence over the same period of time.

The national homicide rates derived from the *UCR* are superimposed on Figure 8.1 for comparative purposes. While *causality* cannot be inferred, the two functions are nonetheless significantly related. One interpretation would suggest that the rising homicide and hockey statistics reflect the changing values and norms of their common cultural background.

The Harbinger Hypothesis

A convincing case has been made for the proposition that sports mirror the fundamental beliefs and values of a culture (e.g., E.E. Snyder & Spreitzer, 1979), although this view is not without its dissenters (e.g., J.H. Goldstein, 1985). This perspective would allow that any major changes occurring in society would be reflected in corresponding changes in its sports. Indeed, given widespread public tolerance and the often ineffectual sanctions imposed by sport officialdom for the misbehavior of athletes, it has been suggested (Russell, 1981b) that certain sports may effectively serve as a bellwether of changing trends in criminal violence. In particular, those sports enjoying mass participation and spectator appeal may provide the earliest and most valid signals of social change. They, more than many of the lesser sports they overshadow, provide a larger and more representative sample of societal values. Thus, in a free-wheeling sports subculture where the criminal justice system reluctantly and only rarely involves itself in cases of interpersonal aggression, one might expect to see the first signs of an impending upturn or downturn in the level of violence in society.

A major feature of Figure 8.1 is the striking similarity between the trend of hockey aggression and violent crime over the past half century. They differ mainly in respect to the year marking the upswing in aggression. Significantly, the point of inflection occurs approximately 10 years *earlier* in the sports aggression data offering support for the harbinger hypothesis. Indices of sports aggression, then, may lead other measures of social change.[1]

Comparisons with earlier periods of history can be useful in providing a wider perspective from which to judge the relative significance of current levels of violence. Sports historian Allen Guttmann (1983) offers one such comparison between contemporary sports violence and that occurring during the notorious rule of the Caesars. He concludes, "But we can safely conclude that Roman sports were certainly more violent than those of modern Europe and North America. And they probably surpassed the violence of Latin American sports as well" (p. 17). To be sure, other historical periods and other civilizations have witnessed more (*and* less) violent sports than present-day North Americans. Beyond this, the public record points to unprecedented levels of aggression in hockey and, to the extent that one is willing to generalize, perhaps to similar increases in other sports as well.

The Definition and Measurement of Aggression

Definitions

As noted in previous chapters, there is a considerable diversity of opinion on definitions of many of the concepts of interest to social scientists. Aggression is no exception. Both Bandura (1973) and Zillmann (1979) present interesting discussions of the complexities involved in defining the concept. However, for the sake of providing a common starting point for the chapters to follow, we will adopt a definition that enjoys fairly wide acceptance. R.A. Baron (1977) proposes that "aggression is any form of behavior directed toward the goal of harming or injuring another living being who is motivated to avoid such treatment" (p. 7).

Sports represent a special situation with respect to aggression insofar as competitors in some sports (e.g., boxing) willingly expose themselves to attacks from others during competition. In other sports (e.g., football and rugby), harm or in-

---

[1] The correlation between the *UCR* homicide statistics and NHL violence is .553, $p < .025$. Advancing the hockey data 10 years to adjust for the lag yielded a correlation of .642, $p < .025$.

jury is often regarded as an unfortunate or accidental by-product of rough play, not as a primary goal of the competitors themselves. The defensive tackle in football "intends" aggression but only to a point short of injuring his opponent. What can be said with some certainty, however, is that actions intended to harm another competitor that fall outside of the agreed-on rules of a sport constitute aggressive behavior (Zillmann, 1979, p. 35). This is not to suggest that aggression does not take place *during* play in a variety of sports. The difficulty for the researcher is one of inferring the intentions of individual competitors and quantifying the acts themselves. Much of the ambiguity is removed, however, when one adopts aggressive rule violations as a criterion. Judgments as to intentions and the seriousness of rule infractions are left to the "experts" (i.e., referees and umpires). To the extent that the experts' judgments are sound, measures of aggression can be derived in several sports. Thus, a cross-check in lacrosse, an illegal tackle in soccer, and the ever popular fistfight in ice hockey all provide potentially valid representations of aggressive behavior.

The reasons for athletes' aggression vary. Even so, the basic distinction between *hostile* and *instrumental* aggression proposed by Buss (1961) allows for their classification. Hostile aggression refers to actions intended to harm another person who has angered or otherwise provoked an individual. Instrumental aggression is aggression that serves as a means to achieve a particular goal. The target may be a stranger or even someone the attacker respects. The impersonal attack itself is usually designed to injure or otherwise impair the performance of an opposing player or team.

For example, coaches in some sports routinely designate one or more players whose major function requires them to defend weaker teammates and/or to attack opposing players. The coach may openly order an attack, or his orders may be understood to be operative in certain situations. Can a player with misgivings refuse to obey such an order?

The research program of Stanley Milgram (1974) makes clear the fact that people are far more obedient than most of us would suspect. Subjects in his experiments played the role of a teacher and were told that the experiment required them to punish the learner (actually, an actor) for his mistakes. A sizable majority of the experimental subjects continued to obey orders to ostensibly aggress against another subject with settings of shock that rose to exceedingly high levels (the actor did *not* receive any shocks but only feigned his responses). Despite the fact that they were free to leave at any time and would receive payment for their participation, most of the subjects remained obedient. Moreover, both the trappings of authority and the consequences of disobedience were minimal in the lab setting. In stark contrast, failure to obey the orders of a coach can and has ended careers. The pressures are such that it would be a rare event indeed when an athlete disobeys an order to carry out an act of instrumental aggression. Just how obedient are the rest of us in the workaday world? Speaking Tangentially 8.1 gives us a disturbing glimpse of obedience in the workplace.

****

Speaking Tangentially 8.1: Obedience on the Wards
In the event that some of my more skeptical readers remain unconvinced that the pressures to obey extend beyond the lab or have significant real-life consequences, consider the following study (Hofling, Brotzman, Dalrymple, Graves, & Pierce, 1966).

A total of 22 nurses received a phone call from a man who identified himself as the physician of one of their patients. Each nurse was instructed to administer 20 mgs. of a powerful drug to the patient; the phony physician said he wanted the drug to take effect by the time he arrived at the hospital, at which time he would sign the order. The nurses knew the drug was potentially lethal and the label contained a clear warning that 10 mgs. was a dangerous dose. Nevertheless, 21 of the 22 nurses dutifully proceeded to carry out the caller's instruction to administer the dosage (actually an inert medication had been substituted), being restrained only at the last minute by the researchers. It's something worth thinking about the next time you, or someone close to you, find yourself confined to a stay in the hospital. For my part, I'll be looking for nurse number 22.

****

Instrumental aggression is not uncommon. By one estimate based on the *UCR*, close to 50% of all criminal violence in the United States is undertaken for financial gain (Borden & Taylor, 1976). I would venture to guess that an equally high, or higher, percentage of sports violence is also instrumentally motivated. But what aspects of competition favor the expression of instrumental motives? For example, would losers, evenly matched competitors, and winners differ in their willingness to resort to aggression to attain their ends? Borden and Taylor (1976) had males compete against a consistently *nonaggressive* opponent in a reaction-time task that allowed the winner to shock his opponent with an intensity of his own choosing. (The upper limit was set at a level described as "decidedly unpleasant.") It was prearranged that some subjects would lose on nearly all trials, some would win on half of the trials, and others would win almost all of the time. The higher the subjects set the shock, the more money they could receive on winning trials (i.e., when they had the fastest reaction times). Which condition produced the greatest amount of instrumental aggression? Winning did! Whereas losing and evenly matched competitors maintained a low level of aggression across all trials, winners not only shocked their opponents with greater intensity, but that intensity increased across trials in the competition. It bears repeating that subjects indicated they were fully aware that their money-making actions were discomforting to their opponents.

Measurement

The use of aggressive rule infractions in research is greatly facilitated by the official records of play. Most organized sports keep meticulously detailed and accurate records of competition. In a limited number of sports (e.g., ice hockey, lacrosse, soccer), illegal aggression occurs with sufficient frequency to provide data for testing a variety of aggression-related hypotheses. In the case of hockey, analysis of the underlying structure of awarded penalties reveals eight different types or dimensions of interpersonal aggression (Russell & Russell, 1984). Among other things, the result suggests that an overall index or, better still, a weighted index comprised of only those infractions that are the strongest contributors to the eight dimensions would capture the full range of aggressive actions occurring in the sport.[2]

It must, however, be acknowledged that relatively little research effort has been directed toward establishing the psychometric properties of such archival measures, a criticism that also extends to the full complement of measures used generally in investigations of aggressive behavior (e.g., Geen, 1976). Nonetheless, the archival approach offers the researcher an alternative *behavioral* measure of aggression as well as an increase in the *triangulation* of measurement. Briefly, triangulation refers to the desirability of measuring a concept by a diversity of means, each with different inherent strengths and shortcomings, to better arrive at an understanding of the processes at work (Webb, Campbell, Schwartz, Sechrest, & Grove, 1981, p. 315). The use of a generally superior behavioral criterion of sports aggression is of course, not confined to archival procedures but can also be found in field studies (e.g., Greer, 1983) as well as the social psychology lab (e.g., Zillmann, Johnson, & Day, 1974).

Various paper-and-pencil inventories have also successfully served the interests of sports researchers. Clearly, the most popular of these is the Buss-Durkee hostility scales (Buss & Durkee, 1957).[3] This easy-to-administer inventory purports to tap eight types of aggression: assault, verbal, indirect, irritability, negativism, resentment, suspicion, and guilt. However, despite initial efforts to refine the scales, they remain subject to a strong response-style bias, that of *social desirability* (Russell, 1981a). The fact that subjects can plainly see what the items measure invites respondents, some more than others, to distort their answers in a way that will allow them to be seen in a more favorable light, that is, as less hostile than they actually are.

Other efforts have been directed toward the development of aggression scales specifically for use in sports settings. Butt (1979) has constructed an aggression scale in conjunction with her assessment of aggressive motivation in athlete samples. Similarly, the Bredemeier Athletic Aggression Inventory (BAAGI) represents an attempt to develop an instrument that is sensitive to differences in the ways that athletes typically express their aggression (Bredemeier, 1975).

---

[2] See also the results of a recent replication (Vokey & Russell, 1992).

[3] The scales have recently been revised (Buss & Perry, 1992).

Theoretical Background

Frustration-Aggression

Perhaps the most widely held public explanation for aggression is frustration. Sportcasters feeling the need to offer an explanation in the wake of an outburst of player violence seize on some disheartening aspect of the situation (e.g., the score, a bruising body check, a play that failed) that in some way has thwarted a player's efforts and conclude that aggression was only to be expected. After all, the instigator was frustrated! Their listeners, in turn, mindful of the annoying character of frustrations in their own lives, have little difficulty accepting the sportcasters' explanation as an insightful analysis of human behavior.

Origin and Merits of This View

The frustration-aggression hypothesis was formulated in 1939 by a group of Yale psychologists (Dollard, Doob, Miller, Mowrer, & Sears, 1939). In its original form, it was proposed that any thwarting of one's goal-directed behavior constituted a state that inevitably results in aggression. Frustration, then, leads to aggression, and, in turn, it could be further assumed that any act of aggression was preceded by a state of frustration. For a time, it seemed that human aggression could be accounted for by this simple, straightforward explanation. However, various critics began to point to exceptions that were at odds with the hypothesis. For example, people sometimes show an intensification of effort rather than aggression when they encounter obstacles in their path. Still others regress or revert to behaviors that were more typical of them at an earlier stage in their development (e.g., sulking, pouting). Thus, it became clear that other responses besides aggression can stem from frustration.

On the aggression side of the equation, it is equally clear that aggression is frequently instigated by factors other than frustration. A shove, a verbal threat, or an insult is frequently sufficient to spark an altercation. Furthermore, the enforcer on a hockey team who attacks an opposing player on orders from his coach may never have been provoked by his victim or frustrated in his own play. He is simply obeying orders.

A *revision* of the frustration-aggression hypothesis (N.E. Miller, 1941) cast the part played by frustration in a more realistic perspective. It allowed that "frustration produces instigations to a number of different types of response, one of which is an instigation to some form of aggression" (p. 338). Nonaggressive responses to frustration are not ruled out. Aggression remains, however, as the dominant or most likely response to frustration.

Most of us encounter numerous frustrations every day, yet the average person seldom responds with an aggressive outburst. Under what conditions, then, is frustration most likely to lead to aggression? Two factors in particular determine the likelihood that one will respond aggressively to frustration. These mediating factors are the magnitude of the frustration and the extent to which the individual is arbitrarily blocked in his or her progress toward a goal. Thus, for example, the closer one is to attaining one's goal when thwarted, the more severely one is frustrated and the more aggressive is the response (M.B. Harris, 1974; Russell & Drewry, 1976).

Consider the effects of the severity of thwarting found during a season of play in a senior men's hockey league. Teams occupying first place exhibited very little aggression. In contrast, when teams found themselves in second place (the most severely thwarted), they showed the greatest amount of on-ice aggression with levels steadily declining thereafter as teams occupied third on down to sixth place in the league (Russell & Drewry, 1976).

As previously mentioned, frustrations that occur capriciously or without any apparent justification produce a greater instigation to aggress than frustrations that are justified. Both mediating factors were seen operating on October 15, 1977, when British race-car driver James Hunt lost control of his car in attempting to pass a teammate and left the course. He stepped from his car and knocked an elderly racecourse marshal to the ground. At the time, he had been leading the grand prix race. It must be noted to his credit that upon regaining his composure, Mr. Hunt put his arm around the marshal in a gesture of apology. Thus, the *intensity* of the frustration was extreme; his loss of points in the world championship standings cost him the title for that year. Also, his car left the track for no apparent reason. The marshal could not have chosen a more inopportune moment to offer his assistance.

Competition and the Frustration-Aggression Hypothesis

Although James Hunt's behavior is readily accounted for by the frustration-aggression hypothesis, only a moment's reflection is necessary to realize that most athletes encounter countless frustrations in playing their sport. Yet overt aggression is relatively uncommon in most sports. The pass dropped in the end zone, the 4-foot putt that rims the cup, and the fly ball dropped in the outfield all should see an aggressive outburst by the thwarted athlete, but that seldom happens.

This question has recently been addressed by Leonard Berkowitz (1988, 1989). While not discounting the possibility that aggression has been masked by other nonaggressive response tendencies, he proposes that rather than frustration per se producing the inclination to aggress, it is *negative affect* created by the thwarting that determines aggression. To the degree that frustrations are experienced as unpleasant, they will provide an instigation to aggression. For athletes in the heat of competition, "if they are not experiencing decidedly negative feelings at the time, perhaps rivalry will not activate aggressive inclinations in them" (Berkowitz, 1988, p. 7). Thus, if players are enjoying the contest and/or winning, their inclinations to aggress when thwarted will likely be muted.

Social Learning Theory

A second major perspective from which much of human aggression can be understood is social learning theory (Bandura, 1973, 1986). You will recall that aspects of the theory were discussed in chapter 6 in relation to the mechanisms by which sports heroes influence their admirers. To recap briefly, aggression may be learned from observing others. In particular, the learner notes whether a model's aggression was successful or unsuccessful in helping him achieve a goal and whether the model's aggression was rewarded or punished. Where aggression is seen to be successful and/or meets with approval from others, learning is greatly enhanced. Even where the model's aggression meets with disapproval or punishment, learning may still take place. The fact that the learner is not seen to perform the aggression displayed by the model does not mean that the lesson was not learned. In all likelihood, two lessons were learned. First, the observer encoded the aggressive skills, and second, he learned that it would be unwise to display his newly acquired ability in the present circumstances.

In a typical social learning experiment, children at play observe an adult, either in person or on a monitor, attack and pummel a large plastic Bobo doll for a brief period of time. Other children watch the adult interact with the doll in a nonaggressive fashion. Later in a new setting, those children who observed the aggressive adult behave more aggressively than those who observed the adult interacting in a positive manner. Indeed, the aggressive actions of the youngsters closely resemble the novel forms introduced by the model (e.g., hitting the doll with a mallet). If the model was additionally praised for his or her aggression (by another adult), the aggression later displayed by the children was greater still. Moreover, such learning is far from transitory but can persist for long periods of time. In sum, aggression can be effectively learned by the attentive observer. Social learning theory, then, offers an explanatory framework for understanding the potential effects on actual spectators and television audiences watching sports events that feature aggression.

Interpersonal Aggression

When Push Comes to Shove

How many of us can resist the temptation to respond to the horn blast of a rude motorist with an equally rude gesture, a curse or a blast of our own? Are face-to-face insults or threats any easier to ignore? For most of us, the answer is clearly no. The general tendency is to give tit for tat. Verbally and physically aggressive exchanges, then, are all too easy to start. Would-be aggressors need only insult or shove the object of their scorn to be virtually assured that an altercation will follow. But how vigorous or intense is the response to provocations? Does the pattern of a series of attacks influence the target's pattern of responding?

Investigations of these questions have found that we frequently act according to a norm of *reciprocity*. When provoked, we show a strong tendency to respond with an intensity that matches that of the original attack. Mild insults evoke similar mild insults in return; a strong attack is met by a similarly strong retaliation (Taylor & Pisano, 1971). This tendency to match the intensity of attacks also extends across a series of exchanges. Faced by a tormentor who steadily increases the intensity of his attacks, we follow suit and do likewise. Were our attacker to steadily decrease the intensity of his attacks, we would again match this pattern and decrease the intensity of our retaliations (O'Leary & Dengerink, 1973).

But what if we are confronted by someone making only hollow threats? Are that person's stated intentions a strong provocation apart from what he actually does? Simply put, it seems that intentions may be every bit as important as deeds in predicting the strength of our response to those bent on attacking us. Expressions of an *intent* to do us serious harm elicit equally strong reactions. A strong retaliation, matching intent, occurs quite apart from what the instigator actually does in the situation (Greenwell & Dengerink, 1973). People intending us harm, even though they never follow through, stand to incur a response equal in intensity to that implied in their original threat.

Escalation of Aggression

Many fights are characterized by their small and often trivial beginnings. Two players exchange unpleasantries, then a shove; next, a punch is thrown and a bench-clearing brawl is under way. This tendency for violent acts to have their origins in a difference of opinion or other petty annoyance is a feature of what have come to be known as *escalation effects* (J.H. Goldstein, Davis, & Herman, 1975). An initial provocation draws a slightly stronger response, with that response in turn drawing a further, slightly stronger, retaliation. The result is an upward spiral of increasingly violent exchanges. Many full-blown acts of mayhem stem from just such small, inconsequential beginnings.

Once the fight is under way, there is a certain inevitability to the upward course of aggression. A number of plausible suggestions for halting the upward spiral of interpersonal exchanges have been tested (J.H. Goldstein, Davis, Kernis, & Cohn, 1981). The results are not encouraging. Neither interrupting the antagonists, drawing their attention to their aggression, videotaping them, nor providing them with expectations of a later face-to-face meeting had any noticeable effects on the escalation of hostilities. Providing a "hot line" for subjects to summon the experimenter did, however, reduce the overall intensity of aggression, although escalation effects occurred as before. The success of the hot line in reducing the intensity of aggression is interesting in itself, for although it was readily available, it was never actually used by any of the subjects.

Situational Determinants

The Weapons Effect

A series of experiments investigating the role of aggressive cues in eliciting aggression has implications for those whose sporting interests involve guns or other weapons. Moreover, those who associate with people having such interests should also be mindful of the implications of this research. It has been shown that people who are merely in the *presence* of weapons exhibit increased aggression (e.g., Berkowitz, 1981; Berkowitz & LePage, 1967; Boyanowsky & Griffiths, 1982; C.W. Turner, Simons, Berkowitz, & Frodi, 1977). The original experiment on the topic (Berkowitz & LePage, 1967) provided subjects with the opportunity to aggress (shock) against an experimental confederate in a setting in which a gun had been "carelessly" left lying nearby. From the subject's point of view, the weapon had nothing whatsoever to do with the ongoing experiment. Subjects in a control condition underwent procedures that were identical except that a badminton racquet rather than a gun had been left in the laboratory. Briefly, subjects in the presence of the gun acted more aggressively toward the confederate than subjects in the presence of the badminton racquet.

A gun, and weapons in general, are presumed to be rife with aggressive cues as a result of their long-standing associations with injury and killing. The classical conditioning theory of learning seems best suited to account for the way in which weapons acquire aggressive cue properties. From the perspective of the Pavlovian model, initially neutral objects gradually acquire aggressive cue value through repeated pairing with anger arousal and violent images. The end result of this extended learning process is that persons and objects long associated in our experience with anger and aggression come to serve as conditioned stimuli capable of eliciting aggression from those in their presence. This capacity of aggressive cues to *elicit* aggression has prompted Berkowitz (1981) to rephrase the cliché "it's the finger that pulls the trigger" to reflect the fact that it is often instead "the trigger that pulls the finger." While research on the weapons effect is not without its critics (e.g., Buss, Booker, & Buss, 1972; Page & Scheidt, 1971), a review of this literature has concluded that overall the phenomenon is well established and reliable (C.W. Turner et al., 1977).

It follows from the foregoing that the playing equipment in a number of sports is rife with aggressive *object* cues (Berkowitz, 1974). Beyond this, however, the sports equipment itself (e.g., bats, lacrosse and hockey sticks, etc.) can sometimes serve a double purpose, a fact that has not escaped the attention of the legal system. Following a 1976 brawl in Toronto's Maple Leaf Gardens, two Philadelphia Flyers hockey players were charged with possession of a dangerous weapon (i.e., a hockey stick) for a purpose dangerous to the public peace (Barnes, 1983, pp. 100–101). The latter function speaks to a separate issue, that is, the *availability* of weapons.

Availability

An important distinction should be made between the *presence* of weapons and their availability. One might think that if guns are available they can and, on occasion, will be used (e.g., Kellermann & Reay, 1986). In a situation that turns ugly, the outcome is likely to be far more serious with weapons present than without weapons being available to those involved, that is, deaths rather than injuries, bruises rather than bruised feelings. However, in the case of violent encounters among *strangers*, recent evidence suggests otherwise (Kleck & Mcelrath, 1991). Weapons seemingly reduce the likelihood of attack and injury, although once an injury is sustained, the probability of death is increased. The overall net effect of guns being available apparently does not appreciably increase the probability of a victim being killed. It will be interesting to follow the results of replications that will almost certainly follow these surprising findings.

Wright, Rossi, Daly, and Weber-Burdin (cited in Zimring, 1985) provide a sobering statistic. These authors estimate that there are between 30 and 40 million revolvers in the hands of private American citizens. Are weapons also available to those attending sports events? Sociologist Irving Goldaber estimates that among sports crowds in U.S. metropolitan centers, 0.5 to 2 percent are carrying concealed weapons (Benagh, 1978). Thus, in a typical World Series crowd of 60,000, we might expect to find anywhere from 300 to 1,200 dangerous weapons. Elsewhere, hooligan elements among European soccer fans have arrived at matches with an impressive array of weapons that included truncheons, heavy chains, starting pistols (Williams, Dunning, & Murphy, 1984), and darts. The aggression-eliciting capacity of the weapons themselves only adds to whatever potential for harm they pose to public safety.

Drugs and Aggression

Alcohol

Rates of alcohol consumption among athletes and their fans vary dramatically from culture to culture and from one sport to another. The hallmark of a good rugby player, in addition to any playing skills he may possess, is his ability to consume inordinate amounts of alcohol. His stature is further enhanced by an ability to tell raunchy stories and sing naughty ditties (Kevin Young, 1988). Alcohol is also prominently featured in the diet of the professional hockey player (Houston, 1979). At the other extreme, one would not expect alcohol to play any significant role in such sports as body building, gymnastics, swimming, and speed skating where the athletes and their following for the most part abstain.

The source of present-day concerns with the effects of alcohol is to be found in the Judeo-Christian tradition. Any preacher worth his salt has at one time or another proclaimed the evils of Demon Rum. Certainly, their sermons were prophetic insofar as they pointed to the social tragedies of alcoholism and the continuing carnage on our highways. It was a small and logical enough step to also conclude that the disorderly behavior of people was *caused* by alcohol. Indeed, today's common wisdom would hold that the more people drink, the more unruly, belligerent, and hostile they become. This popular assumption of a causal link between alcohol and aggression finds general support in recent reviews on the question (e.g., Bushman & Cooper, 1990).

The proposition that alcohol is responsible for social disorder is not without a substantial amount of indirect correlational evidence, particularly from the field of criminology. For example, a review of 10 studies revealed that among murderers, slightly more than 50% had been drinking prior to their offense (MacDonald, 1961). Drinking has similarly been shown to be involved in rape (Johnson, Gibson, & Linden, 1978). Alcohol has also been held largely responsible for hostile outbursts among fans at various sporting events. For example, British inquiries into soccer hooliganism (e.g., J.M. Williams et al., 1984) note with dismay the drunkenness of many of the younger fans and lay much of the blame on alcohol for the disturbances that have marred the sport in recent years.

British perceptions indicting alcohol as a fundamental cause of crowd disorders are shared by their North American counterparts. Cavanaugh and Silva (1980) asked Buffalo Sabres hockey fans to rate the importance of 14 factors they thought contributed to spectator violence. Alcohol was ranked third, with contentious decisions by referees and the age of fans named as the first and second most important reasons. Quite apart from what the facts of the matter might be, the important point to recognize is that public perceptions of crowd violence attribute the major portion of blame to alcohol. The response of sport and government officialdom and their proposed solutions to the problem will therefore likely be predicated on this causal assumption.

Just how strong is the connection between alcohol and aggression? An overview of early studies that investigated the question reveals a mix of findings. As with most social phenomena, the underlying dynamics often turn out to be somewhat more complex than a commonsense explanation would allow. For example, R.M. Bennett, Buss, and Carpenter (1969) found that physical aggression was unaffected by alcohol consumption. Such findings undoubtedly square with the experiences of many of us in observing that people at social functions usually become more sociable and mellow as the evening wears on. While the paradox is puzzling and far from resolved, a series of controlled experiments has brought a degree of order to the topic.

The work of Stuart P. Taylor and his colleagues at Kent State University (e.g., Jeavons & Taylor, 1985; Taylor & Gammon, 1976; Taylor, Gammon, & Capasso, 1976; Taylor & Leonard, 1983) has highlighted the importance of situational variables in determining whether or not intoxicated people act aggressively. Taylor et al. (1976) noted that an important difference between previous studies showing that alcohol led to an increase in aggression and those studies that failed to show any link was the degree of *threat* present in the situation. Specifically, the earlier studies (e.g., R.M. Bennett et al., 1969) did not provide an opportunity for the "victim" to retaliate against the aggressor. The intoxicated subjects were, in effect, socializing in a nonthreatening situation.

In examining the role of threat, Taylor et al. (1976) had subjects engage in a reaction-time task in which the loser on each trial was shocked at a level of intensity ostensibly chosen by the opponent. A no-threat condition was created for some subjects by having them overhear their opponent explain to the experimenter that they did not wish to hurt anyone and planned therefore, to simply push the number 1 button (minimal shock) on all trials. Subjects assigned to the threat condition did not receive such assurances from their opponent.

The results are shown in Figure 8.2. As can be seen, the level of aggression directed at opponents by intoxicated subjects was strongly influenced by the degree of threat present in the situation. Intoxicated and sober subjects did not differ in their aggression under nonthreatening circumstances. However, under threatening circumstances both sober and inebriated individuals exhibited an increase in aggression. In the case of intoxicated subjects, the increase was dramatic. A review of these contending views prompted Taylor and Leonard (1983) to conclude that "the data strongly suggest that the aggression evidenced by intoxicated persons is a joint function of the pharmacological state produced by alcohol and situational factors" (p. 94).

There *are* circumstances, however, in which intoxicated persons may display aggression even though the situation is nonthreatening (Gantner & Taylor, 1992). Certain conditions, though, must be met. These include a general absence of aggression-inhibiting cues such as others conveying their peaceful intentions and/or a strong desire on the part of the intoxicated individual to defeat a competitor. Lacking reassurances regarding the intentions of other people or a strong attitude of rivalry may in such circumstances lead to aggression by those in a state of intoxication.

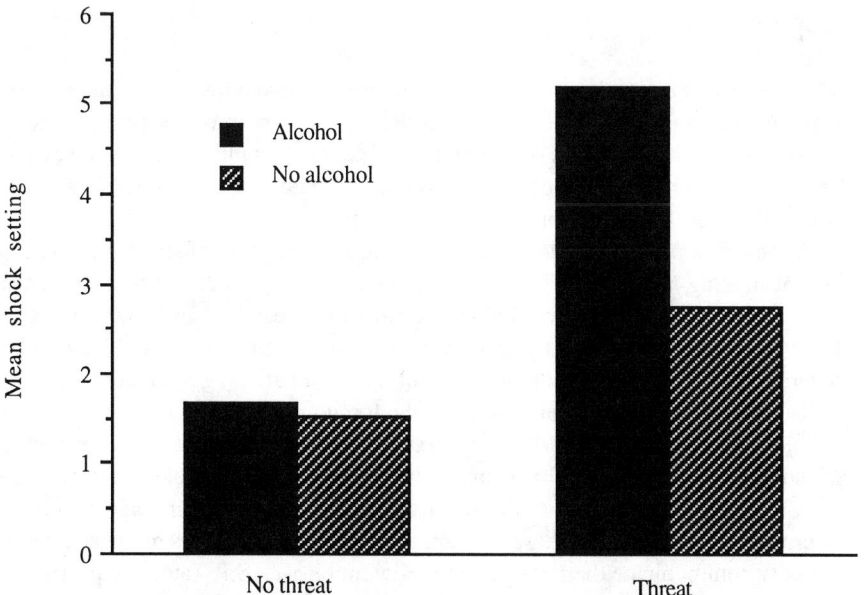

FIGURE 8.2 Shock as a function of alcohol and threat (adapted from Taylor et al., 1976).

The "expectations" that we hold regarding the effects of alcohol or drug use may also, to a considerable extent, determine and justify our behavior in some social situations (Ferguson, Rule, & Lindsay, 1982; Lange, Goeckner, Adesso, & Marlatt, 1975). People may feel less responsible for their actions and thus more willing to engage in antisocial behavior when intoxicated. This point of view draws support from an experiment by Lange et al. (1975). These researchers found that regardless of whether their (angered) subjects had ingested alcohol or not, those who believed they had consumed alcohol were more aggressive than those who believed they had consumed a nonalcoholic drink. Alcohol, then, may serve as an excuse or justification for aggression in some instances.

Not only do the expectations of the drinker determine aggression, but also alcoholic beverages themselves differ in their effects. In a comparison of distilled spirits (e.g., bourbon) with brewed drinks (e.g., beer) subjects served the distilled beverage administered shocks of longer duration to a bogus partner than those who had consumed an equivalent amount of beer. Furthermore, the importance of expectations is once again seen in the result that those served a placebo drink they believed to be alcohol were more aggressive than those who consumed a drink they believed to be beer (Pihl, Smith, & Farrell, 1984). One interpretation of these results is based on cultural expectations whereby the general public has long associated the drinking of hard liquor with a macho, tough-guy image. On the other hand, beer drinkers are usually depicted in fun-filled and congenial surroundings. By this explanation, subjects were behaving in ways entirely consistent with how one is expected to behave under the influence of these two types of beverages.

Applications

The overwhelming majority of studies of aggression have been attempts to identify the factors that instigate aggression. Relatively few have sought to identify the conditions that lead to a *reduction* in interpersonal conflict. However, several alcohol studies have been designed to assess strategies for the control of aggression, strategies that are adaptable to real-life situations.

A recurring problem for sports officials and the operators of sports facilities is that of making alcoholic beverages available at sports events in a way that does not appreciably increase the likelihood of disturbances. The problem is not one that can be easily solved. Any application of research findings would have to be regarded as a first approximation to a solution. There are no guarantees.

Two points in particular emerge from the foregoing. The first to note is that alcoholic beverages differ in their aggressive effects. Second, the creation of a friendly, relaxed, and nonthreatening physical environment for drinking is an equally important consideration. Social threats, however, may remain. It seems impractical to suggest that those who appear threatening to others might somehow publicly communicate their nonaggressive intentions (cf. S.P. Taylor et al., 1976).

Another plausible strategy, that of making a nonaggressive norm salient, is suggested by the work of Jeavons and Taylor (1985). The strategy, of course, hinges on the assumption that the intoxicated person is actually capable of processing the available information. This is not a widely shared view. One opinion holds that an intoxicated individual is unable to process information regarding socially appropriate behavior because of the disruptive effects of alcohol. There is good reason to reject this view. It has been shown that telling intoxicated individuals that others in their circumstances typically behave peaceably (i.e., making a nonaggressive norm salient) dramatically reduces their aggression. Moreover, this reduction occurs in a competitive situation in which they face repeated provocations. Seemingly, intoxication does not produce deficits in information-processing capabilities. Those who are intoxicated can foresee the consequences of their actions and can exercise restraint in response to social cues (Jeavons & Taylor, 1985). One means of forestalling disturbances in drinking areas, then, lies with the possibility of offsetting "aggression-instigating cues" by the introduction of "salient aggression-inhibiting cues" (p. 101).

A further strategy for averting or defusing aggression by intoxicated persons calls for the intervention of a third party. As S.P. Taylor and Gammon (1976) have demonstrated, those who are intoxicated are responsive to the "coaxing, cajoling and reasoning" of a peacemaker even under conditions of extreme provocation (p. 928). Third parties have also been found to be successful in reducing the aggression of sober individuals (Borden & Taylor, 1973). Thus, an additional control measure may be available in the form of security personnel acting as intervention specialists, specifically trained for their task.

Of course, one can always ban alcohol at sports sites. Short of that, the studies described in this section offer several promising strategies for the introduction of alcohol without appreciably increasing the risk of crowd disorders. The suggestions, however, are tentative, and it remains a question for applied research how best to put them into practice.

Marijuana, Diazepam, and Caffeine

The effects of several other drugs on aggression deserve comment if for no other reason than the fact of their widespread use among the general public. The use of marijuana is controversial from several standpoints, none of which I would want to minimize. However, its effects on aggression appear benign. In an experiment that used the competitive-reaction time paradigm (S.P. Taylor et al., 1976), the effects on the aggression of subjects who had ingested a small dose of marijuana were found to be negligible. In contrast, those who were given a large dose displayed a slight *decrease* in aggression.

Diazepam (valium) and caffeine produce effects that are opposite to those of marijuana. Diazepam ranks among the most commonly prescribed drugs in North America as a treatment for anxiety. It is noteworthy that physicians prescribe the drug far more often for women than they do for their male patients. However, the effects on both sexes are similar; diazepam increases the aggression of males and females (Gantner & Taylor, 1988).

An interesting piece of evidence on caffeine effects is provided by a study of 14 adult males who were long-term patients in a psychiatric facility (De Freitas & Schwartz, 1979; see also Ferguson et al., 1982, and S.L. Taylor, O'Neal, Langley, & Houston Butcher, 1991). The researchers surreptitiously switched the patients to decaffeinated coffee for a 3-week period, after which they reverted back to regular coffee. A double-blind procedure was used whereby neither the ward staff nor the patients knew of the changes in beverages. The nursing staff made routine patient evaluations at four points—just before the introduction of decaffeinated coffee, 1 week later, 3 weeks later when the decaffeinated period ended, and sometime after regular coffee was once again made available. The results were persuasive. The introduction of decaffeinated coffee was followed by decreases in anxiety, tension, irritability, and hostility. All of the earlier gains, however, were lost with the reintroduction of regular coffee. In passing, it is worth noting that the authors' case for caffeine being a cause of hostility would be strengthened considerably had they been able to include a control condition in the design of their study.

Anabolic Steroids and Aggression

The use of anabolic steroids by athletes marks a sad page in the history of sport. Their use has resulted in scandal and, quite likely, personal harm to individual users. Notwithstanding the question of their illegality, controversy has swirled around two major issues, the effects of steroids on performance and the potential for physical and emotional harm. The evidence bearing on both issues was reviewed in 1984 by Haupt and Rovere. An updating of research findings in this rapidly expanding field suggests that major psychiatric symptoms may accompany the use of anabolic steroids. For example, Pope and Katz (1988) conducted clinical interviews with 41 football players and bodybuilders who were users of anabolic steroids. Various syndromes were exhibited during steroid use "including manic episodes, major depression, and even delusions and hallucinations" (Pope & Katz, 1990, p. 28). Our present interest, however, is in the relationship between steroids and interpersonal aggression.

The suggestion of a link between steroid use and aggression is not new. Indeed, one writer (Wade, 1972) claims that German troops in World War II were given steroids to increase their aggressiveness in battle. The review of Haupt and Rovere (1984) also notes that many athletes report an increase in aggression while on steroids. They note further that this and other symptoms disappeared when the athletes discontinued their use of anabolic steroids.

A recent case study approach by Pope and Katz (1990) is revealing. In-depth examinations of three men with no previous records of psychiatric symptomology were conducted in the aftermath of their having committed separate crimes of violence, including murder. All three men were heavily involved in a weight training regimen in which they followed the common practice of "stacking" several drugs. While acknowledging the limitations of a case study approach, the authors nonetheless go on to conclude "that anabolic steroids may cause some law-abiding and psychiatrically asymptomatic individuals to develop manic and psychotic symptoms, culminating occasionally in violent crimes" (p. 30). Pope and Katz further speculate that anabolic steroids are contributing to a greater range of social ills involving interpersonal violence than previously recognized. To this point, their role may simply have been overlooked.

Environmental Influences

Aggression is also influenced by a number of environmental factors. Remember (or imagine) if you will the last time you sat crowded together with thousands of screaming spectators at a sports event on a smoggy day when the temperature was in the 90s (30° Celsius). You are also aware that a number of your fellow spectators would benefit from a shower! Under this set of not-too-unusual circumstances (i.e., crowding, noise, high temperatures, and noxious odors), it should surprise no one if spectators' moods and dispositions toward one another took a turn for the worse. Although these and other environmental factors obviously operate in various combinations to influence spectators and athletes, they will be considered individually in the sections to follow.

When the Action Heats Up

What is known about the relationship between temperature and aggression? Throughout the riot-torn decade of the 60s in the United States, it seemed apparent to the press and the public mind alike that ghetto violence was most likely to occur on days when temperatures were extremely high. The observation gradually took form as the *long, hot summer hypothesis,* linking high temperatures to violence. Archival research has generally confirmed the association. For example, increases in temperature in Houston, Texas, were accompanied by parallel increases in the frequency of violent crime, that is, murder and rape (C.A. Anderson & Anderson, 1984), with a similar pattern also being reported for Dallas (Harries & Stadler, 1988).

The picture, however, remains unclear at this point in our discussion insofar as other weather factors change or covary with temperature rises (e.g., barometric pressure, humidity, wind, etc.). Additionally, air-conditioned bars may attract record numbers of patrons anxious to escape a heat wave. Consequently, it could be argued that alcohol rather than temperature plays the major role in any increase in violent crime. As a result of this *confounding* of factors and the use of correlational analyses, one cannot say with certainty that high temperatures per se are the cause of violence. Instead, we look to controlled lab experiments to isolate temperature from the influences of other factors in order to establish causality.

One would have to characterize the results of early investigations of this question as "mixed." Some experiments showed the predicted increase in aggression with increases in temperature. Other investigations revealed that subjects instead became *less* aggressive at high ambient temperatures. The confusion persisted until Robert Baron proposed a resolution of these seemingly incompatible and perplexing findings. In a series of experiments (e.g., Baron & Bell, 1976; Baron & Ransberger, 1978), he was able to show that temperature is indeed associated with aggression. However, the shape of that relationship is *curvilinear* rather than linear. That is, as temperatures rise steadily upward aggression also increases, but only to a point. As temperatures soar to extremely high levels (e.g., above 100°F), aggression starts to turn downward. Over the full upper range of temperature, its relationship with aggression is best described by an inverted-U curve.

Baron's explanation requires that we complicate matters slightly by taking into account the other influences that generally accompany exposure to high temperatures (i.e., stress, anxiety, fatigue, odors, etc.). These additional influences impinging on the individual have been combined under the label *negative affect*. In sum, the model suggests that aggression initially increases with increases in negative affect. Up to some indeterminant point, the individual's dominant response to rising temperatures is aggression. However, as temperatures increase ever higher, a point is reached where aggression is superceded at the top of one's response hierarchy by other responses, such as *escape* from an extremely aversive situation. Thus, as oppressive levels of negative affect set in, aggression is no longer the dominant or most likely response, and aggression is therefore seen to decline.

Neither the escape hypothesis nor the curvilinear model itself has gone unchallenged (C.A. Anderson & DeNeve, 1992). Field studies using police and weather office records have found virtually no evidence of a downturn in aggression at extremely high temperatures (e.g., C.A. Anderson & Anderson, 1984; Harries & Stadler, 1988). In general, they conclude that a straight line or linear increase in violent crime (e.g., aggravated assault) accompanies increases in temperature. There is only a faint indication of a leveling off or downturn, that occurring at temperatures of approximately 100°F (40°C; Harries & Stadler, 1988).

A great many sports are, of course, played under very hot conditions. However, can we say with any certainty that the aggression of athletes is also apt to increase on such days? Evidence from several seasons of major league baseball indicates that as the temperature rises, so too do players' tempers. Reifman, Larrick, and Fein (1991) tallied the number of batters hit by a pitch and the temperatures at game time for 826 contests sampled across three seasons of play. Their analysis revealed that as temperatures rose, so did the number of batters who were hit. Several rival interpretations—such as pitcher wildness, the result of fatigue or sweaty palms—were ruled out as explanations for the relationship. Incidentally, within the range of temperatures that seldom exceeded 100°F, the relationship was linear.

To return to the original question of whether interpersonal violence can be expected to increase under hotter conditions, the answer is a qualified yes. Whether excessively high temperatures produce a downturn in aggression thereafter is a matter of continuing debate and a topic for future research (see C.A. Anderson & DeNeve, 1992, vs. Bell, 1992).

Noise

Noise is an inevitable accompaniment to the vast numbers of people who assemble to witness many of our more popular sports. Before, sometimes during, and after the athletes perform crowds roar their approval or disapproval of what they see. In sports such as auto racing, the roar of engines easily drowns out the noise of racing fans.

It should first be noted that noise is physiologically arousing (Markovsky & Berger, 1983), a state that is generally regarded as conducive to aggression (Branscombe & Wann, 1992a; Rule & Nesdale, 1976). As regards aggression, experiments have consistently shown that people exposed to noise behave more aggressively than others not subjected to noise (e.g., Donnerstein & Wilson, 1976; Geen & McCown, 1984).

Noise is not, however, uniformly negative in its effects on people. Whether it proves to be disruptive or relatively benign depends on several features of the noise itself. In particular, the effect of noise in increasing aggression is more pronounced with individuals who are already experiencing a state of anger arousal. An additional determinant of the level of resulting aggression is whether the noise is controllable or uncontrollable. Where individuals lack control or are unable to terminate loud noise, their aggression is substantially greater (Geen & McCowan, 1984). A further factor mediating the effects of noise is its predictability. When the onset of noise occurs at regular intervals, it has less of an impact than noise occurring at irregular, and hence unpredictable, times. Overall, it may be assumed that noise can be a contributing factor in hostile outbursts among athletes or fans. Of course, its role will be greater in situations where the protagonists are already angry, perhaps by having witnessed an altercation or a controversial decision.

The Cover of Darkness

In many of our social settings, levels of illumination are purposely kept low, often with a view to creating a more relaxed environment in which inhibitions are lowered. Prosocial interpersonal behaviors are, as a result, thought to be facilitated in bars, at parties, and in the bedroom. However, in acting as a general conditioned disinhibitor, darkness may at the same time be responsible for an increase in antisocial behaviors.

Powerful banks of lights illuminate the playing surface at indoor sports events and those staged outdoors after sunset. Generally, the front rows of spectators are brightly lit, whereas those people furthest removed from the playing area watch in relative darkness. The question is whether poorly lit areas at sports sites increase the likelihood of disturbances. The best available evidence (Page & Moss, 1976) suggests that our inclinations to aggress increase under the cover of darkness.

The reasons, however, are somewhat speculative at this point. It may be that feelings of anonymity give rise to aggression as might the depersonalizing of a potential victim whose human qualities are only dimly revealed to a would-be aggressor. These questions remain a fruitful topic of investigation, one that is greatly in need of further research. We might also ask if the fact of aggression being increased by darkened surroundings possibly extends to dark colors (see Speaking Tangentially 8.2).

****

Speaking Tangentially 8.2: Are There Aggressive Colors?
What do you associate with black? Does it not conjure up thoughts of foreboding, darkness, evil, and death? It does for most cultures; an exception is the Chinese, for whom white serves this function. This widespread recognition of black as the color of evil and death stimulated Mark Frank and Thomas Gilovich (1988) to ask whether people wearing black are seen as more evil and aggressive. Of course, an even more intriguing question is whether those wearing black are "black-hearted," that is, whether they actually behave more aggressively than others.

Naive subjects who were unfamiliar with football and hockey rated National Football League (NFL) and National Hockey League (NHL) uniforms on a series of scales. The uniforms in both leagues that were predominantly black were judged to be more malevolent (i.e., bad, mean, and aggressive) than uniforms of lighter colors.

The authors sought answers to their second question in the records of the NFL and NHL for all seasons dating back to 1970. Using aggressive penalty indices in both sports, teams wearing black uniforms were found to have been penalized for greater yardage and spent more time in the penalty box, respectively, than teams wearing uniforms of other colors.

Several explanations for these interesting findings have no doubt already occurred to you. You might for example, suggest that a team's defensive play is judged to be more aggressive when team members wear black. Actually, a test of this suggestion found support. Knowledgeable college students and experienced football referees served as raters. Staged videos of a defensive team in action was rated by the referees as more aggressive and somewhat dirtier when the team wore black in contrast to a white uniform condition. Analyses of the student ratings yielded similar results. An especially critical finding was that referees were more inclined to penalize the team in the black version (i.e., they would call a tighter game).

A further possibility might also have occurred to you. Perhaps donning a black uniform causes players to seek out more aggressive situations. Such appears to be the case. Teams of subjects attired in uniforms—ostensibly to facilitate team cohesion—chose to compete in aggressive activities (e.g., chicken fights, dart-gun duel) more often when they wore black uniforms.

Thus, the results of this intriguing investigation suggest that teams in black uniforms incur an excess of aggressive penalties for two different reasons. First, they appear to be inclined to seek out opportunities for aggression; second, game officials enforce the rules of play more strictly. Incidentally, lest you think that black uniforms helped the fortunes of NFL or NHL teams, those attired in black fared no better in the win column than those wearing other colors.

****

Density and Crowding

Whether or not you have stood jam-packed on the terraces at a soccer match or moved slowly with a capacity crowd exiting from a football game, it is easy to appreciate that some people have fairly strong feelings about being in densely packed crowds. While some take no notice, others express irritation, even hostility, at finding themselves in the middle of large crowds. As with other situational factors, the answer to the question of whether people's feelings of being crowded makes people more hostile is complex.

Before proceeding, a distinction should be made between crowding and density. Crowding is an unpleasant state experienced by an individual as a result of being spatially restricted. Density refers instead to the extent that people are physically concentrated within a given area. Crowding, then, is a subjective feeling of discomfort arising from a *perception* that there are just too many people present for our liking. We may, for example, actually enjoy being packed in a capacity crowd at a sports event but later feel intensely uncomfortable and crowded riding a bus home after the event. Even so, the concentration of the sports crowd and those on the bus may be equal.

It has long been recognized that the interpersonal distances at which people interact and their tolerance of crowding vary considerably across cultures. Residents of high-density U.S. neighborhoods feel less able to control their social circumstances and exhibit symptoms of physiological and psychological stress (Fleming, Baum, & Weiss, 1987). On the other hand, people living in one of the most densely populated areas on the planet, Hong Kong, show little in the way of negative effects that might be attributed to their living conditions (Mitchell, 1971).

In addition to cultural differences, there are also important sex differences in the response to crowding. When females are crowded together, they tend to describe the experience in positive terms. In general, they see it as a rich social occasion. However, when men are crowded, there is an opposite reaction. Males see crowded situations as personally threatening and find the experience to be generally aversive. Under such conditions males become somewhat distrustful and hostile toward one another (e.g., Freedman, Levy, Buchanan, & Price, 1972). Marked differences in the developmental processes through which males and females are socialized are presumed to create different interpretations of and expectations regarding the close presence of others.

Something of the complexities underlying the relationship between density and sexual composition in relation to interpersonal processes are seen in a study by J.E. Marshall and Heslin (1975). Their findings were just the opposite of those reported by Freedman et al. (1972). They found that females working together liked each other *less* under crowded than under uncrowded conditions. Males, on the other hand, liked each other *more* when crowded. In an interesting sidelight, both males and females expressed a greater liking for one another in the crowded, mixed-sex condition.

In speculating on the reasons for their discrepant results, J.E. Marshall and Heslin (1975) see the far greater *time* required for their experimental task (1 1/2 hours) as a critical factor. They reason that the initial hostility of males gradually gives way to the development of a team spirit and an active striving to achieve task goals. Women initially respond positively to the intimacy and warmth of being crowded with one another. The structure and length of the task, however, require them to eventually relinquish the experience of intimacy and instead "focus on leadership and achievement" (p. 958). The ambivalence they feel toward their own success, achievement, and each other's abilities makes "the close proximity uncomfortable for them" (p. 958).

Personality differences are also involved in determining the response to close interpersonal distances. In this regard, the reactions of men to invasions of personal space by women are interesting, being in part mediated by personality factors. Men identified as physically *assaultive* generally require greater interpersonal distances between themselves and an attractive female than do nonassaultive men. On the other hand, men who are dispositionally *shy* do not differ from nonshy men under conditions where the woman wears conservative attire (i.e., a dress). But when approached by the same model wearing skimpy attire (i.e., a swimsuit), the nonshy men tolerate much closer, near-collision approaches; shy men, however, keep her at even greater distances (Russell, Huddle, & Corson, 1988). Inasmuch as people requiring a larger personal space also react more strongly to intrusions, the results of crowding may be more serious in the case of particular individuals, that is, those already dispositionally assaultive. The reactions of individuals to crowding, then, are apt to be mixed and dependent on their cultural heritage, sex, personality, and length/type of group activity, among other factors.

Ions

Another environmental factor that is not widely recognized as influencing our behavior is the balance of ionization in the atmosphere. Atmospheric environments vary in the extent to which the air molecules carry a preponderance of positive or negative electrical charges. It has long been thought that positive ions exert adverse effects (Charry & Hawkinshire, 1981), whereas negative ions are regarded as generally beneficial. Many sports are played in settings that can be expected to have a concentration of positive ions. Air-conditioning equipment, automobile emissions, crowds, and winds, all are recognized as sources of positive ions. The question is whether or not the atmosphere in which some sports are played might be contributing to the negative moods (e.g., Russell, 1981c) and overt hostility that sometimes occur at sporting sites.

Until quite recently, support for these ideas has been based on a mix of meteorological studies and sheer speculation. The strong winds that occur in various parts of the world, the Santa Ana winds of California, the Chinooks of the Northern Rockies, and the Sharav in Israel, create environments with a surplus of positive ions. Researchers have noted that increases in various social indicators (e.g., homicides, suicides, depression) coincide with the onset of these winds. While supportive of the notion that positive ions are generally harmful, such data is nevertheless correlational and confounded by several additional meteorological variables. As winds spring up, temperature, humidity, and barometric pressure also undergo dramatic changes. Any one, or a combination, of these influences could just as easily be responsible for any changes observed in the general population. It clearly remained for a controlled experiment to systematically examine the effects of ions in isolation from other covarying influences.

One of the earliest experiments (R.A. Baron, Russell, & Arms, 1985) assessed the impact of negative ions on mood and physical aggression. Part of the design took account of an individual differences variable, the Type A/B personality distinction. You will recall from the previous chapter that among other characteristics, Type A individuals are impatient, hard driving, and somewhat hostile. The popular view of ions would predict that people overall, and especially Type A's, would be less aggressive in a "beneficial" negative ion environment. The results, however, did not support this view. Whereas Type B's were unaffected in their behavior by negative ions, those subjects identified as Type A's showed an *increase* in overt aggression.

Negative ions have also been found to intensify one's existing feelings toward a stranger (R.A. Baron, 1987). If subjects saw that they shared many of the same attitudes with another individual and were thereby disposed to like him, such feelings were enhanced in a negative ion environment. Otherwise, if they held few attitudes in common and were thus inclined to dislike the other subject, their feelings of dislike were intensified. One might cautiously extend these findings to suggest that where hostilities exist or are fostered among rival factions in a crowd, negative ionization may exacerbate an already unfriendly situation. Just as clearly, negative ionization might also increase goodwill among those who find themselves among friends.

In concluding this section, I would draw your attention to the fact that my coverage of environmental factors is far from exhaustive. Discussion has been confined to those factors that have more immediate implications for sports. Other environmental factors have weaker ties to sports aggression, some of which are supported by research and others of which qualify only as myth. For example, foul odors (Rotton, Frey, Barry, Milligan, & Fitzpatrick, 1979) and air pollution (Rotton & Frey, 1985) also provide conditions that favor aggression. On the other hand, absolutely nothing out of the ordinary happens on nights when the moon is full (see Speaking Tangentially 8.3).

****

Speaking Tangentially 8.3: The Moon Made Me Do It!
Among a sample of Canadian university students, approximately 64%, men and women alike, believe the full moon influences human behavior (Russell & Dua, 1983). A truly astonishing array of behaviors has at one time or another been attributed to lunar cycles, including births, deaths, sexual power, epilepsy, somnabulism, pyromania, alcoholism, mental illness, accidents, suicides, and aggression. However, when carefully designed and con-

trolled studies are conducted, they fail to support any suggestion of lunar influence (see a review by Rotton & Kelly, 1985). But how are sports related to this lunar literature?

Sports have on two occasions (Russell & deGraaf, 1985; Russell & Dua, 1983) provided an alternative to the common practice of using homicide rates in testing the merits of a lunar-aggression hypothesis. In these studies, aggressive penalties in ice hockey (e.g., fighting, charging, etc.) were classified according to the synodic and anomalistic cycles. Basically, the synodic cycle refers to the phase of the moon (i.e., new moon, first quarter, second quarter, full moon), whereas the anomalistic cycle refers to the distance between Earth and its moon, called perigee at its closest point, apogee at its farthest distance. Despite a number of tests and organizing the data in various ways, there was simply no hint of a lunar-aggression relationship across two full seasons of play. Thus, as popular and attractive as fanciful lunar theories may be, we are required to look to more down-to-earth explanations for an understanding of human behaviors.

****

Coping Strategies

If violence is generally deplored and a concern of most people, how are we able to suspend our abhorrence when we participate in or watch sports with violent content? Surely the infliction of harm on another person whether by our own hand or by someone else should cause us distress. What set of dynamics, then, sometimes enables us to accept that which is normally unacceptable in ordinary, everyday circumstances?

A good part of the explanation is to be found in self-regulatory mechanisms that operate to ensure behavior that conforms to our personal standards for acceptable, socially responsible conduct (Bandura, 1973, 1983). Anytime we fall short of our standards, the result can be *self-censure*, an especially effective form of punishment for unacceptable behavior. It is noteworthy that in the case of a few individuals, this same self-regulatory mechanism can instead reward aggressive actions. Athletes in certain sports may come to value and glorify violence to such an extent that interpersonal mayhem becomes a source not of shame but of personal pride. For example, some individuals within the subcultures of hockey (M.D. Smith, 1983), prison populations (Toch, 1984), or educational settings (Olweus, 1978) who are directly or vicariously embroiled in violence may derive feelings of enhanced self-worth and prestige from their involvement.

A self-regulatory mechanism does not operate uniformly in all circumstances to internally control behavior. It is subject to a variety of influences that can neutralize or disengage the self-censuring consequences we might normally suffer for our aggression. This disengagement of internal controls will be greatest where the causal connection between the aggression and its consequences for the victim is thoroughly obscured. Some of the specific means by which people can avoid negative self-evaluative consequences for their aggression are outlined in the sections to follow.

Moral Justification

Aggression that would be reprehensible under ordinary circumstances may be construed as "right" in the service of higher moral values. For example, if one's disorderly activities can be seen as an effort to preserve or even advance national honor, then others sharing those sentiments are less likely to condemn the activity. English soccer hooligans have with some regularity characterized their conflicts abroad in nationalistic terms. J.M. Williams et al. (1984) describe the behavior of British fans in Madrid for a World Cup match against Spain. Rival English and Spanish fans baited each other with chants about ownership of Gibraltar and the Malvinas, the islands over which England and Argentina had fought the Falklands War of 1982. Just before the mounted police rode in to disperse the demonstrators, the English were heard provoking the Spaniards by singing renditions of "Rule Britannia" and "You'll Never Take Gilbraltar" (p. 104). On an earlier excursion to Northern Spain,

> a drunken expedition of about 10 fans set off at 3 a.m. to scale a steep hill which overlooked the village. A British flag was staked at the summit and cries of 'England! England!' interspersed with National Front slogans, were probably audible for miles around. (p. 82)

Cloaked in the mantle of nationalism, they fully expect that others will see their misguided behavior as a praiseworthy expression of patriotism.

Palliative Comparisons

Another common means of exonerating oneself for aggression is to cite instances of more extreme aggression committed by others. "The brawl at last night's game was a tea party compared to the one last month in _____." Thus, one's actions are made to seem almost benign by comparison.

Euphemistic Labeling

Aggressive acts can also be made to appear less serious through the use of euphemistic descriptions. Various phrases are used by sportscasters to describe for their listeners the effects of a particularly vicious tackle or a fighter being knocked unconscious. The downed athlete is described as "knocked out of his socks," "rang his chimes," "had his numbers knocked off," or "cold-cocked." These characterizations engage faintly amusing imagery and in so doing make light of the incident. Bobsledders who adopt the "Kamakazi position" (head first) in making their run down the Cresta course in St. Moritz refer to those occasions when their chin hits the ice as "the Cresta kiss." Such labels trivialize the incident and draw attention away from the fact that the athlete may have sustained a serious injury. Hunters in my part of the world similarly prefer to speak of "harvesting" the deer and elk population each fall rather than killing them. Labeled in this fashion, one gets the impression that they are performing a public service. In each case, the reality of what has happened is softened and is thereby made less troubling.

Misconstruing the Effects of Aggression

Yet a further means by which those witnessing violence avoid self-reproach is seen when the results of a violent act are downplayed or ignored altogether. Injured athletes are often described as able to "walk off" their injury or just shaken up. Although sportscasters were scarcely able to avoid discussing the potentially career-ending injuries to quarterback Joe Thiesman and boxer Sugar Ray Leonard, they seldom make more than passing reference to the legions of lesser known athletes who have sustained often life-long injuries. Equally insidious are the cumulative effects of irreversible brain damage frequently incurred and seldom recognized, even by those engaged in combatant sports (Levin, Eisenberg, & Benton, 1989; Russell, 1991). Protected in these ways, the public and those involved in high-risk sports can view their activities as relatively safe.

Displacement of Responsibility

If responsibility for our aggression can be attributed to others, we hold ourselves much less accountable for our actions (Milgram, 1974). The team goon ordered by his coach to assault an opposing player avoids negative self-evaluations inasmuch as a legitimate authority implicitly assumes responsibility for his deed. He might remind himself that, after all, he was only carrying out orders.

Diffusion of Responsibility

When a number of people share in committing an act of aggression, each individual can regard his responsibility for the outcome as but a fraction of those who participated. Individual participants in a sports riot may feel they had little part in the violence given that many others were also involved. As one of the 1,000 or so celebrants who burned and looted in a celebration riot, they bear but 1/1,000th of the responsibility for the destruction—not a matter worth losing sleep over! Obviously, were they to commit some of the same destructive acts on their own, this means of escaping the self-recriminating consequences of their actions would be unavailable.

Dehumanization of Victim

Self-absolving mechanisms that are associated with the victim's status also provide means whereby normally reprehensible behavior can be made more acceptable. While human interactions call for the observance of fair and compassionate behaviors toward one another, this understanding is sometimes waived in instances where members of a rival team are relegated to a subhuman status. Once divested of human qualities by derogatory labels and descriptions, a group can be attacked with few qualms. The aggressors can take a measure of comfort from their having aggressed not against their fellow man but against lower life forms (e.g., savages, Neanderthals).

For example, subjects in an experiment overhearing others being described as a "rotten bunch" were found to be more aggressive toward that group than those who heard humanizing remarks. Similarly, when responsibility for punishing the group was shared with others, shock levels were again set higher (Bandura, Underwood, & Fromson, 1975).

Attribution of Blame

Of course, if one can make a case for a fight being instigated by the other fellow, then one's actions must by contrast be defensive in nature and not at all troubling. The course of most violent encounters involves an escalating spiral of exchanges between the parties. The protagonist can usually characterize some defensive action on the part of his victim as having provoked the dispute. If the aggressor is successful in convincing others with this ploy, then the intended victim got only what he deserved.

The processes by which Dr. Jekylls are transformed into Mr. Hydes does not take place overnight. Rather, changes in the levels of an individual's aggression or that tolerated by the general public occur very gradually, to borrow a term from psychophysics, by just unnoticed differences (JUDs). Thus, people gradually become disinhibited in their aggression both individually and as spectators. One becomes desensitized to current levels of aggression such that incrementally higher levels can be introduced and tolerated. The self-censure that might formerly have followed from being a party to this new level of aggression fails to occur. What was previously unacceptable becomes acceptable.

Suggested Readings

Baron, R.A., & Richardson, D.R. (in press). *Human aggression* (2nd ed.). New York: Plenum.
    The ideal starting point for students of aggression, this book provides a careful examination of the biological, social, environmental, and individual determinants of human aggression.

Brain, P.F. (Ed.). (1986). *Alcohol and aggression.* London: Croom Helm.
    An advanced reference source in which experts review the research pertaining to many of the basic issues currently being debated by those investigating the effects of alcohol.

Geen, R.G. (1990). *Human aggression.* Pacific Grove, CA: Brooks/Cole.
A primer that provides a broad introduction to the basic findings on human aggression.

Goldstein, A.P., Reagles, K.W., & Amann, L.L. (1990). *Refusal skills: Preventing drug use in adolescents.* Champaign, IL: Research Press.
This little book is a dandy primer for those venturing into the field of study regarding drugs. In addition to providing an authoritative introduction, it describes a program that may in many cases head off drug use by those populations at risk.

Megargee, E.I. (in press). Aggression and violence. In H.E. Adams & P.B. Sutker (Eds.), *Comprehensive handbook of psychopathology* (2nd ed.). New York: Plenum.
This is easily the best single-chapter source for an overview of what we currently know about the topic of human aggression.

9

Catharsis Through Sports: Fact or Fiction?

Among the most pervasive and persistent beliefs surrounding sports is the notion that participation in aggressive sports affords athletes the opportunity to get rid of their aggressive impulses. Merely watching others act aggressively is also presumed to provide spectators with similar opportunities to give vent to their accumulated frustrations and pent-up hostilities. Additionally, some writers have chosen to define catharsis even more broadly to include predictions that a reduction in physiological arousal will occur as a result of participating in or observing aggressive activities (Hokanson, 1970; Quanty, 1976). These cathartic beliefs are the subject of this chapter with regard both to their historical origins and the scientific evidence attesting to their validity.

Those Who Believe

Some indication of the extent to which these cathartic beliefs have currency is seen in the responses of 525 University of Lethbridge students to the statement "Participating in combatant or aggressive sports is a good way for people to get rid of their aggressive urges." Males and females alike expressed 63% agreement with the item. A sample of older men ($N = 84$) attending a local ice hockey game indicated 75% agreement with the same question (Russell, 1983b). However, a sex difference was revealed in another university sample. Biaggio (1987) found that females provided a stronger endorsement of hostility catharsis than did males.

Cathartic beliefs were also assessed by Michael Tarnok (1984) in an honors thesis at New York University. Interviews ($N = 99$) with New Yorkers who were approached "in the Rockefeller Center area, a Long Island warehouse, and along a grocery food route covering the five boroughs" revealed 48% agreement with the item "A sporting event is a place where I can let myself go, feeling relaxed afterward." A neutral category was included and endorsed by 34% of the respondents. Had a forced choice format (e.g., agree-disagree) been used instead, one can predict that approximately 65% of Tarnok's respondents would have endorsed the item, a figure virtually the same as in the Lethbridge sample. Finally, neither the age nor sex of those interviewed was related to agreement with the question.

Interviews ($N = 400$) with spectators at a professional wrestling card (Bratton, Clark, Dyer, Harding, & Roberts, 1978) included a question asking them to rate the importance of each of 18 possible reasons for their attendance. The only

"cathartic" reason—"I can release my aggression (hate) at Stampede Wrestling"—
was ranked 11th overall. Interestingly, married spectators rated it as a less important reason than either singles or those checking their marital status as "other."
However, males and females judged the reason to be of equal importance.

Many educators apparently subscribe to cathartic beliefs. In a survey of school
teachers ($N = 137$), J.C. Bennett (1988) indicates that a "sizable percentage" expressed support for the proposition that aggressive sports provide cathartic benefits for children. Teachers under the age of 25 expressed stronger support than
their older colleagues, with the young males giving the strongest endorsement of
all to the catharsis item.

An overview of sex differences in cathartic beliefs presents a mixed picture.
Whereas women expressed stronger cathartic beliefs in Biaggio's (1987) study,
J.C. Bennett (1988) found the greatest support for the concept among a group of
young men. In other studies, males and females appear to share equally in the belief that cathartic benefits result from observing (Bratton et al., 1978; Tarnok,
1984) or participating in aggressive sports (Russell, 1983b). At the same time, it
appears that a majority of people overall (i.e., perhaps as many as two thirds) believe a cathartic experience can be achieved through participation in combatant
sports or by merely observing interpersonal aggression among athletes.

Opinions on the issue abound. In the field of education, many school systems
appear to have uncritically embraced the cathartic view in the process of planning
their athletic and recreational programs. The voices of earlier critics have gone
largely unheeded. For example, as early as 1969, Nighswander and Mayer sound-
ed a note of caution in making the following observation:

> Although many parents, educators, counselors, and psychotherapists en-
> courage children to participate in aggressive activities as a way of coun-
> tering aggressiveness, it has been indicated in a number of research stud-
> ies that such cathartic activities often tend to increase aggressiveness
> instead of decrease it. (p. 465)

Referring specifically to football, J.C. Bennett (1991) further contends that the
presumed benefits of catharsis provide a convenient, although ill-founded, justification to educators for maintaining interscholastic football programs.

Therapeutic catharsis also occupies a central position in many forms of modern
psychotherapy (e.g., Bach & Goldberg, 1983; Nichols & Zax, 1977). Holt (1970)
presents a strong case for the free expression of anger to the extent that it facilitates
a basic restructuring and clarification of the events/circumstances that led up to an
individual's original state of anger. In a therapeutic context, the client's interpretation of a situation, his expression of feelings, and the changes sought are thought to
be personally beneficial. In the interests of providing a balanced view of the role of
catharsis in various therapies, the reader is referred to an eloquent discussion and
defense of the concept put forward by Novaco (1975; 1986, pp. 16–21).

Something of the attraction of clinicians to catharsis and its presumed therapeutic role in clinical practice is seen in two examples. Psychiatrists Proctor and

Eckerd (1976) enthusiastically extol the cathartic value of aggressive sports and recommend that patients attend violent sports to fulfill their "psychic needs" through a cathartic experience. The logic of the cathartic position is presented in a whimsical analogy:

> People's emotions are similar to steam locomotives. If you build a fire in the boiler of a locomotive, keep raising the steam pressure and let it sit on the track, sooner or later something will blow. However, if you take it and spin the wheels and toot the whistle, the steam pressure can be kept at a safe level. Spectator sports give John Q. Citizen a socially accept-able way to lower his steam pressure by allowing him to spin his wheels and toot his whistle. (p. 83)

Yet another therapist sees catharsis working in the interests of his patient on the golf course:

> In golf his primitive impulses to violence reappeared and he said that he ac-tually felt "crazier" on the golf course than he had been during some phas-es of his serious mental illness. To him the only pleasure derived from golf consisted in the moment when he struck the ball and all his viciousness, bit-ter aggression and latent sadism found release. (Oberndorf, 1951, p. 83)

With any professional group, it is to be expected that opinion will be sharply divided on many of the major issues. Opinions on the merits of a hostility cathar-sis hypothesis within the psychological community are no exception. In a survey of North American psychologists, Biaggio (1987) found greater support for the concept among psychologists who had not been involved in research in recent years; their colleagues who were active researchers expressed less support. More-over, her sample of university students expressed considerably greater support for catharsis than did their psychology professors.

Cathartic ideas also circulate as matters of opinion in legal circles. Barnes (1983) observed that the prosecution of hockey players for engaging in fist fights is unlikely inasmuch as it

> is often claimed that such combats are not a cause of serious injuries and serve as a safe escape valve for players' frustrations. Without such a means of release, it is claimed that players might resort to serious attacks using sticks or other equipment. (p. 122)

Writing in the *Wisconsin Law Review* (Kuhlmann, 1975), a legal commentator ar-gued that "spectators find healthy ventilation for their own violent emotions in watching violence on the playing field. From a public policy standpoint, the net result could be positive." Against a background of widespread public acceptance of cathartic beliefs, one must assume that the weight of these arguments in legal decisions is not inconsequential.

Whether or not these beliefs are founded in fact has far-reaching implications for the planning of sports and recreational programs in community, educational, correctional, and other institutional settings. If, as a majority seems to believe, combatant sports serve the prosocial function of providing an outlet for aggression, then a strong argument can be made for their inclusion in various programs. There are also implications for parenting. Are overly aggressive children better-off in a sport where they can work off some of their aggression, or would it be better to direct them into a nonaggressive activity?

Support for the cathartic view would further provide a justification for media violence and its continued promotion. In sports, as elsewhere, violence might be seen in a more positive light, other arguments notwithstanding (e.g., injuries, the development of antisocial attitudes and values, etc.). Otherwise, if cathartic hypotheses have failed to find support in the scientific community, then the case for the promotion of sports featuring interpersonal aggression must rest on other, less defensible grounds such as entertainment or profits (see Speaking Tangentially 9.1).

****

Speaking Tangentially 9.1: Does Violence Sell?
Sexually titillating themes have long found favor as a successful marketing tool in the advertising and entertainment industries. But are violent themes equally good box office? Can the violence in certain sports be defended on the basis of its being what the fans want and will pay to see?

Western Hockey League records provided the data for tests of the relationship between excessively violent games and subsequent attendance (Russell, 1986). Attendance at the next home game following each team's two most violent games during the season were compared to attendance following each team's two most peaceable matches. Several analyses failed to reveal any association between violence levels and the number of fans passing through the turnstiles. In ice hockey, at least, the promotion or tolerance of player aggression cannot easily be defended on either entertainment or economic grounds.

****

Clearly, there is a division of public and professional sentiments on the question. But catharsis is not a recent invention nor even an invention of this century. Before considering the evidence for and against the concept, we would do well to briefly review its origins and thereby perhaps better understand why it is so deeply rooted in the public consciousness.

Roots of Catharsis

The attraction of catharsis is best understood against the background of its early emergence in philosophical thought and later adoption by 20th-century theorists of human behavior. In tracing the course of cathartic ideas, it should be noted that the list of those embracing the concept are numbered among the most eminent and influential scholars of their day. This fact alone may account for much of the concept's current popularity. Early mention of catharsis is to be found in the writings of Aristotle, who observed that those witnessing the expression of "tragic" feelings in the Greek tragic theater would themselves be purged of the same emotions, for example, pity, fear (Berczeller, 1967; Goodman, 1964; Scheff & Bushnell, 1984). While aggression was never specifically mentioned by Aristotle, it has generally been assumed that he would have viewed it in similar terms.

More recently, catharsis reappears as a central concept in the Freudian perspective. Freud proposed a death instinct fueled by a continual welling up of destructive impulses. Freud's pessimistic prognosis for mankind was a future in which we are doomed to repeat our history of wars and terror. Such hope as there is lies in our being able to redirect our aggression into relatively safe channels. Various forms of competition, including sports, offer one such alternative. British psychotherapist Anthony Storr (1968) reflects the Freudian position in concluding, "It is obvious that the encouragement of competition in all possible fields is likely to diminish the kind of hostility which leads to war rather than to increase it—rivalry between nations in sports can do nothing but good" (pp. 158–159). However, in all fairness it should be noted that Dr. Storr no longer subscribes to this view (Personal communication, September 7, 1992).

The Freudian view of catharsis was later given formal expression by the Yale group of psychologists (Quanty, 1976) in their influential book *Frustration and Aggression* (Dollard, Doob, Miller, Mowrer, & Sears, 1939). Appended as a corollary to the frustration-aggression model was the following: "The expression of any act of aggression is a catharsis that reduces the instigation to all other acts of aggression" (p. 53). However, the effects predicted by Dollard et al. are short-lived and over the long run may actually contribute to an increased likelihood of aggression through a process of learning. As they suggest, "presumably this reduction is more or less temporary, and the instigation to aggression will build up again if the original frustration persists. Also the repetition of a mode of release may produce learning of it" (p. 50). Thus, the concept again found a place as a central tenet in a major theoretical work.

Perhaps the greatest impression on the public mind came with the publication of Konrad Lorenz's (1966) *On Aggression*. A best-seller, this engaging volume presents the views of ethology, a European tradition of inquiry involving the systematic observation of lower organisms in their natural habitat. One of the more contentious implications of their work is the suggestion that vestiges of the rigid, stereotyped sequences of behavior (i.e., "fixed action patterns") observed on the part of lower species extend to humans. You will recall the ethological case for interpreting the home field advantage as an example of "territorial" defense, an argument evaluated in chapter 2. More central to the present discussion, however, is the part played in the model by a cathartic process thought to be associated with fixed action patterns of aggression. In freely extending the model to the human level, one is asked to imagine a reservoir that is continually being filled with aggressive energy. It follows from this hydraulic analogy that it would be in the best interests of all concerned for people to periodically discharge this energy into safe channels. Otherwise, dangerous levels may build up to the point where aggressive energy could spill over or break through the dam with devastating consequences for those unfortunate enough to find themselves in its path. International competition in the conquest of space, debates, and sports are suggested as providing mankind with potentially safe outlets. With reference to sports, Lorenz (1966) comments:

> While some early forms of sport, like the jousting of medieval knights, may have had an appreciable influence on sexual selection, the main function of sport today lies in the cathartic discharge of aggressive urge; besides that, of course, it is of the greatest importance in keeping people healthy. (p. 242)

Far less well known are the more recent opinions of ethology's two leading figures. In a *Psychology Today* interview, Lorenz qualified his earlier position stating, "Nowadays, I have strong doubts whether watching aggressive behavior even in the guise of sport has any cathartic effect at all" (R.I. Evans, 1974, p. 93). Citing the example of crowd disorders at soccer matches, Nikolaas Tinbergen (1968) sees an "inflammatory effect" (enhancement) as often dominating a "waning effect" (cathartic) in determining the postmatch behavior of fans (p. 1418).

In summary, it should surprise no one that cathartic beliefs are deeply held and widespread among the general public. The names highlighted in the brief sketch above are historically numbered among the most authoritative analysts of behavior (Lorenz and Tinbergen are Nobel laureates). A notable exception to this imposing array is Charles Darwin, who on the next-to-last page of his monumental work *The Expression of the Emotions in Man and Animals* offers a dissenting opinion in observing that "he who gives way to violent gestures will increase his rage" (Darwin, 1872/1965, p. 365). While the stature and influence of earlier proponents of catharsis may in large measure account for the concept's current popularity, the critical question to which we now turn is whether such beliefs are justified on the basis of research evidence.

For the most part, theories that posit a cathartic mechanism fortunately lend themselves to predictions that can be tested under controlled conditions. Indeed, in recent decades an enormous amount of research has been conducted in which the results have had a direct bearing on the concept of catharsis. By far, the greatest number of investigations have been set in the social science laboratory, a lesser number being carried out in complementary field settings. Of these, a relatively small number have in one way or another involved sports. It is these studies that will be emphasized and their findings integrated with the results of a far larger number of nonsports investigations.

The organization of the sports aggression literature that bears on the catharsis question will consider first those investigations involving sportspeople who are active *participants* in sports that feature interpersonal aggression. A review of the effects on spectators of *observing* aggression follows. Finally, the special cases of *fictional* aggression and *media* presentations of sports aggression are examined for their role in possibly providing viewers with a cathartic experience.

Catharsis: One on One

> Rockne: Every red-blooded young man in any country is filled with what we might call the natural spirit of combat. In many parts of Europe and elsewhere in the world this spirit manifests itself in continuous wars and revolutions. We have tried to make competitive sports serve as a safer outlet for the spirit of combat. I believe we have succeeded."
>
> From the movie *Knute Rockne: All American* (Warner Bros., 1940), starring Pat O'Brien, Ronald Reagan, and Donald Crisp

A variety of approaches and methodologies have been used in exploring the effects on athletes of their participation in aggressive sports. These range from static comparisons of those active in aggressive versus nonaggressive sports to controlled laboratory experiments. The former design, of course, is subject to a selection bias whereby those attracted to aggressive sports may at the outset be more/less aggressive than those choosing to participate in nonaggressive sports. Whatever the outcome of such studies, the results may just as easily be attributed to initial differences in temperament rather than to influences arising from the sport in which subjects have chosen to participate. Designs yielding more definitive results ideally would provide for the random selection and assignment of subjects to the sports being compared.

Static Comparisons

Notwithstanding a selection bias, it might be argued that cathartic effects would be seen in generally lower aggression scores on the part of sportspeople generally and especially those engaged in contact sports where cathartic opportunities abound. Using a *behavioral* measure of laboratory aggression (i.e., shock), Zillmann, Johnson, and Day (1974) compared nonathletes with athletes in noncontact sports (swimming, tennis) and those participating in the contact sports of football and wrestling. The three groups did not differ in their aggression. In another study, LeUnes and Nation (1982) compared introductory psychology students who had never "lettered" in a sport with those who had discontinued their football "careers" after high school and members of a university football team. Again, the groups did not differ on a measure of anger. Finally, a preseason comparison of two tennis squads and a noncompetitive student sample failed to reveal any differences in aggression (Ostrow, 1974).

Occasionally, comparisons of this sort show sports participants to be higher on aggression than others (e.g., Thirer, 1978). Even within a relatively homogeneous sports setting, high school football players scored higher on measures of direct and indirect hostility than a sample of physical education students whose temperament might be thought to resemble that of the football players (Patterson, 1974). Thus far, little can be said to favor catharsis. What support there is, is left to two studies that used a projective measure of aggression.

To be sure, some static comparisons do provide evidence for a cathartic interpretation. For example, TAT aggression scores were reported to be lower among college boxers than among participants in cross-country, wrestling, or a nonsports control group (Husman, 1955). Similarly, TAT aggression was found to be lower among police officers who chose boxing as an activity than among their fellow officers who chose other, nonviolent activities (Atkins, Hilton, Neigher, & Bahr, 1972). However, in both studies the boxers scored higher on a companion measure of guilt. Inasmuch as those experiencing high levels of guilt are generally less aggressive than individuals with few feelings of guilt (Knott, Lasater, & Schuman, 1974), there is a strong possibility that guilt rather than catharsis was responsible for any reduction in aggression (cf. Quanty, 1976, p. 117). In summary, findings from static comparisons are difficult to interpret. Yet despite their design limitations, or perhaps because of them, they fail to provide any clear pattern of support for a catharsis position.

Before-After Comparisons

A decidedly improved research design with which to test cathartic effects involves pre- to posttreatment comparisons of aggression among subjects (randomly) assigned to an aggressive activity with control subjects assigned to a neutral activity condition. A number of investigators have used variations on this basic design in tests of a catharsis hypothesis. Two investigations have examined the potential cathartic benefits of vigorous motor activity. In the first of these (Ryan, 1970), subjects were required either to pound with a rubber mallet or to remain inactive over the same period of time. When later provided with the opportunity to aggress, subjects in the two groups did not differ in the levels of aggression (shock) they directed toward an experimental confederate. Subjects in a second study (Hornberger, 1959) were required to hammer nails. Compared with an inactive control group, those hammering nails were subsequently found to be more *verbally* aggressive. But might it be the case that verbal aggression itself acts as a safety valve to relieve pent-up hostility?

This view has been expressed by Narancic (1972), who sees the function of curses acting "as a lightning rod to conduct away 'bad blood' and very often serve to prevent more serious encounters" (p. 208). Narancic also foresees difficulties for the sportsman if his inclination to curse is repressed: "If the swear word becomes a whisper and is pushed back into the throat psychological complexes have to look for another channel" (p. 210). In a test of the effects of verbal aggression, Loew (1967) had subjects recite aggressive words aloud. Compared to controls who recited neutral words, the verbally aggressive group later acted more aggressively toward a peer. Thus, it appears unlikely that athletes who swear in competition are realizing a reduction in their hostility through a cathartic discharge of their emotions. Likely just the opposite is occurring (see also Ebbesen, Duncan, & Konecni, 1975).

Several other studies have attempted to track the course of player hostility over a full season of competition. In one investigation (Ostrow, 1974), the hostility of noncompetitive control subjects was compared to that of two intercollegiate tennis teams, one of which was an alternate squad whose members competed little, if at all. Perhaps because of their frustration with not making the first team, members on the alternate team showed the only change in hostility, an increase from preseason to postseason play. In a similar vein, college football players designated as redshirts (i.e., inactive for a season) were found to be higher on hostility than their teammates, a result the authors also attribute to the frustrations arising from an inactive status (Nation & LeUnes, 1983b). In another field study, Patterson (1974) compared the hostility scores of physical education students and football players over a season of play. Whereas the physical education students remained unchanged, the hostility of football players underwent a significant increase to the end of their schedule. Finally, collegiate wrestlers have also been found to show a marginal increase in aggression over a season of competition (Husman, 1955).

Two studies point to a reduction in aggression as a result of aggressive behavior. Young boys diagnosed as aggressive threw darts at photographs of people considered to be significant in their lives (Kidd & Walton, 1966). Following four weekly therapy sessions, the authors report a decrease in the youngsters' hostility toward authority figures and peers (7% of the target choices). However, hostility toward the remaining 93% of the targets (i.e., parents, siblings, teachers) was unchanged over the course of the program. In an exploratory study (W.R. Johnson & Hutton, 1955), the House-Tree-Person test was administered to a small sample ($N = 8$) of college wrestlers at three points in time. From well before the start of the season until just before their first match, the men showed an increase in intrapunitive aggression. From the prematch to the morning following their bout, "aggressive feelings" were greatly reduced irrespective of whether they had won or lost their match. Unfortunately, the lack of a control group in both studies severely weakens whatever support they might otherwise have provided for a cathartic interpretation of the results.

Let the Record Speak for Itself

The question of catharsis has also been addressed through the use of sports records (e.g., newspaper summaries, league records, etc.). These *archival* investigations have a lengthy history in sports studies reaching at least as far back as Triplett's (1898) classic study of competitive bicycle racing. The use of historical records has allowed researchers to assess the results of participation in aggressive sports over a much greater span of human history and across a wider variety of societal forms than would otherwise be possible. In the context of the present discussion, one might expect the record to show interpersonal aggression declining from the early through to the later stages of an aggressive contest. Whatever pent-up frustrations and hostility an athlete brings to his event, relief is only as far away as his first scrap. A review of ice hockey records provides an evaluation of this prediction. Five independent analyses of league records reviewed by Russell (1981b) and a further study (Harrell, 1981) provide a consensus that interpersonal aggression increases over the course of a game. Alternatively, one might suggest that more time and opportunities are needed for aggression to be successfully vented than that afforded by 60 minutes of playing time. However, when the time frame is expanded, we find that aggression also increases with the number of times any two teams have met over the season (Russell, 1983a).

For the balance of this section, we turn to two large-scale investigations of the effects on societies engaged in the promotion of aggressive sports. The first of these studies was reported by anthropologist Richard Sipes in an important and widely cited article (Sipes, 1973). He determined the degree to which past societies were involved in conflicts (e.g., war, revolution) *and* the extent to which combatant sports were featured in these same societies. The cathartic view, stressing the beneficial role of aggressive sports in reducing levels of aggression, stood to be upheld if a negative relationship resulted between the two measures. However, a *positive* correlation was found; that is, as societies were found to be increasingly involved in combatant sports, they experienced correspondingly higher levels of inter- and intrasocietal violence. While causality cannot be inferred from this association, and the study is not without its critics (e.g., Eibl-Eibesfeldt, 1979), against the background of the foregoing review it would to this point appear unlikely that the promotion of violent sports serves the best interests of societies, past or present.

Would combatant sports played at an *international* level before the eyes of the world perhaps achieve cathartic goals? While the Olympic Games are promoted on the basis of their fostering goodwill among the athletes and nations they represent, critics point to the themes of nationalism and militarism that have dominated successive games. Do the Olympics serve the interests of world peace by providing an occasion when international tensions can be lessened and mutual regard enhanced among nations? More specifically, can existing tensions and hostilities among nations find a release through participation and/or the witnessing of Olympic events?

Keefer, Goldstein, and Kasiarz (1983) extended the work of Sipes (1973) in asking similar questions about Olympic participation in combatant sports and national involvement in war. In more recent times, nations have individually expressed the extent of their interest in combatant sports through their choice of the events in which they plan to compete. All sports were initially classified as either contact or noncontact. Next, archival sources provided data on the extent of Olympic involvement by participating nations as well as details of their military engagements. The principal findings included *positive* relationships between involvement in wars and both a preference for combatant sports and sending larger teams to the games. (The latter analysis included a correction for population sizes.)

Again, although the relationship cannot be assumed to be causal or inevitable, the evidence is consistent with the results of Sipes's (1973) investigation. As Keefer et al. (1983) point out, the relationship between time at war and a preference for combatant sports may have come about as a result of the games being staged amid a climate of rivalry (rather than competition), hostility (rather than friendship), nationalism (rather than internationalism), and militarism (rather than pacifism). However, I would echo the authors' optimistic conclusion: "The Olympic ideal referred to by Coubertin is not beyond our grasp. It may only require a change in the way international athletic competition is conceived and presented, rather than any change in the competition itself" (p. 191).

Other archival studies have tested the catharsis model on an equally grand scale. The intensity and diversity of destructive means in wartime are virtually unlimited. This being the case, wars provide an ideal opportunity for a people to experience catharsis. One of the predictions that follows from the catharsis model would see a reduction in societal violence in the immediate postwar years.

The monumental work of Archer and Gartner (1984) in developing the Comparative Crime Data File (CCDF) provided for just such a test. Briefly, the CCDF includes the official records of crime and violence from 110 nations for the period 1900–1970. Using combat deaths per million population as a reflection of a nation's wartime experience with violence, the postwar homicide rates of countries with high levels of combat deaths were compared with those suffering the loss of relatively fewer troops. Countries experiencing the greatest levels of involvement with wartime violence were found to have experienced *increases* in postwar homicides even greater than those with fewer combat deaths per capita. Moreover, both defeated and victorious nations saw homicide levels rise in the aftermath of conflict. However, it was the winning sides that experienced the steepest increases. Thus, evidence amassed on a global scale involving the most extreme violence has failed to yield any semblance of support for cathartic notions.

Is It Catharsis or Learning?

The work of sociologist Terry Nosanchuk (Nosanchuk, 1981; Nosanchuk & MacNeil, 1989) in investigating the effects on aggression of participation in the martial arts identifies an important caveat to the foregoing. His principal finding of increased years of participation being associated with decreases in aggression modifies a conclusion that participation in a combatant sport must necessarily produce a more aggressive individual. The philosophical underpinnings taught during training in the traditional *dojos* can apparently bring about a fairly basic restructuring of cognitions such that nonviolent options and solutions to problems are increasingly preferred at the expense of violent ones. This occurs despite the acquisition of lethal skills.

Further support for the suggestion that the philosophical component of traditional martial arts training can reduce the aggression of its students comes from the work of Trulson (1986). Juvenile delinquents were individually assigned to participate in one of three training conditions: (1) the traditional Korean martial art of Tae Kwon Do, (2) a modern version of the training which de-emphasized the philosophical component, and (3) a control condition in which the delinquents maintained contact with the instructor while engaging in sports activities.[1] The groups met three times a week for a period of 6 months. The results strongly support the reasoning developed above. Students of the traditional form of Tae Kwon Do showed decreased aggressiveness, whereas those for whom the philosophical teachings had been deemphasized showed a major increase in aggressiveness and, I might add, an increase in their delinquent activity. Control subjects remained unchanged over the course of the program. Students trained in the traditional manner also showed an increase in social skills and self-esteem, along with lowered anxiety.

Inasmuch as combatant sports are apt to be with us for some time to come, it is interesting to speculate that integrating peaceful philosophies with training in other aggressive sports might yield similar results. On a more ominous note, however, many of the martial arts imported to North America have been basically altered from their original forms in Asian practice (Back & Kim, 1984). Nonviolent philosophies play little or no part in such training.

Summary

In the foregoing, the concept of catharsis was discussed and evaluated specifically in regard to aggressive interactions in sports. Investigations testing the catharsis hypothesis in sports have generally failed to provide support for this widely held belief. Rather than athletes in aggressive sports experiencing a discharge of pent-up hostility through their participation, the opposite frequently occurs. Although athletes engaged in sports featuring interpersonal aggression will sometimes show no change in their aggressivity, more often the result is an *increase* in the hostility of those involved. Aggression begets still more aggression.

Catharsis in the Stands

The other side of the catharsis coin proposes that those who merely observe and vicariously experience aggression are likewise afforded opportunities to give vent to their aggressive inclinations. Thus, spectators attending any one of a number of sports containing episodes of interpersonal aggression would be predicted to leave the venue more serene than they were prior to the event. Writing in 1929, Brill saw the benefits of spectatorship extending beyond the football grounds into the community and home. In a passage that hints at the then private matter of domestic violence. Brill unreservedly declares the following:

---

[1] There is no indication that subjects were assigned randomly to the conditions of the experiment.

On the other hand, through the operation of the psychological laws of identification and catharsis, the thoroughgoing fan is distinctly benefitted mentally, physically and morally by spectator-participation in his favorite sport. And his wife might find him a much less pleasant animal to have around the house, when he was there, if he did not absent himself from time to time to let off the accumulated steam of ancient instincts. (p. 430)

The cathartic value of spectatorship is further proclaimed:

He will purge himself of impulses which too dammed up would lead to private broils and public disorders. He will achieve exaltation, vicarious but real. He will be a better individual, a better citizen, a better husband and father. (p. 434)

Brill makes no mention of women possibly enjoying similar benefits.

Was Brill's Optimism Misplaced?

A series of field studies conducted in numerous sports over the past two decades has produced a consistent pattern of findings. By and large, studies in this tradition have involved the use of subjects who were real-life fans in actual attendance at sporting events.

Two early investigations (Kingsmore, 1970; E.T. Turner, 1970) produced conflicting results. Using a Thematic Apperception Test measure, Kingsmore (1970) found that spectators showed less extrapunitive aggression after observing the matches on a professional wrestling card. A self-report measure also revealed a decrease in aggression among the wrestling fans. However, neither measure yielded any pre- to postgame differences among spectators attending a professional basketball game. On the other hand, E.T. Turner (1970) found increases in aggression (i.e., the frequency of aggressive words elicited by projective measures) among college students watching football and basketball games. No changes were found among those attending an amateur wrestling card.

The catharsis hypothesis was further tested by J.H. Goldstein and Arms (1971), who used a superior design and, importantly, avoided the use of ill-suited and questionable projective measures of aggression (e.g., Anastasi, 1988). Their study was conducted on the occasion of the Army-Navy football game held annually in Philadelphia. Following a *random* procedure, a sample of men entering the stadium was intercepted individually and asked to complete several scales from the Buss-Durkee Hostility Inventory (Buss & Durkee, 1957). An equivalent sample of males was approached at the conclusion of the contest. The same procedures were followed at an equally competitive but nonaggressive intercollegiate gymnastics meet that served as a control event.

It will be recalled from the previous chapter that social learning theory (Bandura, 1973, 1986) would predict a general increase in fan hostility as a result of lowered inhibitions arising from the observation of aggression on the gridiron. On the other hand, the frustration-aggression hypothesis (Berkowitz, 1965, 1969) would predict that only those fans supporting the losing team would be thwarted and therefore likely to exhibit an increase in hostility. The cathartic view, of course, holds that *all* spectators will be *less* hostile following the observation of player aggression regardless of their allegiances. The results best supported the social learning view insofar as fans of *both* the Army and Navy teams showed an increase in hostility from before to after the contest. For men watching the gymnastics meet, there was no change in hostility over the course of the program.

As with most field investigations, it is often difficult to control for a number of extraneous factors that later become plausible rival explanations for whatever differences might occur. Such was the case in the Philadelphia study. In addition to differences in crowd size and norms governing spectator behavior, one event was held indoors; the other exposed fans to the vagaries of the weather. Perhaps more important, it can confidently be assumed that an indeterminate percentage of the subjects arrived for the football game somewhat intoxicated and became increasingly so as the game progressed. For those inebriated men who interpret their circumstances or those of the players with whom they identify as somehow "threatening," an increase in hostility is to be expected (e.g., S.P. Taylor, Gammon, & Capasso, 1976). One might also question whether the graduate student interviewers were able to faithfully follow the randomization procedure of approaching every *N*th male who passed their station. They might be forgiven for thinking they had miscounted if the upcoming *N*th male is huge and mean-looking, instead seeking the cooperation of the *N*th plus one male. Flushed with success in the pretest phase, their newfound confidence perhaps allowed them to approach designated men in the postevent stage irrespective of appearances. Assuming that huge and ominous looking men are in fact, mean, several such departures from the script could create significant pre- to posttest differences. It has also been suggested (Mann, 1974) that the overall increase in hostility might just as reasonably be attributed to the spectators' disappointment and annoyance with a dull, lopsided contest (Navy 27, Army 0).

The merits of these and other rival explanations were tested in a replication conducted with Canadian university students serving as subjects (Arms, Russell, & Sandilands, 1979). Males and females were assigned randomly to either pre or postevent conditions at ice hockey, a professional wrestling card, or the control event, a provincial swimming meet. Once again, there was a general increase in hostility on the part of those attending events featuring interpersonal aggression. Insofar as the procedure involved the random assignment of (sober) students to the experimental conditions, the rival explanations advanced to account for the Goldstein and Arms (1971) results seem far less probable. Moreover, the outcome of the final match on the wrestling card hung in the balance until the final seconds when the forces of good overcame the forces of evil. Mann's (1974) suggestion that the Philadelphia results might have come about because of a mismatch thereby appears less plausible.

Several other studies have addressed the question of spectators' reactions to aggressively toned sports events. In the first of these, Herrmann (1977) assessed the reactions of 205 German fans to soccer matches. He concluded that "latent tension is neither repressed [gebunden] nor channeled but rather intensified and activated" (cited in Guttmann, 1986, p. 156). Elsewhere, University of Arizona basketball fans displayed an increase in hostility over the course of regular league games (Leuck, Krahenbuhl, & Odenkirk, 1979). A similar result was reported by Harrell (1981) in his analysis of spectator reactions to 14 World Hockey Association (WHA) games in Edmonton.

A supplemental analysis of Harrell's (1981) data revealed an intriguing finding. He found that spectators who were more "tolerant" of aggression (i.e., frequently attended WHA games) showed a decrease in hostility over the first two periods of play. Those attending infrequently showed an increase in hostility. Although Harrell used frequency of attendance as his operational definition of *tolerance*, the same measure also satisfies a definition of *desensitization*. Individuals exposed to prolonged episodes of violence may as a result be less responsive to future violence (e.g., Björkqvist, 1985; M.H. Thomas, Horton, Lippincott, & Drabman, 1977). However one chooses to account for the decline in hostility, Harrell's finding is important in raising the possibility that an individual differences variable may mediate a cathartic response.

Finally, Sloan (1979) noted a sex difference in the response of Notre Dame students to an amateur boxing card. Whereas women became more angry over the course of the evening, men showed no change. However, spectators at Notre Dame football and basketball games displayed general increases in hostility from before to after these contests. In short, spectators viewing sports in which interpersonal aggression is featured more often than not exhibit like behavior; they, too, become hostile. The reactions of spectators appear to closely track the outbursts of aggression by athletes.

Russell (1981c) undertook a period-to-period examination of the course of spectator hostility at an especially violent hockey game and a relatively peaceful game. Fan hostility at the violent game increased from pre- to postgame levels; no change occurred at the peaceful game. Overall however, the pattern of change was found to be curvilinear. As seen in Figure 9.1, spectator hostility increased through the first two periods, declining thereafter. This inverted-U function is centered over the second period during which most of the 184 minutes in aggressive penalties were awarded. (The league average for the season was 56 minutes.) Spectator arousal followed a similar course, a finding of some importance inasmuch as a heightened state of physiological arousal is generally seen to facilitate aggression. However, it is not by itself either a sufficient or necessary condition for aggression. It is also noteworthy that both the hostility and arousal functions began to show signs of decline at the conclusion of the match, a central point of the discussion to follow.

A Digression

I am occasionally asked to speculate about the wider repercussions of a violent contest being staged in a community, especially the suggestion that it contributes

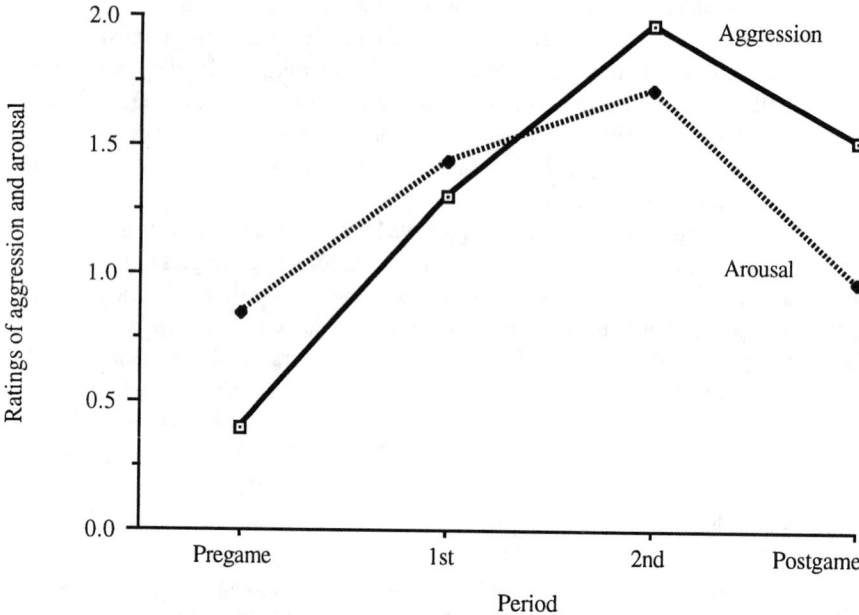

FIGURE 9.1 Spectator aggression and arousal at a violent game (adapted from Russell, 1981c).

in some way to violence in the home. Fortunately, a recent study (White, Katz, & Scarborough, in press) allows me to do more than just speculate that violent sports events have their counterpart in domestic violence. Following *wins* by the NFL Washington Redskins, the emergency wards of Washington, D.C.–area hospitals reported increases in admissions for women who were victims of gunshots, assaults, stabbings, and falls. The authors favor an explanation whereby power motives are enhanced through identification with the winning hometown Redskins (see also Tesler & Alker, 1983). Another explanation would implicate physiological *arousal* carried over from sports events as a contributor to later outbursts.

In the short run, the sheer passage of time works to reduce earlier levels of heightened hostility for those leaving the sports venue. While we don't follow our subjects home or even into the parking lot to observe postgame aggression, evidence would suggest that most highly aroused individuals return to their normal base rate in fairly short order once they leave the event (e.g., Zillmann & Bryant, 1974). However, if a fan were to ruminate or dwell on the episode that originally angered him (e.g., a controversial call by the referee, heckling by rival fans, etc.), a high level of arousal might be maintained for hours, days, or perhaps longer. Later provocations that might under normal circumstances be ignored or resolved peacefully may in the case of highly aroused individuals precipitate an altercation. It seems reasonable to infer, for example, that an indeterminate amount of domestic violence is exacerbated or instigated with the return of a family member still fuming from watching a sport in which violence was prominent. The Roman Emperor Nero is a case in point. Returning home late from watching the chariot races in the Circus Maximus, he was berated by his wife Poppaea; he promptly kicked her to death (H.A. Harris, 1972, p. 215).

However, high levels of anger arousal can be maintained for much longer periods of time and action taken well into the future when individuals continue to dwell on the event that originally angered them. A recent shooting death and suicide by a 28-year-old Montreal man will serve to illustrate the point.

> What appears to have been a simmering grudge over a lost pool game came to a bloody end early Sunday when a man shot and killed a neighbor, wounded the neighbor's common-law wife, then turned the gun on himself during a police car chase. ("Grudge Over," 1990)

An interview with a relative of one of the victims revealed that the perpetrator had remained angry for *8 months* after he lost a pool game at a nearby bar.

Spectatorship Through the Electronic Media

Although large numbers of spectators are subject to a variety of important influences—some good, some not so good—while physically present at sports contests, vastly greater numbers are also open to influence through the medium of television. One might suggest, however, that because viewers are physically distanced from the play and generally isolated from other fans, the effects may differ in strength or form from those observed with stadium spectators. As a consequence, the section to follow will specifically examine the question of whether this subset of the spectator experience affords a cathartic reduction in hostility.

Particularly brutal scenes from the award-winning movie *The Champion* have been used extensively (e.g., Berkowitz, 1965; Berkowitz & Geen, 1966) in a series of experiments designed to assess the role of aggressive cues in eliciting aggression from viewers. Actor Kirk Douglas plays the part of an aging prize fighter who is beaten unmercifully in the final scenes by a young challenger. Typically, the experimental design called for subjects to be randomly assigned to conditions in which they were either angered or not angered by a confederate before seeing the short, five-minute film clip. Immediately thereafter, subjects were provided with an opportunity to aggress (shock) against the confederate-subject with whom they had viewed the film. The same procedures were followed for control subjects who saw an equally arousing but nonaggressive film. Generally, exposure to the boxing film resulted in increases in aggression, especially among subjects who had initially been angered.

Parenthetically, the aggressive cues in the film proved to be highly effective in drawing aggression from aroused subjects. For example, when the confederate was simply introduced to subjects as *Kirk* Anderson, he was aggressed against more than when he was introduced as *Bob* Anderson (Berkowitz & Geen, 1966). As weak a link as sharing the first name of the actor portraying a boxer may appear to be, it was nevertheless sufficient to elicit higher levels of aggression. Indeed, even an introduction in which the confederate was identified as a physical education major with an interest in boxing (as opposed to a speech major) produced comparable results (Berkowitz, 1965). (The powerful role of aggressive cues in eliciting aggression was illustrated in chapter 8 in a description of the weapons effect.)

Would scenes of either a violent hockey game or fast-paced competitive play provide a cathartic experience for viewers? Fourteen-minute videotapes of a fight-filled game and a spirited, skillfully played game sequence (devoid of aggressive incidents) were shown individually to males who had earlier been angered or treated politely by a confederate (Russell, Di Lullo, & Di Lullo, 1989). Following a showing of their assigned film, subjects completed a set of scales designed to assess their current mood state. They also had an opportunity to aggress against the confederate by refusing to help him with his research, thereby delaying his graduation. Was there evidence of catharsis? In a word, no!

Compared to control subjects who worked on a jigsaw puzzle, only *increases* in aggression resulted, and these were confined to angered subjects viewing the film of hockey brawls. Subjects in that condition reported a heightened aggressive mood state and, further, directed more aggression toward the experimental accomplice. Viewing fast-paced, competitive hockey action does not appear to increase viewer aggression. Moreover, the films of nonviolent, competitive play and hockey brawls were judged by independent raters to be equally entertaining. In this case, violence added nothing to the entertainment value of competition. The observation of aggression, then, presented in isolation from other aspects of a competitive sport, increases rather than decreases viewer aggression.

A concluding investigation (Josephson, 1987) in this series of examples used Canadian second- and third-grade boys as subjects. Prior to the experiment, teachers made ratings of the aggression that each youngster characteristically exhibited during the school day. High and low aggressive groups of boys were then shown either a nonviolent or a violent television film. Those assigned to the nonviolent condition watched a very exciting "boys' motocross bike racing team" in action. Boys assigned to the violent condition instead watched a film that featured excessive police violence. The partner of an officer who had been slain by a group of snipers joined an elite Special Weapons and Tactics (SWAT) unit. Together, they set about to avenge the death of their fellow officer, shooting or knocking out all of the snipers.

After viewing their assigned film, the boys were taken to the gymnasium for what was described as a second study, one that called for them to participate in a game of floor hockey. During the games, trained observers recorded all instances of interpersonal aggression (e.g., elbowing, tripping, name-calling, pushing, poking, pinching, and sitting on another boy). Those boys who had been identified as aggressive by their teachers showed an increase in aggression as a result of seeing the violent police film. Boys identified as nonaggressive did not show comparable increases in aggression. It appears that those who exhibit strong aggressive tendencies on a day-to-day basis are more likely to respond with aggression to violent television programming than those with weaker tendencies. Thus far, it does not appear that television provides a special circumstance in which catharsis is somehow able to find expression.

In the Company of Others

Continuing in this research tradition, Dunand, Berkowitz, and Leyens (1984) took into account the *social context* in which aggression is observed. Subjects in this experiment watched either Kirk Douglas in *The Champion* or an equally arousing but nonaggressive track film, *Bannister Wins the Mile*. During the showing of the films, individual subjects were seated alongside another (confederate) subject who watched either passively or in an "active" condition, making enthusiastic comments about the film. Watching the boxing film predictably produced more subject aggression than watching the mile run of Dr. Roger Bannister. More interesting, however, was the finding that the greatest amount of aggression was shown by those who viewed *The Champion* in the company of an actively involved co-spectator (see also Russell & Pigat, 1991). Only a small step is required to generalize this finding to the television room in our homes, the movie theater, or spectators in the stands at a sports event. Seemingly, the behavior of those with whom we watch televised sports can significantly affect our actions over and above the influence attributable to the event itself. Furthermore, the social environment created by coviewers—passive or otherwise—does not appear to provide a situation in which a cathartic process can be seen to operate.

Other social and contextual factors are, of course, at work simultaneously to worsen or soften the impact on individuals viewing televised sports violence. For example, the current status of the viewer's relationship with other co-viewers, the presence of alcohol, and interruptions in the flow of programming—all can determine to some degree the nature and/or intensity of individual responses to media coverage of sports. The research of Worchel, Hardy, and Hurley (1976) provides a case in point. These investigators demonstrated that the interruption of full-length movies by commercials, far from providing a welcome interlude, instead increases the aggression of viewers. Even greater increases in viewer aggression occur when commercial messages are interspersed throughout a violent film. Of course, in real life the impact of interruptions may be lessened insofar as many people turn to other matters during the commercial segments (i.e., letting the cat out, eating, or attending to pressing bodily functions). Thus, media viewing takes place in a complex social setting in which many competing influences interact to shape our responses.

The catharsis/enhancement issue has also been examined by means of showing violent sports films to *groups* of subjects, a procedure that provides a closer approximation to real-life theater audiences. As was noted earlier, arousal is generally thought to facilitate aggression (e.g., Branscombe & Wann, 1992a). As a consequence, a common experimental practice is to insult or otherwise anger half of the subjects prior to exposing them to the films. In the series of investigations to follow, subjects were not deliberately angered. Assembling subjects in this way for the purpose of viewing a film more faithfully reflects the character of audiences generally and thereby enhances the external validity (e.g., Cook & Campbell, 1979) of whatever findings emerge. That is to say, one is not required to generalize very far afield in order to conclude that results from this more realistic research setting apply to similar settings in the real world. However, the downside to this less sophisticated design is that this gain may be at the expense of internal validity inasmuch as the results are likely to be subject to any number of rival interpretations.

Briefly, subjects were shown films with violent content including fight sequences in ice hockey (Celozzi, 1977; Eastwood, 1974); football (Lennon & Hatfield, 1980); and a basketball game in which the visiting team was attacked by hometown fans (Thirer, 1978). Once again, cathartic effects were not in evidence. Pre- to post-film comparisons revealed either no change in subjects' hostility (Eastwood, 1974; Thirer, 1978) or a significant increase (Celozzi, 1977; Lennon & Hatfield, 1980).

Field Studies

On a grander scale, several studies have examined the effects of televised sports violence on members of the general public. In this regard, Senator Edward Kennedy has been credited with an interesting statement to the effect that televised games of the NHL Boston Bruins are followed by increased violence in youth hockey leagues throughout the viewing area (Donner, 1990, p. 158). Evidence of such widespread media influence was sought by Richard Goranson (1982), a York University psychologist, who examined the relationship between levels of aggression in televised NHL games and that occurring on the following day in minor hockey. Obviously, a cathartic reduction was one of several possible outcomes.

The penalty records for each of 45 Toronto Maple Leaf games were compiled, as were the comparable records of 1,202 amateur games played in the television broadcast area. Essentially a zero correlation resulted, this despite a careful examination of the influence of numerous other variables that could conceivably mask a relationship. However, Goranson's (1982) findings are deserving of even closer scrutiny. One suggestion in particular arises from the work of D.P. Phillips (1983, 1986). In similar investigations of the impact of media violence, Phillips has consistently found that the effects on the public peak 3 days after the televised event. Although the reasons for the 3-day lag are unclear at present, the effect is stable and could conceivably be found in Goranson's data or with similar designs. But now I will describe the innovative research program of Phillips.

Using official U.S. government figures (i.e., death certificates), Phillips has found increases in the numbers of homicides, suicides, and automobile fatalities following major media stories of dramatic events that correspond to each tragedy (Phillips, 1983, 1986). For example, the fictional suicide of a popular soap opera heroine is followed shortly thereafter by an increase in suicides among young women in the general population.

Media critics have typically focused their criticism on programs featuring war, police/gangster excesses, violent cartoons, and deranged killers running amok in a community. Rarely are questions asked regarding the effects of violent content in sports programming. One might ask, for example, if a football game or prize fight can be shown to have a direct, widespread, and harmful impact on the viewing public? That is, is there actual concrete evidence of serious harm beyond that shown to occur in the social laboratory? Phillips (1983) says the answer is yes.

All heavyweight championship fights during the period 1973–1978 were examined in relation to U.S. homicide rates in the 10 days following their televised broadcasts. Homicides were found to increase by 12.5% on the third day and 6.6% on the fourth day following the fights. Also, it seems that the steepest rise in homicides occurs after the most heavily publicized fights. Perhaps the most intriguing result of all was the finding that the homicide victims resembled the loser of the title fight in several basic ways. That is, following a loss by a young white fighter, there was an increase in the homicides of young white males. When a black contender lost, the incidence of homicides rose among young black males.

An interesting link with Phillips's (1983) results is seen in one of the experiments in the Berkowitz series (Berkowitz & Geen, 1966). Confederates introduced as having the same first name as the eventual *loser* in the film *The Champion* subsequently attracted the greatest amount of aggression from subjects. Phillips's results, of course, leave unanswered the further question of whether the murderers also resemble the winners of the various title fights. Thus, it would appear that championship prize fights do not indiscriminately cause an increase in homicides but rather selectively harm members of specific subgroups in a population, notably those who resemble the losing fighter.

As a footnote, mention should be made of Phillips's (1983) supplemental finding that homicides decrease *slightly* on the day of the (football) Super Bowl and the following day, rising to peak again on the third day. It should be emphasized that this pattern, while suggestive, fell short of statistical significance. It must also be pointed out that some critics have expressed reservations regarding the conclusions reached by Phillips (e.g., J.N. Baron & Reiss, 1985; Freedman, 1984). Baron and Reiss, for example, provide an in-depth evaluation of the program, concluding "that imitation effects attributed to mass media events . . . are statistical artifacts of the mortality data, the timing of media events, and the methods employed in past research" (p. 347). However, a recent study that used more sophisticated statistical analyses, in the main confirmed Phillips's findings (T.Q. Miller, Heath, Molcan, & Dugoni, 1991). For a review of this fascinating research program and a rebuttal to his critics, see Phillips (1986).

When Aggression Is a Spoof

From time to time it has been argued that watching aggression that is stylized or fictional may be especially conducive to a cathartic response (Noble, 1975). Cartoons, roller derby, professional wrestling, and other theatrical forms serve to illustrate this category of aggression. It goes without saying that if the viewer believes in the authenticity of what he or she is seeing—quite apart from the objective reality of the situation—then that aggression should more correctly be described as realistic. For example, while regular wrestling fans are not especially skeptical, university students attending a professional wrestling card overwhelmingly saw the ring action as a sham (Arms et al., 1979). So dubious were they, in fact, that several planned analyses comparing believers with nonbelievers had to be abandoned. Even so, you will recall that in this same study a general increase in hostility was found among those students watching the wrestling matches.

In another experiment (Berkowitz & Alioto, 1973), the fictional nature of a wartime documentary was created by means of instructions that preceded the film. Some subjects were told that the film they were about to see was a Hollywood reenactment; others were led to believe that they would be seeing actual footage from the battlefield. Both versions resulted in increases in aggression. A similar test using full-length movies was conducted by Worchel and his colleagues (1976). The first film depicted realistic aggression (*Attica*) and the other, fictional aggression (*The Mouse That Roared*). Both produced equal increases in viewers' aggression.

In a final example (Russell, Horn, & Huddle, 1988), the combatants were females. Men were individually assigned to watch either a 20-minute film clip of a ladies' professional wrestling match, a segment in which actresses wrestled topless in a makeshift mud pit, or a no-film control condition. The principal finding was an increase in hostility on the part of men watching both versions of stylized aggression. In summary, it would appear from these and other studies that there is not a special case to be made for fictional aggression somehow creating conditions that are conducive to a cathartic experience. Rather, as with realistic aggression, hostility is likely to be enhanced by fictional depictions of interpersonal conflict.

Conclusion and Implications

Despite the general popularity of cathartic beliefs, participants and spectators in sports show little evidence of experiencing anything resembling a cathartic response to aggression. Rather, just the opposite usually occurs. With few exceptions (e.g., Freedman, 1984), this conclusion is consistent with those reached in other reviews of the sports (Goranson, 1978; Peper, 1980; Russell, 1983b) and nonsports literature (Geen, 1983; Geen & Quanty, 1977; Geen, Stonner, & Shope, 1975; Goranson, 1970; Quanty, 1976; Walters, 1966). The conclusion of Goranson (1978) aptly sums up the sports research on vicarious aggression catharsis: "I think that this is one of the rare occasions in behavioural research where an unqualified conclusion is warranted. The observation of violence does not reduce aggressiveness" (p. 12). I can only add that a belief that *participation* in aggressive sports acts to reduce aggressiveness is similarly unsupported by research. Neither can we look to the media or fictionalized portrayals of sports aggression to provide a unique set of conditions under which catharsis is somehow able to operate.

If the widespread belief that sports offer participants and spectators opportunities for a cathartic venting of aggression is largely myth, can there be any harm in people retaining the belief much as they do superstitions? I think there *is* cause for concern and a case to be made for actively dispelling cathartic beliefs. While a belief that the number 13 causes misfortune may present difficulties for those managing skyscrapers, and a few others, the problems are not serious and can be easily resolved. On the other hand, actions taken on the basis of cathartic beliefs can have far-reaching and serious consequences for individual well-being and the success of institutional programs.

Notably, some parents holding unchallenged cathartic beliefs may enroll or keep their children in aggressive sports, confident that the sport is managing, and providing an outlet for, their child's aggression. From the parents' perspective, the sport can be expected over time to moderate their youngster's aggressive tendencies. However, as the evidence indicates, their sport-as-therapy prescription is unlikely to produce the desired outcome. Problems of aggression management are better dealt with by qualified clinicians (see, e.g., A.P. Goldstein & Keller, 1987; Novaco, 1986).

A general acceptance of cathartic notions can further be expected to influence the choice of activities to be included in community, educational and other institutional programs. When it comes to a choice, should the prison recreational program feature volleyball or boxing? Obviously, boxing should get the nod if you believe it will serve as a healthy outlet for the inmates' aggression. Better their aggression be discharged in the ring than in a riot! Again, the results could be terribly disappointing.

Finally, the assumption of cathartic benefits provides a convenient justification for the aggressive content in sports and portrayals of violence in media programming (Novaco, 1986). Richard Walters expressed this point well in summarizing his early review of the aggression literature as follows:

> The highly consistent evidence from studies of aggressive models by Bandura, Berkowitz, Walters, and others suggests that the catharsis doctrine is not merely mistaken, but its promulgation can lead to the defense of mass-media content that has socially harmful effects. (Walters, 1966, p. 71)

I agree.

An Exception to the Rule?

Is there a case *for* catharsis? The answer appears to be a qualified yes. Cathartic effects have been reported with some consistency, albeit under a fairly limited set of circumstances. Those circumstances typically involve a situation where an angry individual is provided with the opportunity to immediately aggress directly against the person who has just provoked him. Under these and certain other conditions, an aggressor may subsequently be found to be less aggressive (e.g., Doob & Wood, 1972; Konecni, 1975; Konecni & Doob, 1972).

It may be that Plato (in *The Republic*) was the first to get it right. In the course of providing a valuable methodological critique of human aggression research, Konecni (1984) draws our attention to Plato's advice for men made angry:

> "If one man is angry with another, he can take it out of him on the spot, and will be less likely to pursue the quarrel further." . . .Thus, the *performance* of *aggressive* actions, provided that one is *angry*, against the *anger instigator*, will decrease the probability of further *violent actions*. (p. 30)

However, extending these circumscribed findings to make a case for catharsis acting in general circumstances to reduce interpersonal aggression presents some obvious difficulties. Those party to most altercations in sports (as elsewhere) are caught up in a series of exchanges: provocations—aggressive response—retaliation—retaliation to the retaliatory attack, and so on. What happens all too often is an upward spiral of aggression, with neither party able to extricate himself easily from the exchanges. While escalation effects may begin over petty issues, the final level of hostilities is out of all proportion to the magnitude of the original provocation (J.H. Goldstein, Davis, & Herman, 1975; J.H. Goldstein, Davis, Kernis, & Cohn, 1981). The point to be emphasized is that in real life the "action" is not suddenly frozen in time following our attack on the person who provoked us. It is unlikely that the individual we attack will "learn his lesson" and walk away. Rather, he will attack us in turn, probably with even greater force. We, of course, usually feel compelled to respond at least in kind. So, while we may experience a catharsis of aggression in that brief moment before a retaliation occurs, a retaliation is almost certain to follow on the heels of our attack. In short, the special circumstances under which a cathartic effect can be demonstrated are embedded among other behavioral sequences (e.g., an escalation of hostility), which simply override any tendencies for aggression to be reduced.

A Postscript

There is, of course, every reason to continue research on catharsis. As Murray and Feshbach (1978) conclude in their aptly titled article *Let's Not Throw the Baby Out With the Bathwater*, it would be premature to abandon efforts to specify the conditions that facilitate catharsis. As their own work shows, *fantasy* aggression may decline following aggressive behavior. The special importance of this finding lies in the possibility that lowered levels of aggressive imagery may, in turn, lead to a further decline in aggressive behavior. The implementation of most proposed "solutions" to real-world violence are often forestalled by various social, economic and political practicalities. As a consequence, it behooves us to explore fully every avenue that could conceivably lead to promising strategies that give hope to reducing conflict on all levels. Catharsis may yet play a role.

Suggested Readings

Konecni, V.J. (1975). Annoyance, type and duration of postannoyance activity, and aggression: The "cathartic effect." *Journal of Experimental Psychology: General, 104,* 76-102.
   This classic experiment is the starting point for anyone planning to undertake experimental research on catharsis.

Novaco, R.W. (1986). Anger as a clinical and social problem. In R.J. Blanchard & D.C. Blanchard (Eds.), *Advances in the study of aggression* (Vol. 2, pp. 1–67). New York: Academic Press.
   The topic of catharsis is reviewed in the context of a comprehensive discussion of the role of anger in clinical and social settings.

10

Spectatorship and Crowd Behavior

One of the more intriguing actors present at a sports event is the spectator. The spectators' role in aiding or hindering athletic performance has been highlighted in earlier discussions of social impact theory, the home field advantage, and social facilitation (chap. 2). However, if we redirect our focus away from the influence that spectators have on athletes to consider instead the behavior of spectators themselves, we find that the available evidence on most questions is fairly limited. Even within the broader context of collective behavior, the dynamics underlying the various behaviors of crowds are only partially understood despite a great amount of speculative theorizing over the better part of a century (see, e.g., Lang & Lang, 1961; Milgram & Toch, 1969; R.H. Turner & Killian, 1972; K. Young, 1946). Of course, evidence relating to the behavior of the subset of sports crowds is even more sparse.

I have chosen to limit coverage in this chapter to five major aspects of spectatorship from among a larger number of topics that have traditionally attracted the interest of social scientists. These include the motivational question of why people attend a sports event, the composition of audiences, and aspects of the spectator experience itself. Additionally, two of the more sinister forms of spectator behavior, panics and riots, will be discussed in conjunction with the factors thought to underlie their occurrence.

Motives for Attendance

Not everyone comes to see the game. For some, the contest merely provides the setting and opportunities for the expression of other motives. The social contacts provided by the crowd itself suggests a reason for people to attend. This very point was elaborated by William McDougall (1908) in developing his case for the existence of a gregarious instinct in humans. The question he posed at the turn of the century certainly argues convincingly for the view that we are social creatures. (However, additionally labeling the observed behavior as an "instinct" creates a tautology that adds nothing to our understanding.) McDougall asks his readers, "What proportion of the ten thousand witnesses of a football match would stand for an hour or more in the wind and rain, if each man were isolated from the rest of the crowd and saw only the players?" (p. 74). We would guess very few in 1908, fewer today.

Editorial comments appearing in *Cricket* during the 1880s deplored the fact that many of those in attendance at the Eton-Harrow match knew nothing about the game (Sandiford, 1982). In particular, it seems that thousands of ladies had turned the event into a fashion show. Among contemporary events, the Epsom and Kentucky derbies appear to have suffered similar fates.

Other motives for attendance also found expression at the medieval tournaments where knights practiced their lethal skills. A 13th-century narrator is quoted in his advice "to a young man eager for seduction" (Guttmann, 1981, p. 15):

> These tourneys, I repeat, provide
> A fitting field for you who would
> Learn the delights of womanhood.
> For many a fancy wench abounds
> Round and about the tilting grounds;
> Gaily they flock from far and near.

From antiquity to the present, then, spectators have attended sports events for a variety of reasons, only one of which is to observe the skill of the athletes.

Those who have studied crowd behavior (Mann & Pearce, 1978; Mehrabian, 1976; Sloan, 1979) note the strong attraction of people for the company of others who share similar interests. Mehrabian (1976) sees our attendance at sports arenas as "conducive to socializing; it may lead to the development of new friendships or the renewal or intensification of old ones" (p. 284). The case for the socializing function of spectatorship draws indirect support from data provided by spectators at Australian football league games. Interviews revealed that only 20% came alone; the remainder were in the company of friends or relatives (Mann, 1977, cited in Mann & Pearce, 1978). Virtually the same ratio was noted in marathon queues for tickets to Melbourne football matches (Mann, 1969). Elsewhere, 26% of the celebrants at Ohio State's 1974 football victory over the University of Michigan were alone (Aveni, 1977), whereas only 15% of those attending a Canadian ice hockey game arrived unaccompanied (Russell, 1992b).

Of course, these figures are, at best, only suggestive of an affiliative motive for attending sports events. Moreover, if such a motive *is* operating, it may not produce the socially enriching experiences suggested above by Mehrabian (1976). Several studies (e.g., Arms et al., 1979; Russell, 1981c) note that the quality of spectators' moods (e.g., "social affection") instead deteriorates during a sports event. These findings may, however, be confined to hockey, wrestling, and similar combative sports. Other types of spectator sports may prove to be more conducive to forging friendships and fostering harmonious relations.

The relative importance of spectators' motives for attending a sports event is seen in the results of a recent field study (Russell, 1992b). Following a random sampling procedure, teams of carefully rehearsed student interviewers approached adults at Western Hockey League (WHL) games. The 5-minute interview asked how frequently they attended WHL games and sought ratings of the strength of their reasons for attending. Although men and women were equally motivated to attend a hockey game, they did so for somewhat different reasons. Males rate their interest in watching "good, skillful hockey" and "fights" as stronger reasons for attending than do females. On the other hand, women attend out of a stronger desire to "please someone else."

Spectators' frequency of attendance was also related to their reasons for attending. People who regularly attend games rate "to support the team" and "good, skillful hockey" stronger than those who attend less often. Those attending infrequently rate "to please someone else" and "nothing better to do" as more important than do regulars.

In sum, the major reason for attendance overall is the opportunity to witness "good, skillful hockey" (i.e., the sport being played at an elite level). This finding reflects, after all, what the sport is supposed to be all about. In this regard, G.J. Smith (1976) found that adults select their sports hero/heroine largely on the basis of ability. A strong reason for WHL attendance may therefore be to see the skillful play of the game's future stars.

Two other important reasons for attending deserve comment. A social motive (i.e., "to meet people") and the opportunity "to watch the fights" were rated as average in strength. Interestingly, those who attend in anticipation of fights erupting are to be found largely among the young, single adult males.

The motivations for attending can be expected to vary from sport to sport and also with the importance of an event, such as the Olympic games (Mashiach, 1980). Included among other reasons for attendance is the venue's traditional role in providing an agreed-upon site for those planning to stage a disturbance. Rival groups of supporters can create disorder under the watchful eye of an interested media. These acts of *outlawry* (Mann, 1979) characterize only a few sports, notably soccer. In such instances, the contest itself is often of secondary interest to the contending groups. Of course, particular individuals may attend for other, entirely anomalous reasons (see Speaking Tangentially 10.1).

****

Speaking Tangentially 10.1: The Rainbow Man
The motives for attendance are diverse and multiple. Consider the example of Rollen Stewart, otherwise known as the "Rainbow Man," who is one of several individuals who travel to major (televised) sports events for the sole purpose of getting their religious message on camera. After receiving a call from the Lord in a Pasedena motel, Rollen converted all of his worldly possessions into cash; he doesn't believe in banks. Since 1977 his 50-week-a-year-job as a "cheerleader for Christ" has taken him to a royal wedding, beauty pageants, and cameo appearances at the Indianapolis 500, football, basketball, and golf. Not easy work considering the travel, figuring out camera angles and dodging security guards all the while concealing his multicolored wig and "John 3:16" banner. His motive for attendance is singular; he readily admits that he doesn't care who wins or even who plays ("Rainbow Man," 1987).

****

Turning to more general considerations, there is evidence (e.g., D.F. Anderson, 1979) to suggest that for some, spectatorship may serve as a substitute for participation in sports. Interviews with residents of a metropolitan area in the United

States were classified as either "nonfans," "spectator fans," or "participant fans," the latter being actively engaged in their favorite sport rather than merely watching. Nonfans, however, reported greater participation in sports than did respondents classified as spectator fans. Moreover, G.J. Smith, Patterson, Williams, and Hogg (1981) found that 88% of their sample of truly dedicated fans actively participated in sports on a weekly basis. Taken together with Anderson's results, it would seem that the dedicated fan is actively involved in recreational activities; those who can be described as "casual" spectators likely participate less than nonfans.

Crowd Composition

In the introduction to *Sports Spectators*, Allen Guttmann (1986) expresses his dismay at the lack of basic information about the sorts of people who in the modern era "pushed through the turnstiles and took their seats in the grandstands and the bleachers" (p. 1). Scholars have instead chosen to focus their efforts largely on studying the causes, and means of controlling, sports-related violence. He takes issue with this disproportionate emphasis in arguing as follows:

> Important as these questions are, they are not the *only* ones worthy of sustained attention. It is also important to ask just who the spectators were and how they behaved when they *weren't* rioting. It is important to ask about the political functions of spectatorship, about the social role of the spectators, about their gender and social class, about the relationship between the "active" participation of the athlete and the "passive" participation of the fan. (p. 2)

Finding myself persuaded by Guttmann and not wishing to perpetuate this imbalance, I have attempted to bring together in this section the descriptive findings of several relevant investigations. It is to these studies of crowd composition that we now turn.

It is stating the obvious to point out that various sports attract spectators of different stripes. It is equally obvious that the spectators at any single sports event are far from homogeneous. Across sports, audiences can be expected to differ in terms of such factors as age, male/female ratio, socioeconomic level, race, ethnic background, personality, and so on. Not surprisingly, the *behaviors* exhibited by spectators at different sports are also diverse. For example, Wray Vamplew (1980) has contrasted crowd disorders at British sports events during the Victorian era and documented the excesses of drinking and gambling among soccer fans, behavior not particularly in evidence at cricket matches. At the same time, Vamplew acknowledges that situational factors such as physical constraints (standing vs. seating accommodations) and the "nature" of the sport itself may also have been contributing causes of the disorders that marred soccer matches of the day.[1]

---

[1] Soccer matches are described as inherently more "explosive" than cricket matches.

Since the days of Rome's Circus Maximus, a facility that accommodated 250,000 spectators, arrangements have been made to ensure divisions by social class. The knightly tournaments of 16th-century Britain similarly saw stands and pavilions constructed for the benefit of spectators, with the choice vantage points made available to the upper classes. The arrangements included a gallery specially set aside for the ladies (Guttmann, 1981). The practice has its modern-day counterpart in the private boxes and suites available in domed stadia for those of privilege.

The composition of sports crowds can further be expected to differ with the importance, venue, or timing of the event. For example, major events such as the annual Superbowl game (football) or baseball's World Series attract many people who rarely if ever attend games during the regular season. There has also been a long-standing recognition that the composition of crowds varies with the workweek. Explanations cited by Sandiford (1982) for the disruptive behavior of British cricket fans in 1887 were generally in agreement that a cricket crowd was not responsible for throwing bottles onto the field. Rather, the culprits were a "holiday crowd"! Then, as now, in the aftermath of disorder, the genuine fan is differentiated from "an unruly element," "a small minority," or "visitors bent on disruption." Apologists are quick to point out that the *true* fan would not discredit his team or sport by his behavior.

Who's at the Track?

The question of crowd composition has been examined in only a handful of investigations. The most comprehensive of these is Rosecrance's (1986) study of those who play the ponies. His classification system deserves to be summarized in some detail.

John Rosecrance, an inveterate horse player for over 30 years, benefited from his insider status in developing a typology of those at the track. Interviews with 95 racetrack gamblers at Hollywood Park and Santa Anita provided the groundwork for classifying players according to five categories.

1. Pro (5%): Professional handicappers are those who devote all of their time and energy to the practice of their craft. They earn their livelihood at the track and only receive recognition as a pro after at least two or three years of sustained winning. Their strategy for success stresses objectivity and generally excludes elements of luck, hunches, emotion, sentimentality, or desperation from their wagering decisions. Typically pros dress conservatively at the track, remain outwardly calm during the running of a race, and regard complaining over the outcome as bad form.

2. Serious player (10%): Serious players have made a full-time commitment to their occupation, often leaving the security of a regular job to indulge their passion. They are often poor losers, maintain less control over their emotions and are inconsistent in their betting strategies. Rosecrance observes that the compulsive gambler, unsuccessfully chasing pro status and constantly searching for funds to wager, can be found in this category.

3. Bustout (5%): Players identified as bustouts support their track activities largely from temporary, menial occupations (e.g., dishwasher, washroom attendants). They are chronically broke, having previously exhausted all lines of credit. They often cannot afford the price of admission to the grounds and instead wait until after the seventh race when the gates are opened. Even the cost of the *Racing Form* may prove prohibitive. They will ask departing patrons for their copy or rummage through the wastebaskets. Rosecrance found that bustouts are surprisingly knowledgeable about handicapping but do badly at the payout window because of "inappropriate betting strategies and poor money management" (p. 90). Compulsive gamblers enjoy a dual classification, being found among both bustouts and serious player categories.

4. Regular (45%): Pensioners, or those with jobs whose hours of work allow them to attend the races, make up this major category of player. The older punters are typically conservative and bet chalk (i.e., the favorites). These players regard their activities as meaningful, with their day at the track adding a certain zest to the other wise drab days of retirement.[2]

Other regulars who are "flexibly employed" augment their income from generally low-paying jobs (e.g., gardening, taxicab driving). Of all the categories of horse players, they are the most vocal, rooting on their choices and booing the losing jockeys. This flexibly employed segment contains a disproportionate number of Blacks and Mexican-Americans, who usually bet the long shots as a wagering strategy.

5. Part-time player (35%): Part-time players include those whose jobs allow them to attend only on weekends. The majority are white-collar workers, many of whom have aspirations of becoming regular players upon their retirement. While most are satisfied with their present jobs, a minority express dissatisfaction, feeling that the responsibilities of their jobs keep them from adequately analyzing the races.

Rosecrance has identified several additional elements among those to be found at the track. These include *regular* fans and *occasionals*, the latter group attending only infrequently. Neither type regards themselves as horse players. Additionally, note is taken of those involved with the actual staging of the races (i.e., *insiders*), among whom are the jockeys, owners, and track officials. This classificatory system lays an important groundwork for future comparative studies of the players among racetrack and other betting crowds.

A final "nagging" question, unanswered by Rosecrance, concerns that group of racing fans who leave the track each day as winners. Speaking Tangentially 10.2 identifies the qualifications necessary for membership in this elite circle.

****

Speaking Tangentially 10.2: Win, Place, or Show
What sort of abilities does it take to pick the winners at the racetrack? Ceci and Liker (1986) studied punters at Brandywine raceway in Delaware in an effort to identify the fac-

---

[2] The elderly horse players themselves provide an additional off-track category for their less fortunate cronies whose domestic obligations keep them from the track: honey dos— "Honey do this, Honey do that"!

tors involved in successful betting decisions. They initially divided a sample of men who closely followed harness racing into "expert" and "nonexpert" groups. The experts were those able to pick the top horse, according to actual post-time odds, in 9 out of 10 races and the top three finishers in at least five of the races. While the nonexperts demonstrated far less handicapping expertise, they nonetheless performed above a chance level.

What were the critical factors that distinguished between the successful and not-so-successful handicappers? They were found to be equal in virtually all respects: age, experience, socioeconomic status, and intelligence. There was, however, one major difference. The experts used more *cognitively complex* decision-making strategies. Simply put, the complex reasoning required for successful handicapping does not derive from experience, IQ, and so on, but rather from an ability to process available information "using a mental model that [contains] multiple interaction effects and nonlinearity" (Ceci & Liker, 1986, p. 255). You will recall that cognitive complexity was described in chapter 5 and identified as a critical attribute of leaders required to perform well under stress.

****

Who Watches High School Football Games?

Crowd composition was also the focus of an investigation of those attending high school football games in the biethnic city of El Paso, Texas (Freischlag & Hardin, 1975). Methodologically, the study is especially noteworthy. The potentially biasing effect of a selection factor as a rival explanation for their findings was virtually ruled out at the outset. Few potential spectators to these games, where crowds averaged 1,850, were barred from attending for financial reasons or because of conflicts with jobs. At each stadium, an inexpensive ticket provided admission to *all* seats. Additionally, the games were played in the evening, after normal working hours. In effect, nearly anyone who wanted to attend could do so.

The distribution of spectators by social class did not differ from the general population of El Paso. However, among spectators social class was itself related to their *ethnic* backgrounds with Mexican-Americans being overrepresented in the lower strata. The social class of spectators was, however, unrelated to whether they chose to sit in peripheral or more central seating locations.

The major thrust of the study involved comparisons of the academic achievement of student spectators with students at large and also in relation to where they chose to sit in the stands. To their credit, Freischlag and Hardin (1975) verified the self-reports of grade point averages by means of school records. Students attending the football games differed from the general population of students insofar as the distribution of their grades was leptykurtic; that is, a heightened peak centered over the average B and C grades. Noticeably absent from the stadia were A and F students. Furthermore, the academically superior students were found to sit in more central locations. Among those seated in the peripheral sections, only 37% had A and B grades, whereas nearly two thirds of those in the central sections were A and B scholars.[3]

---

[3] This pattern of voluntary seating by students in accordance with their grades is reminiscent of an early classroom study by Coleman Griffith (1922).

At Ringside

The composition of crowds attending a professional wrestling card has been investigated by Bratton and his students (Bratton et al., 1978). Interviews were conducted with equal numbers of male and female fans of Stampede Wrestling, a weekly event on the Calgary sports calendar. Analyses of demographic data revealed that 46% of those in attendance were married, 36% were single, and 18% "other." The distribution by age was as follows: under 18 (24%), 19 to 30 (39%), 31 to 45 (23%), and over 45 (14%). Education was distributed in a pattern not unlike that found generally in the province, that is, junior high school (29%), senior high school (36%), trade/technical school (13%), some college (12%), and university (6%). Spectators at the matches additionally described themselves as predominantly Protestant (55%), with a further 20% indicating ties to the Catholic church and 13% indicating "other." Thereafter, 5% had no religious affiliation, and the balance were distributed across Jews (3%) and Mormons (2%). However, actual church attendance was an entirely different matter. Only 10% indicated that they attend church regularly, 39% occasionally attend, and fully 47% never manage to find their way to a church.

The answers to several more probing questions asked in the Bratton et al. (1978) interviews provide a glimpse of the psychological makeup of a wrestling audience. First, they would appear to be strongly attracted to the sport, a majority stating that they preferred to watch wrestling over other sports. Regarding their own participation in sports, 40% indicated an active involvement. Finally, what sort of wrestling did they most enjoy? Wrestling action described as *brawling* and *bloody* was preferred by 83% of the respondents. To a companion question, 63% stated that they enjoyed *clean* and *scientific* wrestling.

While demographic information on the composition of crowds in attendance at various sports is an important first step in developing an understanding of crowd behavior, such data may be specific to a particular time period or geographical region. For example, in recent years we have witnessed a sharp rise in the popularity of professional wrestling. Slick media promotions and its faddish appeal to those in the higher social strata may have altered the traditional demographic profile of wrestling audiences. For these reasons, our ability to generalize may be somewhat restricted.

The Spectator Experience

Just as athletes are influenced by spectators, so too are spectators influenced by what they see. Audiences are not somehow immune to personal influence as a result of the events they witness. We saw in the previous chapter that in the case of observing combatant sports, spectators frequently experience an increase in hostility as well as changes in a number of other emotional states. The results of observing sports action may be transitory, long-term, or trivial, or they may have major consequences for observers and those with whom they are involved on a day-to-day basis.

There is a commonly recognized tendency for people to establish bonds, however tenuous, with successful others (e.g., the firm that employs them, social organizations, the regiment). One of the clearest expressions of this tendency is to be found in sports and to a considerable degree characterizes the passionate loyalty of some fans to an athlete or team. The nature of that bond has been described by Mann (1974): "That loyalty to a sporting team involves the kind of emotional reaction ordinarily associated with defense of self and family testifies to the role of the team as a kind of reference group" (p. 37).

We see, for example, that fully 98% of males identified as deeply committed sports fans report being either somewhat or very upset following a loss by their favorite team (G.J. Smith et al., 1981). A loss by a college football team has further been shown to result in partisan spectators estimating a greater likelihood of war erupting in the Persian Gulf, as well as the anticipation of a greater number of allied casualties (Schweitzer, Zillmann, Weaver, & Luttrell, 1992). By contrast, males anticipated doing better on an anagrams task and expected to enjoy greater success in their attempts to date attractive women after their basketball team won (Hirt, Zillmann, Erickson, & Kennedy, in press). Spectatorship, then, can produce changes in our emotions, judgments, motivations, and behaviors.

The behavioral consequences for those of us who strongly identify with a team are varied. Among other things, intense loyalties can influence our evaluation of others (Branscombe, Wann, Noel, & Coleman, 1992); increase physiological arousal (Branscombe & Wann, 1992a); and affect our self-esteem (Branscombe & Wann, 1992b). The direction of such changes, of course, depends on whether *our* team wins or losses. The two topics selected to illustrate that broad range of influence involve changes in our day-to-day activities as well as shifts in our underlying motivations. Both arise as a result of *successful* performances by our favorite team.

The BIRG Phenomenon

Success in sports is generally equated with winning, failure with losing. Robert Cialdini and his colleagues (Cialdini et al., 1976) sought to examine the effects that associations with "success" might have on the individual. They reasoned that football fans would show by their overt behavior a tendency to seek to share in the good fortune of their team. Such behaviors, intended to establish links with successful others, are collectively referred to as the "basking in reflected glory" (BIRG) phenomenon. As a special form of personal image management, fans vicariously share in the triumphs and defeats of their favorite team. Wins see them attempt to draw closer to their team; losses encourage a distancing from those who have fallen short of success. In effect, our team's triumphs become our triumphs, and as we shall see shortly, our team's failures become *their* failures.

What aspects of fans' observable behavior could conceivably be affected by their team's success? Cialdini et al. (1976) reckoned that one's affiliation with a winning team might be publicly expressed in several ways, one of which was the wearing of

team-related apparel (e.g., school sweatshirts, scarfs, buttons) during the days immediately following a victory. The prediction was formally tested at five major U.S. colleges, each with a nationally prominent football program. Support for the BIRG phenomenon was forthcoming insofar as students wore more team-related apparel on
Mondays following a weekend victory than they did on Mondays following a loss.

A second study was undertaken in an attempt to expand the empirical base of
support for the phenomenon. Students at Arizona State University were contacted
by telephone and asked to describe the results of either a football game their
school had recently won or a game the team had recently lost. Students describing
an Arizona win used the personal form of the plural pronoun *we* more often than
did their fellow students asked to describe their team's loss. The interviewers
were typically told, *"We* beat Houston, 17 to 14" or *"They* lost to Missouri, 30 to
20" (Cialdini, 1985, p. 167). The impersonal form *they* serves to distance or otherwise dissociate the fan, in his own eyes or those of others, from the team's failure. There was even a tendency for the BIRG phenomenon to be stronger when
students thought the caller represented an independent survey agency than when
they thought the survey originated on campus.

A variation of the telephone survey (Cialdini et al., 1976) involved having the
students take a test of general information before being asked to describe a recently won or lost game. The test was rigged to ensure that some of the students
would themselves experience failure. In contrast to students who were allowed to
experience success, those who had just failed used the plural *we* more often in describing a recent team victory. This same group seldom used *we* in their descriptions of a defeat. On the other hand, students who were successful on the test used
the pronoun *we* equally often in describing their team's victories and defeats.

Lee (1985) conducted a replication that additionally examined the impact of
personal success/failure on memory for details of their university's recent basketball *losses*. Subjects who ostensibly had just experienced success on a quiz tapping their knowledge of obscure university facts recalled more details of the basketball games than those for whom a failing experience had been arranged. Lee
explains this interesting result in terms of a threat-induced denial of knowledge.
That is, those for whom university affairs were salient engaged an ego-protective
mechanism whereby they dissociated themselves from a mediocre team showing.
In the case of low-saliency subjects, they feared compounding their earlier failure
by giving further incorrect answers. Lee additionally found that students experiencing success used *we* more often when the performance of the basketball team
was salient to them than when it was an unimportant matter. There was a slight
tendency in the opposite direction for those experiencing failure to use *we* less often when the team's record was salient than when it was nonsalient.

As with any behavioral disposition, fans are going to differ in the strength of
their tendencies to BIRG or to cut-off reflected failure (CORF). Wann and
Branscombe (1990a) reasoned that those with close ties to a team would be more
strongly affected by their team's success or failure than those with weaker allegiances. Their study of Kansas University "Jayhawk" basketball revealed that the
strength of fans' identification was indeed a factor that determined their reactions

to victories and defeats. Those with strong ties to the team showed a greater tendency to BIRG following Jayhawk wins than those who only weakly identified with the team. Those whom Wann and Branscombe describe as die-hard fans were, additionally, less prone to CORFing following Jayhawk losses. Rather, it is the fair-weather fans or those who weakly identify with the team who show the strongest tendency to distance themselves from failure.

One suggestion that emerges from the above is that the success enjoyed by others with whom we strongly identify may act in ways that offset our own shortcomings. Those fans who are most susceptible to the BIRG phenomenon just may be those who have the poorest self-concept. As Cialdini (1985) reasons, "deep inside is a sense of low personal worth that directs them to seek prestige not from the generation or promotion of their own attainments but from the generation or promotion of their associations with others' attainments" (p. 168). Cialdini's interpretation is intriguing and suggests several testable hypotheses.

Cialdini's (1985) conclusion is challenged by a view that instead sees close ties to a sports team acting as a buffer against feelings of alienation and depression (Branscombe & Wann, 1992b). Support for this position is seen in the responses of students to several standardized measures. In general, those who identified most strongly with teams were also those with higher self-esteem and lower feelings of depression and alienation. The authors note, however, that the correlations, although significant, were weak.

BIRG and Attribution Theory

The BIRG phenomenon has more recently been extended to attribution theory (Burger, 1985), a topic featured in chapter 3. If people draw close to winners and distance themselves from losers, then the attributions made for a team's victory should be similar to those typically made by the fan for himself when he experiences success (i.e., internal attributions). With the passage of time a selective forgetting process is thought to occur whereby self and team-flattering reasons (e.g., the home team's outstanding play) are increasingly recalled at the expense of situational reasons such as "Our opponents had an off night." Inasmuch as the BIRG phenomenon has more recently been characterized as a "cutting-off-reflected-failure" process (Snyder, Lassegard, & Ford, 1986), fans are better described as actively distancing themselves from home team defeats. As a result of connections to the team being severed, attributions for a team loss would not be predicted to become more situational over time as they do in the individual case. Burger tested these predictions by phoning students on the morning following a basketball game that their university had won or lost. Additionally, other students were phoned 4 or 5 days after the two contests and were asked why they thought the team had won or lost the game. The results were revealing.

First, the BIRG phenomenon was found to be alive and well. Once again, students used the pronouns *we* and *us* to describe the reasons for a win by their team, avoiding the use of these pronouns after a defeat. This difference in *we* terms held even for the two groups of individuals called several days later. More important, Burger found the predicted increase in internal attributions from the morning after a victory to the time when students were called some 4 to 5 days later. By contrast, those in the immediate and delayed conditions following a loss by the team offered more (internal) dispositional reasons overall for their team's defeat than did those phoned after a victory. However, there was no evidence of an increase in dispositional attributions from the immediate to the delayed conditions following a loss. Thus, attributional effects of the BIRG phenomenon are enhanced over time following observed success, whereas its impact tends to remain constant for fans who have distanced themselves from the team following a loss.

In addition to our emotional states, overt behaviors, and attributions, can our basic motivations similarly be altered by the changing fortunes of our favorite team in competition? In the case of power motivation, the answer would appear to be yes.

Power Motives

One among a number of human motivations is a desire for power. Numerous sports are rife with power cues, not the least of which are the cues provided by the all-powerful victors of a competition. The basic question for Tesler and Alker (1983) was whether the power needs of individual spectators are affected by the outcome of a contest. These investigators chose college football as the setting for assessing the impact of winning and losing on spectators' power motivation. But first, a word about power itself.

An initial distinction between the *image* of power and *actual* power should be kept in mind. An increase in the image of power is seen in the activities of fans following their team's victory (i.e., the BIRG phenomenon). However, an equally important question remains. Would a desire for actual power also be increased by the spectator experience and, if so, under what conditions?

Tesler and Alker (1983) distributed advertisements for a paid position as an experimenter to football fans entering the stadium before a game. Those interested were asked to phone for details that same day. They reached an answering machine that described two available positions. The first (Position A) required the individual to judge the performance of experimental subjects. Those judgments, then, would form the sole basis for determining whether or not the subjects received rewards (actual power). The second (Position B) was described as one in which the individual would appear to make the decision but actually the person hired for Position A would have the final say (image of power). These procedures were followed at two home games, one a victory, the other a loss. How did a hometown win (high power) and a loss (low power) influence spectators' choice of experimenter roles?

As can be seen in Figure 10.1, most of those who had just witnessed a victory by their team chose the power position. Spectators whose team had just suffered a defeat instead chose the position that provided only the illusion of power. However, these effects on power motivations arising from vicariously experiencing

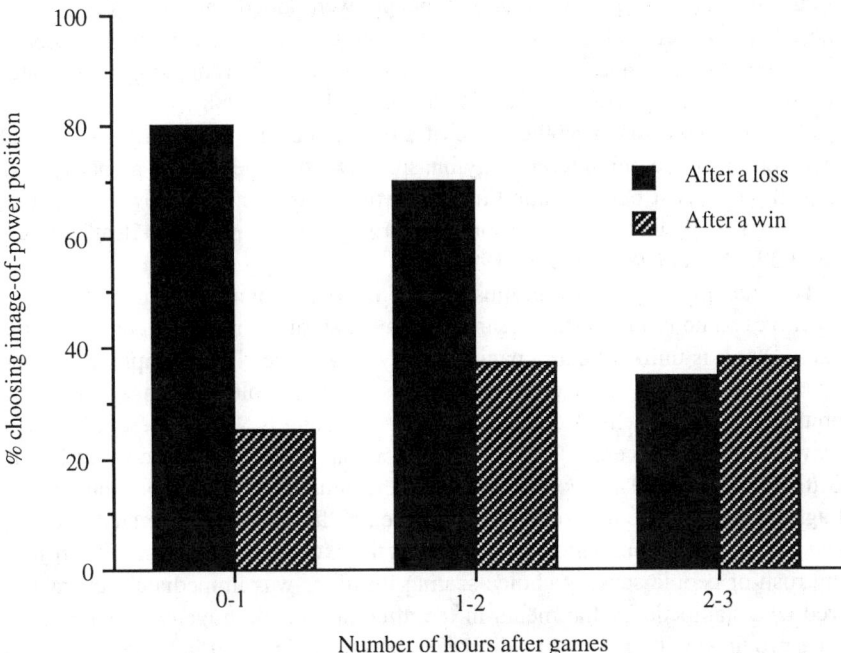

FIGURE 10.1 Percentage choosing image-of-power position (adapted from Tesler & Alker, 1983).

success or failure tend to be fairly short-lived. Two to three hours after the game, fans of winning and losing teams are indistinguishable in terms of their power preferences. As Tesler and Alker (1983) suggest, intervening experiences and competing interests erode the influence of game outcome in fairly short order. The authors also leave us to ponder the lingering question of the football players themselves and their power preferences having just won or lost a game.

Panics

In the remaining sections we will consider two of the more destructive types of crowd phenomena—panics and riots. Although rare, panics are nonetheless an important form of crowd behavior to study if for no other reason than the death and injury that frequently accompany their occurrence. In sport, the interest in panic is largely restricted to *unorganized* groups such as audiences at various sports venues or celebrants gathering in the aftermath of a team victory. To be sure, panics in *organized* groups (e.g., a military unit) are equally important, although a somewhat different set of factors is thought to predict their occurrence (Schultz, 1964b).

It is also useful as a first step to make a distinction between *exit* panics and the far less common *entry* panics (Mann, 1979). An exit panic was reported to have occurred in Katmandu, Nepal. Ninety people were killed and dozens injured as they fled a soccer stadium that was in the path of a fast approaching hail storm. The 30,000 soccer fans streamed toward a single exit; the remaining seven gates had been locked by stadium officials ("Nepalese Look," 1988).

Harlem, New York, was the scene of a recent entry panic. A large crowd had gathered outside a neighborhood gymnasium awaiting the start of a charity basketball game. Just before game time, the crowd was "funneled down a flight of stairs to a single entrance." The forward surge crushed 8 people to death and injured 29 ("Six at City College," 1991).

The example I've chosen to illustrate the internal dynamics of an entry (or acquisitive) panic is a doubtful one that displayed all of the requisite conditions for panic. Yet it is unlikely that a panic actually took place. The example is also instructive in drawing attention to the media's dominant role in defining and interpreting such events. In December of 1979, 11 young rock fans were killed in a crowd attempting to enter Cincinnati's Riverfront Coliseum for a concert by the British group *The Who*. Foremost among the situational factors present on that tragic occasion were unreserved seating (i.e., a "first come, first seated" policy) and an inadequate number of doors to admit the expected 18,000 fans. The resulting rush of people seeking choice seating locations was immediately characterized as a stampede by the media in the aftermath of the tragedy. Their readers were provided with images of a disorganized, chaotic mass of individuals bent on getting the best available seats with total disregard for each other's safety. The "magnetizing effect" of the music on a crowd described as barbarians who "stomped 11 persons to death [after] having numbed their brains on weeds, chemicals, and Southern Comfort" (Royko, cited in N.R. Johnson, 1987b) was seen as yet a further cause. To the media, the general public, and some scholars, the elements of an entry panic were plainly present.

However, sociologist Norris Johnson (1987b) reached a different conclusion. After a thorough examination of police and media records and interviews with many of those involved in the event, he concluded that panic did not cause the tragedy. In fact, he uncovered numerous examples of helping behavior. The social norm of the strong helping the less able prevailed (e.g., men helping women, adults helping children) despite the threat posed by the forward surge of people. Groups of people who had arrived together remained relatively intact throughout the ordeal, with very few indications of a breakdown in social order. It would appear that the "stampede" and the "panic" were media creations for which fictional explanations were then provided.

Norris Johnson (1987a) reached a similar conclusion in the cases of two other "panics" that occurred in the Cincinnati area, the 1977 Beverly Hills Super Club fire that claimed 160 victims and the 1985 run on the Home State Savings Bank. In summarizing his analyses he comments, "Ruthless competition did not occur," and further, "I was struck not by the breakdown of social order but by its strength and persistence; not by the irrational, individual behavior of popular myth, but by the socially structured, socially responsible, and adaptive actions of the affected" (p. 180).

The lesson to be drawn by students of collective behavior is clear. Because the media are among the first to arrive on the scene (academics are probably last) and because press deadlines cannot wait on the careful analyses of qualified experts, the media boldly assume responsibility for identifying and interpreting these events for the general public. Unfortunately, the label they pull, almost from thin air, may be inaccurate and entirely misleading. The same might be said of their explanations. With regard to exit or entry panics in general, Johnson concludes that "documented cases . . . are surprisingly scarce in the literature" and in fact, "panic occurs very infrequently" (N.R. Johnson, 1987b, p. 371). Panics, then, should only be labeled as such when the conditions for a panic have been met according to the best available evidence.

There is general agreement among theorists (e.g., Foreman, 1953; Schultz, 1964a, 1964c) that *three* conditions must be present in order to label a crowd action as a panic. First, the crowd must be in a state of intense fear. The fear itself may result from an actual danger or a danger "perceived" as imminent. It may later be apparent to an official inquiry that, in retrospect, crowd members were not personally endangered in the circumstances preceding a panic. Nonetheless, it is the crowd's perception of danger, justified or not, that is a determining factor in the crowd's response. It is also important to note that while fear is a necessary condition for panic to occur, it is by no means a sufficient condition. In some circumstances, intense fear may instead lead to inaction or resignation to the situation, especially if there appears to be no means of escaping the danger. However, if an escape route exists and is taken by crowd members, then the second of the conditions for panic is met, namely, flight behavior.

When a crowd flees a source of immediate danger, it is more accurately described as flight behavior even though individuals are terrorized and flee in a frantic and chaotic fashion. Such was the case when an unknown person discharged a tear-gas canister in the stands during a high school football game in Gaffney, South Carolina ("175 at Football Game," 1986). The spectators poured onto the field. Later, 175 people were treated at the local hospital for minor injuries and exposure to the gas. However, the event lacked the third and necessary ingredient for panic, that of a restricted avenue of escape.

The stage for panic is fully set when the design or operation of a sports facility is such that it cannot accommodate the rapid and disorganized departure of those who have gathered to witness an event. Escape routes may be too few, too precipitous, poorly lighted, or inadequately signed. As ludicrous as it seems, authorities have been known to lock exits to prevent entry by those who might sneak in without a ticket. To the degree, then, that frightened spectators are impeded in their hasty and disorderly flight from danger, panic can be said to be present.

Panic in the Laboratory?

On the surface, it might seem that experimental investigations of panics are not really feasible on methodological, if not ethical, grounds. Despite the difficulties of such research, a small number of imaginative experiments have been conducted in lab settings (e.g., Klein, 1976; Mintz, 1951; Schultz, 1964a, 1964c). The starting point for any discussion of the factors involved in panic is the classic research of Alexander Mintz. Particularly interesting is his design of a clever analogue intended to represent the essential elements of a panic situation.

A large, specially constructed bell jar into which water could be introduced at a controlled rate served this purpose. Subjects were each given a string attached to a cone in the jar. Groups of subjects then had the task of removing their cones one at a time through a narrow neck before the rising water got them wet. Success required that subjects place the group interest ahead of personal gain and take turns to ensure an orderly and speedy removal of all cones. Any departure from this strategy produces a jamming of cones in the neck. The "threat," of course, comes from the rising waters, whereas the "costs" are financial for those unable to extricate their cones in time. Subjects were rewarded for successful escapes and fined on trials when they failed. A principal finding was that in the absence of a reward structure, there was little evidence of jamming.

But wait just a darn minute, you say. How can you equate being burned to death in a stadium fire with getting your cone wet? Good question, and certainly one that has been asked before. The answer will depend on your willingness to generalize from the social lab setting to real-life events. For some, their misgivings stem from what appears to be a lack of external validity (Campbell & Stanley, 1966) in the design. Yet, *if* the researcher has successfully identified and represented in the simulation just those key variables that underlie the behavior of interest—in this case, panic—then insights into the dynamics that are involved may well be forthcoming.

The Bradford Fire

Perhaps the clearest example of a sports panic in recent years comes from British football. A horrific stadium fire on the soccer grounds at Bradford, England, in May of 1985 resulted in 57 deaths and over 200 injured. The grounds were packed with approximately 10,000 excited supporters, many of whom had come to see their team receive the championship trophy for having won the third division of the English professional soccer league. As a result of their victory, the club was to be elevated to the second division for the first time in 37 years.

Shortly before halftime, smoke was seen rising from under the stands. The soccer match continued, and spectators made no effort to leave the site, nor did anyone attempt to fight the fire. Only when flames were seen some 2 minutes later did several constables begin to direct people away from the area and onto the soccer pitch. Four minutes after the first hint of danger, the fire had spread up the back of the stands and engulfed half of the stadium roof. A minute later, the entire stand was an inferno. While many fans escaped to the playing field, others attempting to leave by the exit gates found themselves trapped. The gates had been locked to prevent unauthorized entry by late arrivals (I. Taylor, 1987). The horror of the tragedy was brought home to millions of viewers in Europe and elsewhere by Yorkshire Television who recorded the entire sequence of events.

According to reports (Lewis & Veneman, 1987; I. Taylor, 1987), the flames were fed by paper and rubbish that had been allowed to accumulate under the grandstand for over a decade. Some 6 months earlier, the chief fire officer had issued a warning that the wooden stand, built in 1908, was a fire trap. No action was taken.

As N.R. Johnson (1987a) points out, true panics are rare. In most cases, the term *panic* describes the behavior of only a section of the crowd. More often, the elements of both flight *and* panic are seen to occur in the same historical example. While many at Bradford fled unimpeded onto the pitch, others in the same crowd fell in passageways or otherwise found the escape routes blocked.

The writer was indirectly involved in one such real-life example where the reaction of some spectators who were impeded was panic; for others, flight from danger would best describe their experience. The writer was consulted by the prosecution in a Louisiana case, *Delores Lucas v. The Parish of St. Bernard*. The plaintiff had been seated at ringside during the final match of a professional wrestling card. The featured tag team used a scaled-down version of a flamethrower as part of their act. While making their way to the dressing room following a controversial win, one of the wrestlers discharged the flamethrower in the direction of his detractors in the audience. Those in the immediate vicinity scattered to avoid the flames, many stumbling and falling in their attempts to beat a hasty retreat. In the melee that followed, enraged fans hurled chairs in the direction of the ring, one of which struck and seriously injured Ms. Lucas. The grounds for the damage suit alleged negligence on the part of those staging the card for, among other things, not providing adequate security personnel. Two off-duty policemen hired for the evening were guarding a coffee counter at the time of the incident. Also, the availability of portable chairs that became weapons in the hands of provoked patrons was cited as negligence in the case. For your interest, a generous out-of-court settlement was reached in the case.

An important point emphasized by Mann (1979) is that many panics could be averted with planning for a worst-case scenario. The dilapidated stands at Bradford, with their accumulation of combustible trash, was a tragedy waiting to happen, as it ultimately did. Elsewhere, exits are locked. Finally, it is disconcerting to learn that months after there was a decision in the case, the tag team noted above continued to use the flamethrower in their act (personal communication, Gary Dragon, May 23, 1988). I would echo Mann's suggestion (1979, p. 352) to his readers that they take a critical look at the design and operation of the civic facilities in their own communities. The modern arena in my city, built in 1975, is a veritable death trap. The narrow, precipitous, and reversing stairwells can, at best, accommodate only an orderly evacuation of spectators.

Perhaps precisely because panics are rare, architects, builders, and managers of entertainment facilities regard panics as too remote a possibility to be taken seriously or to plan for. Contractors typically do little more than meet construction code standards. Such codes are intended to ensure an *orderly* exit of people in an emergency but seldom make sufficient allowances in design for a stampede. As Mann (1979) has summarized, "in many, if not most, cases, entry and exit panics can be blamed on the ignorance of authorities and officials who create the physical conditions for panic" (p. 348).

The emotional state of the crowd itself is a further consideration in contingency planning. Sports events do not exert equal effects on the spectators they attract. At some (e.g., ice hockey, professional wrestling) the quality of mood of those in attendance generally deteriorates over the course of the event; that is, the spectators become less socially affectionate, more hostile and fatigued (e.g., Arms et al., 1979; Russell, 1981c). Additionally, contact sports such as hockey produce heightened states of physiological arousal, particularly at games featuring excessive player violence. On those rare occasions when spectators are suddenly threatened with personal danger, sports crowds that are already highly aroused and fatigued (Foreman, 1953) can be expected to behave less adaptively (i.e., chaotic flight) than those crowds not already aroused and hostile. As noted elsewhere (chap. 2), increasing levels of arousal improve one's performance but only to a point. At extremely high levels of excitation (Bindra, 1959), the quality of people's actions deteriorates. This curvilinear relationship between levels of arousal and performance—an inverted-U function—provides the prediction that a shout of "Fire!" in an audience will often produce erratic flight behavior, the more so among audiences that are hostile and highly aroused. Authorities would do well to take extra measures with crowds likely to be volatile and extreme in their reactions to particular sports events.

Riots

Riots are also a rare but nonetheless worrisome aspect of sports. Certainly, the potential for riots exists in any sport that attracts a large following. Once again, you are reminded that social scientists seldom agree on a definition of the behavior they are attempting to understand; riotous behavior is no exception. A general definition suggested by Bittker (1970) will serve as a starting point. He defines a riot as "an uncontrolled violent disorder involving groups of people whose participation in the disorder may or may not include a shared sense of social, economic, or political oppression" (p. 166). Darrow and Lowinger (1968) define a riot simply as "aimless behavior involving disturbances or turmoil." In addition to these general definitions, a number of distinctions among *types* of riots will be considered shortly within the framework of a major classification system. First, however, an overview of the riots that have occurred in a single sport provides a sense of scale.

Riots have periodically marred football (soccer) throughout this century. A summary of the major disturbances associated with the sport is shown in Table 10.1. Several points should be noted. Although football-associated riots have taken place in a variety of cultures, their occurrence overall has been relatively

Table 10.1. Deaths and Injuries Associated with Football Disturbances

Date	Location	Deaths	Injury	Date	Location	Deaths	Injury
1902	Glasgow	25	350	1979	Hamburg	1	15
1946	Bolton (UK)	33	500	1979	Lagos	24	27
1957	Florence	—	120	1980	Calcutta	16	100
1959	Naples	—	65	1981	Athens	21	54
1961	Chile	5	300	1982	Moscow	60	—
1964	Lima	350	500	1982	Columbia	24	50
1964	Istanbul	—	84	1982	Algiers	8	600
1966	Cairo	—	300	1985	Peking	??	??
1967	Kayseri	48	602	1985	Bradford	57	200
1968	Buenos Aires	72	113	1985	Mexico	10	30
1971	Glasgow	66	—	1985	Heysel	39	470
1974	Cairo	48	47	1991	Johannesburg	42	42

Source: Adapted from Dunand, 1986.

infrequent. Moreover, some of the tragic events labeled as riots also contained elements that meet the criteria of a panic. Finally, Table 10.1 also provides an indication that riots have become more commonplace in recent decades.

Because riots are virtually unpredictable and occur with little or no warning, research has taken the form of ex post facto case studies. The data for these investigations is usually based on accounts provided by untrained observers, such as media people, police, community leaders, and sometimes a sample of the rioters themselves. Details of the circumstances and the sequence of events are typically obtained by means of interviews or through the archival record (e.g., newspaper stories, police reports, film footage). The lack of reliability of eyewitness testimony from various sources has been well documented in recent years. It is far from clear that even experienced police officers provide eyewitness accounts that are any more accurate than those of civilians (e.g., Yarmey, 1990, pp. 324–325). Because of these and other limitations, it should surprise no one to learn that the dynamics and causal factors involved in riots are, at best, only partially understood.

Many riots, of course, have as their root cause a history of political, religious, class, or racial injustice. From this perspective, when a particular combination of conditions and a precipitating event come together, be it on a street corner or in a stadium, a riot is likely to erupt. The origins of other types of riots are, however, to be found in more immediate causes. One possibility is raised in Speaking Tangentially 10.3.

****

Speaking Tangentially 10.3: Are Spectators *Primed* for Violence?
Are we in some sense primed or made ready for aggression, perhaps, even before we find our seat at a football game or a boxing match? Daniel Wann and Nyla Branscombe (1990b) of the University of Kansas see it as a strong possibility. Their research interests in social cognition have led them to examine the effects of hostile words in activating hostility-

related schemas. (Schemas are simply the set of interrelated beliefs and feelings that one has about something.) To illustrate, subjects made complete sentences from sets of scrambled words that included the name of an aggressive sport (e.g., boxing, hockey); other subjects made sentences from word sets that contained nonaggressive sports (e.g., billiards, golf). Shortly thereafter, both groups were asked for their impressions of Sandy, an individual who had been described to them in neutral terms. Those subjects who were earlier "primed" in the aggressive-sport name condition perceived Sandy to be more hostile and to have a greater interest in aggressive sports than those subjects not primed with aggressive-sport names. The authors emphasize that "individuals confronted with merely names of aggression-related sports will be predisposed to later perceive hostility in other persons" (p. 13). As a further consequence, others may be seen to attend because they like the violence or because they are looking to start trouble. As noted previously in connection with self-fulfilling prophecies (chap. 2), one's expectation of aggression may be sufficient to bring about that very result.

****

The usual starting point for understanding any complex and diverse set of phenomena is the construction of a system of classification. This sorting of various examples of the phenomena into somewhat compatible and logical groupings often provides a clearer overall picture and may suggest fruitful lines of investigation. Just such a classificatory scheme has been developed specifically for sports riots by Leon Mann (1979, 1989).

FORCE: A Typology

In all, five categories are proposed as sufficient to account for the different kinds of riots that have taken place in the realm of sports. These include: frustration, outlawry, remonstrance (protest), confrontation, and expressive. The first letter of each type provides an easy-to-remember mnemonic, FORCE.

Frustration

Fans who have developed close emotional bonds with their team vicariously share in the triumphs, near triumphs, and defeats of those to whom they are devoted. What the team experiences, they experience. As in any close relationship, frustrations can arise from a variety of sources. Those that have the potential to instigate frustration riots include being prevented from seeing one's team in action and seeing the team members being treated unfairly by game or senior sports officials. This distinction recognizes frustrations caused by *deprivation* and those caused by the *perceived injustice* in decisions made by officials.

By deprivation, Mann (1979, 1989) refers to those occasions when spectators are blocked in their attempts to witness, or gain access to, the performance of their heroes. A deprivation riot occurred on July 5, 1978, at a football stadium at Orchard

Park, New York, at the conclusion of a Rolling Stones concert. Approximately 300 of the 72,000 fans in attendance stormed the stage when the group refused to come out for an encore. Stage hands armed with 2 x 4s were able to hold the rioters at bay. The stage for a deprivation riot is also set when sports fans who have waited long hours in anticipation of obtaining tickets discover that none are available.

The second type of frustration riot follows from people's perception that officials have made grossly unfair decisions. These might include the referee's calling a penalty at a critical point in a match, an infraction that had previously been ignored, or a league official's imposing a punishment that by previous standards was unusually harsh. The famous Montreal Canadiens hockey riot of 1955 provides a perfect illustration.

The Montreal riot had its beginning in a decision by Clarence Campbell, president of the NHL, to suspend Maurice "The Rocket" Richard for the balance of the season. The league decision came as a result of Richard's violent assault on an opposing player and a game official who attempted to intervene. The suspension angered most hockey fans across Canada, particularly those in Quebec for whom the Rocket was a personal hero. His loss to the team was felt more acutely because the league-leading Canadiens were but two points ahead of Detroit, a team they were scheduled to play next. Opposition to the decision grew steadily on the day of the game, with demonstrators appearing in front of the Montreal Forum, the site of the game. Not surprisingly, Mr. Campbell became the focal point of the fans' wrath. Intense media coverage on the day of the game centered on the question of whether the president would choose to attend. Unwisely, he did.

Detroit scored their second of four goals just as Mr. Campbell and a police inspector took their seats during the first period of play. Spectators pelted the president with vegetables, bottles, and rubber boots. Before the period ended, Mr. Campbell had been struck by a youth who escaped into the crowd. The approximately 300 Forum employees and others (i.e., policemen, firemen, ushers, etc.) who were responsible for crowd control were scarcely in evidence. By the end of the period, the president was unprotected and surrounded in his box by enraged fans. Thankfully for Mr. Campbell's well-being, a diversion was created. A mindless fan picked that very moment to discharge a tear-gas bomb. The panic that would likely have followed was narrowly averted by the reemergence of the Forum staff, who kept all the doors in the Forum open. Campbell and his party seized the moment to escape to the first-aid center. With the game called and forfeited to Detroit, the highly aroused fans poured out into the street to join the demonstrators. Outside, the crowd turned ugly, and what followed was a night of destruction. A crowd in excess of 10,000 besieged the Forum, hurling bricks and other missiles. Ground-floor stores in the Forum, and later an additional 50 stores along an adjacent street, were damaged and looted. Police finally brought an end to the rioting around 3:00 a.m.

Lang and Lang (1961) concluded from their account of the incident, that responsibility for the actual rioting rested mainly with teenagers. It did appear, however, that the youths were openly encouraged by older adults. Hockey fans, it seems, were only minimally involved in the disorder.

Outlawry

The second type of riot in Mann's (1979, 1989) FORCE classification is outlawry. Riotous behavior of this type, while it may occur at or close to a sporting event, appears to be largely unrelated to the contest itself. Unruly elements come to the event prepared to do battle, actual or symbolic. The sports event is simply the staging ground for conflict. Media attention is guaranteed, as is the enemy of the day (e.g., rival supporters).

Soccer hooligans represent the clearest example from this category. Although soccer hooliganism has been extensively investigated in recent years (e.g., Marsh, 1978, 1982; Moorhouse, 1984; Pilz, 1989; I. Taylor, 1987; Williams et al., 1984; Zani & Kirchler, 1991), there is little agreement on its underlying causes. Opinions range from a view that hooliganism represents a ritualized form of violence where injuries are the exception rather than the rule (Marsh, 1978), to a class struggle (I. Taylor, 1987). In the most general terms, those creating disturbances before, during, or after a match can be described as often unemployed and underprivileged young males (e.g., Zani & Kirchler, 1991).

Remonstrance

Mann's typology recognizes a third type of riot, one that has its origins in a long-standing ideological conflict. The sports event is used merely to showcase a particular social or political cause, a tactic that sometimes leads to violence. The media attention, normally focused on the sports event, is essentially co-opted by the "political" faction. Touring South African sports teams encountered remonstrance riots during the early 1970s. These demonstrations were frequently orchestrated and planned to gain maximum publicity for the antiapartheid cause.

A similar series of planned political demonstrations came perilously close to disrupting the 1988 Calgary Winter Olympics. Members and supporters of the Lubicon Indian band of Northern Alberta had for years tried unsuccessfully to reach a settlement of their land claims with the Provincial and Federal governments. Despite a few anxious moments, their demonstration remained orderly, and the Lubicons were able to present their case to a worldwide Olympic audience. The remonstrance riot that might have taken place, never did.

Confrontation

Confrontation riots have their beginnings long before the actual staging of the sports events. Groups with a history of hostility toward each other meet at the sports site as supporters of teams that in some way symbolize the contending causes. Their long-standing antagonisms have their origins in religious, racial, class, or economic injustice. The sporting event itself provides an opportunity for partisan spectators to turn out and support "their" team. Doing so, of course, places them directly in the path of their traditional rivals (i.e., supporters of the other cause). Not surprisingly, simmering discontent and hatred occasionally erupt in violence.

Scottish football provides the clearest illustration of this category. The sport has been marred throughout the past century by clashes between supporters of the Glasgow Rangers (Protestant) and the Celtic (Catholic) clubs. Few would dispute a conclusion that the ongoing violence between the two factions represents a small-scale reenactment of the "troubles" in Northern Ireland. As a review of this ongoing conflict makes clear, the causes are complex and deeply rooted in the political and economic history of Northern Ireland (Moorhouse, 1984).

Racial tensions found violent expression in confrontation riots in the aftermath of the James J. Jeffries—Jack Johnson world heavyweight championship fight of 1910. Staged in Reno, Nevada, on the Fourth of July, the match pitted the reigning white champion Jeffries against the black challenger. During the 6 months leading up to the fight, there were news stories, almost daily, on the location of the bout, speculation on the outcome, and reports from the respective training camps. It was also evident during this time that support for the two boxers was sharply divided along racial lines.

The fight ended in the 15th round on a TKO when Jeffries's seconds jumped into the ring to assist their helpless fighter, who had been knocked to the canvas for the third time. The controversial underdog, Jack Johnson had become heavyweight champion of the world. Unfortunately, the violence did not end in the ring. An estimated 10 people lost their lives in racial clashes that erupted in many U.S. cities following Johnson's victory ("Bar Fight," 1910).

Expressive

The final category in the FORCE typology is the expressive riot. This type of riot stems from the highly charged emotional state of fans whose team has just triumphed or from the equally aroused state of those whose team has suffered defeat. It is the *extreme* emotional state of fans, irrespective of whether it arose from the joy of victory or the anguish of a defeat, that can lead to uninhibited activities. The unrestrained behavior can itself take any one of a number of riotous forms. Riots arising from a victory celebration gone sour can be every bit as destructive as one instigated by the embittered fans of a losing team.

Mann makes two important points about his category of expressive riots. First, expressive riots do not occur because the fans have been frustrated or somehow thwarted in their quest for victory. Such riots fall into his category of frustration riots. Mann also is clear in stating that expressive riots are strictly *postevent* occurrences.

In this regard, a number of major sports events are traditionally preceded by several days of celebration and high jinks by rival groups of fans. Examples include the week-long festivities leading up to the U.S. Super Bowl and Canada's Grey Cup football championships. Listiak (1974) notes in his analysis of Canadian celebrants that there is an ever present potential for serious riotous behavior. In virtually all instances, however, the considerable tact shown by police in dealing with revelers in all likelihood defuses a multitude of minor incidents that might otherwise escalate. For the most part, police look the other way and informally suspend enforcement of the laws governing misdemeanors.

Examples of postevent expressive riots are relatively plentiful. Following their 1971 victory in the World Series, 100,000 baseball fans celebrated in the streets of Pittsburgh. Unrestrained joy turned to destruction. Cars were overturned, fires were started, and phone booths were destroyed. Others danced nude in the streets, and a dozen rapes were reported ("Pittsburgh Victory," 1971).

The Heysel Riot

The 1985 Heysel stadium disaster in Belgium will serve as a case study that will illustrate several points with respect to the attempts of social scientists to understand the causes of riots. What follows is an eclectic overview of the sequence of events that transpired, one that draws heavily on the work of others (e.g., Dunand, 1986; Lewis, 1989; I. Taylor, 1987; 't Hart & Pijnenburg, 1988; Kevin Young, 1986).

Less than 3 weeks after the Bradford fire, England's Liverpool side were to meet the Italian champions, Juventus, in the final match of the European Cup. The site was Heysel stadium in Brussels. Both clubs were accompanied by large numbers of their fans, who occupied their respective sections at the end of the stadium. Minutes before the match was to begin, Liverpool fans broke through the fencing that separated them from the Italian supporters. These ritualized charges into the rival fans' zone are known as "the taking of the ends." The charging Liverpool fans created panic among the retreating Italians, who were pushed up against a 6-foot-high concrete retaining wall. The wall collapsed. Thirty-nine people were crushed to death, and a further 470 were injured (Dunand, 1986). As with the Bradford fire, television crews were on hand to record the tragedy for millions of viewers worldwide.

A Comment on Causes

As important as the question of causal factors may be, you are apt to be disappointed by the inadequacy of the answer. Largely because of the nature of riots (e.g., their rarity, unpredictability, scale, and many forms), social scientists can provide only tentative answers at this juncture. Considerable evidence exists identifying the factors that facilitate aggression at the individual (chap. 7) and situational (chap. 8) levels. It is this evidence that generally forms the basis for generalizing to exceedingly complex real-life events. Scientists and knowledgeable consumers of scientific findings recognize the dangers inherent in generalizing too freely to phenomena far removed from the original setting and methodology used to produce the findings. With other phenomena, evidence confirming lab results is often forthcoming from field investigations. However, in the case of large-scale phenomena such as riots and panics, their infrequent and unanticipated occurrence make in vitro studies largely impractical.

Further impediments to an understanding of the underlying causes of riots include the fact that riots are multiply determined. Rather than riots stemming from a single cause, a number of factors must be present and occur in a particular sequence. A determination of the factors involved in riots generally has to be made retrospectively on a case-by-case examination of antecedent events.

A further point deserves mention. Although unruly behavior clearly occurred at Heysel stadium, the dreadful toll that resulted is not entirely to be accounted for by psychological or sociological explanations. Had the retaining wall not collapsed, the event would in all likelihood have simply been reported as yet another example of English hooligans on a rampage that resulted in minor injuries to a number of Italian fans. While the English instigated the riot, surely the result was far, far more than any of them had bargained for or would have wished. Or was an engineering variable (i.e., the quality of stadium construction) also causally implicated to a significant degree? Perhaps the severity of a riot should be judged by its features, less so by its consequences?

All this is not to say that research on riots to date has been unproductive. Quite the contrary. Despite the difficulties, a substantial amount of theorizing and empirical findings is available. It is to selected aspects of that literature that we now turn for insights into the processes involved in sports riots. We begin with a theory.

A Social Systems Analysis

Those who have sought the reasons for riots have typically found answers that lay blame to the actions of one or more individuals or some aspect of the situation (e.g., alcohol, frustration over the outcome of a contest). However, a fresh and radically different approach to understanding riots has been proposed by 't Hart and Pijnenburg (1988). These writers have adopted a systems point of view to explain the Heysel stadium tragedy. Their analysis draws heavily on *normal accidents theory* (NAT), developed by Perrow (1984), to explain man-made disasters such as those that occurred at Bhopal (India), Tsjernobyl (USSR), and Cape Kennedy in the case of the *Challenger* tragedy. I should mention that my sketch of their theory is based on a book review by Jacob Rabbie (1989). Why my dependence on Dr. Rabbie? The book is written in Dutch.

Normal accidents theory (Perrow, 1984) advances the proposition that some technological systems are so *complex* and *tightly coupled* or compressed in time that accidents are difficult to avoid and should be regarded as normal. Most high-risk systems have particular characteristics, in addition to their toxic or explosive dangers, that make accidents a certainty. Systems (e.g., a biological lab, oil supertankers, a nuclear power station, *a Cup final*) with an excessive number of components (i.e., officials, spectators, equipment, procedures) may experience two or more failures. The failures *interact* in a way that was not anticipated and for which no provisions have been made.

Staying with a technological example to illustrate Perrow's (1984) term *interactive complexity*, consider two unexpected system failures. Not in anyone's wildest dream would it happen, but failure X started a fire while failure Y shut down the fire alarm. According to the designers of the system, it was almost inconceivable that it could happen, but it did. Adding a backup alarm and an extra sprinkler system might seem an adequate precaution, but this in turn might open up other unanticipated interactions among inevitable failures in the future. The interactive complexity of a technological system, then, is not a characteristic of the operator but rather a feature of the system.

Still, if time allows and if other means to intervene are available, the situation may yet be saved. However, in some high-risk systems there is little or no slack to be had. There is instead *tight coupling*. That is, processes occur rapidly and cannot be terminated, nor can the failed components be separated from the other components. The initial trouble cannot be corrected and will quickly worsen without hope of being stopped, at least for some time. Even an understanding of what the problem is or where it lies may take considerable time. What might have been merely an incident becomes an accident or a catastrophe. Although system-accidents are rare, they are nonetheless inevitable and in the view of Perrow (1984), can be considered normal.

The main thrust of the 't Hart and Pijnenburg (1988) book, then, is that NAT can be extended to account for accidents in *social* systems. Certain complex technological (e.g., nuclear power plants) and social systems (e.g., a Cup final) invite errors and failures. Such system features qualify as "error-inducing systems" in Perrow's (1984) terminology.

To return to the Heysel disaster, 't Hart and Pijnenburg (1988) provide an analysis in which a variety of errors and failures resulted from a faulty organizational structure and policy decisions. Among the organizational shortcomings leading up to the Cup final were the following:

1. The lines of authority and responsibility for public order and safety at the stadium were unclear and open to various interpretations. Those whose roles were never clearly spelled out included the state and municipal police, the minister of internal affairs, the govenor, and the burgomaster. The match organizers, and the international and Belgium football unions, were also somewhat unclear as to their responsibilities.

2. There was not a unified set of regulations governing order and safety to guide the organizers in their preparations for the Cup final. Overall, the regulations of the bodies involved were often noncommittal and overlapping, with omissions and contradictions.

3. Preparatory meetings held in advance of the event were highly selective in terms of those invited to attend. For example, the fire brigade and health services were excluded. Minutes of the meetings were not readily available, resulting in some misunderstanding as to what agreements had been reached. Other decisions were never taken (i.e., what to do about the dilapidated stadium, the availability of alcohol, and the appropriate response to drunken fans).

4. The efficiency with which various organizational elements carried out their responsibilities varied considerably. The lack of control in the selling of tickets by the Belgium football union reflected a sloppy organizational structure. The result was a failure to clearly separate the Juventus and Liverpool supporters from each other and from those spectators who were in some sense neutral. The state police had organizational problems as well in having to prepare for a Papal visit at the same time as the Cup final. Hasty preparations produced an ineffectual command structure.

Note again that no single one of these "failures" was itself sufficient to cause the Heysel tragedy. From Perrow's (1984) perspective, an error-inducing system is characterized by the *combination* of interactive complexity and tight coupling. Errors elicit other errors and are sequentially compounded.

One series of developments, in which each development involved a "failure," illustrates one causal chain leading to the eventual disaster.

1. The lack of foresight by those selling tickets resulted in the Liverpool and Juventus supporters standing close to each other.
2. As a result of inadequate preparations, there was only a handful of state policemen stationed in the corridor separating the two groups.
3. These policemen were insufficiently instructed and did not know how to respond.
4. The police were without leaders. Their commanders were outside the stadium. Moreover, because of faulty communications and a hierarchical command structure, they could not call in reinforcements. As Rabbie (1989) put it, "Out of this confluence of errors, the Heizel drama was born" (p. 55).

The authors ('t Hart & Pijnenburg, 1988) extended their analysis of the tragedy to the quality of the decision-making process during and in the immediate aftermath of the crisis. Failures continued to be revealed in all likelihood making a dreadful occurrence even worse. A few of the flawed arrangements will suffice to provide an overview of the factors that hampered an effective response to the disaster. Foremost among the decision failures was the absence of an overall coordination plan to deal with such emergencies and the lack of contacts between such units as the state and municipal police. Many of the individuals and organizations involved in the crisis had different kinds of information, formed different interpretations of the events that had transpired, and often worked at cross-purposes to one another.

To summarize, the systems approach adapted by 't Hart and Pijnenburg (1988) to the Heysel tragedy has been described and illustrated at some length. However, in addition to giving us a glimpse of the internal dynamics of a developing disaster, the case study has also provided an alternative level of explanation. Rather than seeking personalized explanations (e.g., human error by one or more of the principals), explanations are sought on the basis of tightly coupled, integratively complex systems.

The Role of Personality

As the reader will recall, chapter 7 provided an overview of personality theory and research, some of which related to aggressive behavior. Included among the individual differences variables highlighted were the macho and Type A personalities as well as Machiavellianism. Two other personality constructs, aggressivity and internal-external locus of control, are singled out to more directly illustrate the potential contribution of this class of factors to our understanding of riots.

Stating that the actors in a riot have aggressive personalities does not come as a startling revelation to anyone. However trite the statement may seem, it is nonetheless important that it be reaffirmed and additionally considered for its behavioral implications. What is implied and confirmed by careful investigation is that aggressive individuals have a preference for violent scenes (Lefkowitz, Walder, Eron, & Huesmann, 1973); actively seek out such experiences (Fenigstein, 1979; Russell, 1992b); and respond more aggressively than others (Josephson, 1987; Wilkins, Scharff, & Schlottmann, 1974).

To illustrate, men who scored high on measures of assaultiveness and antisocial tendencies were also those who gave the highest ratings to "I like to watch the fights" as a reason for their attendance at a hockey game (Russell, 1992b). These same males also reported the greatest likelihood that they would actually join in a fight or disturbance should one erupt in the stands. And again, it was the young, single adult males who expressed the greatest enthusiasm for involving themselves in a crowd disturbance.

Finally, those found in the vanguard of a riot likely include substantial numbers of verbally and physically aggressive individuals who are largely unresponsive to those urging restraint and largely unconcerned about what others will think of their actions (i.e., people who score low on a measure of social desirability response style). There is even a suggestion that the efforts of those openly condemning the prospect of a disturbance will instead see their efforts increase the likelihood of violence among such individuals (Russell & Pigat, 1991).

A second personality variable with links to actual riots is internal-external (I-E) locus of control (Rotter, 1966). Its relevance is seen in a study conducted in the Watts district of Los Angeles during the riot-torn decade of the 1960s (Ransford, 1968). Resident male blacks ($N = 312$) who were heads of households were asked, "Would you be willing to use violence to get Negro rights?" A measure of I-E locus of control was found to be related to endorsement of the item. That is, those with an external orientation indicated a greater willingness to resort to violence than did internals. Ransford characterizes externality as a state of *powerlessness* whereby individuals believe they are incapable of exerting control or influence over their circumstances. People who feel powerless to effect change in their lives may see violent means as their only remaining option.

Ransford also assessed two other social factors that were found to be related to a willingness to resort to violence. Both *isolation* from whites (e.g., little contact with whites either at work or in the neighborhood) and *dissatisfaction* stemming from racial discrimination were also associated with endorsing violence. Combining all three factors into two "ideal" types revealed that among those who were not alienated (high contact), had low powerlessness (internal orientation), and had low dissatisfaction, only 12% would turn to violence as a means of resolving injustices. Among those found in the other extreme ideal type (i.e., those alienated, powerless, and dissatisfied), 65% endorsed the use of violence.

These findings are impressive. (However, see the discrepant findings of Forward & Williams, 1970.) Ransford's choice of variables has been shown to sharply distinguish between those willing and those not so willing to engage in riotous behavior. Whether these and/or other individual differences variables predict equally well in a general sports context remains an open question for future research. It may be that these factors contribute to riots only in the cases of those that arise from long-standing grievances and reflect racial, economic (e.g., I. Taylor, 1987), or religious differences (e.g., Moorhouse, 1984), that is, those that would qualify as confrontation riots in the FORCE typology.

Summary

Sports have been marred by spectator violence since earliest times. Depending on what the wisdom of the day saw as the root cause(s) of crowd disruptions, authorities have at various times instituted rules or practices intended to maintain public order. Various tactics have historically included the use of gatemen at sporting events to turn away known troublemakers, segregating the spectators, and raising admission prices to reduce the numbers in attendance and thereby hopefully improve the quality of the crowd. Further attempts at crowd control saw restrictions placed on gambling, alcohol, and weapons (Sandiford, 1982; Vamplew, 1980, 1983).

The effectiveness of solutions to the practical problem of reducing spectator violence is dependent on our understanding of the factors that produce violence in the first instance. In some areas, the causal factors are reasonably well understood (e.g., the observation of aggression and alcohol); in other areas, our understanding is rudimentary. Even so, the fact of aggression being multiply determined makes predictions to specific situations problematic. Of course, the situations themselves differ widely in terms of crowd composition, peoples' motives for attendance, the nature of the sport, official policies, as well as the culture in which the event is staged. The sheer complexity of all this dictates that proposed solutions be carefully tailored to fit the circumstances. Even then, the best thought-out proposal should be regarded as tentative, with a likelihood of success only somewhat above a chance level. Still, the effort should be made. To do nothing at entertainment sites is to invite a repetition of the tragedies at Bradford, Heysel, and Cincinnati.

Suggested Readings

Buford, B. (1992). *Among the thugs*. New York: Norton.
Buford describes his experiences as a member of British hooligan organizations for the better part of a decade. His eyewitness accounts and personal analysis of causes make for fascinating reading.

Canter, D., Comber, M., & Uzzell, D.L. (1989). *Football in its place: An environmental psychology of football grounds*. London: Routledge.
This book draws heavily on a British social science literature in presenting a valuable perspective on soccer violence. A survey of fans' opinions provides some interesting insights into their view of the sport.

Hirt, E., Zillmann, D., Erickson, G.A., & Kennedy, C. (in press). The costs and benefits of allegiance: Changes in fans' self-ascribed competencies after team victory versus defeat. *Journal of Personality and Social Psychology*.
Ed Hirt and his colleagues have demonstrated a range of effects on fans who strongly identify with their team. In the aftermath of witnessing a victory, males predict a better performance of motor skills for themselves and anticipate greater success in their attempts to date gorgeous women.

Kremer, J., & Scully, D. (1991). Psychology and sport: Past, present . . . and future? *The Psychologist: Bulletin of the British Psychological Society, 4*, pp. 147–151.
As their title implies, the authors offer us an overview of the links between the traditional fields of psychology in relation to sport, in addition to charting a future course for the discipline.

References

Adams, J.S. (1965). Inequity in social exchange. In L. Berkowitz (Ed.), *Advances in experimental social psychology* (Vol. 2, pp. 267–299). New York: Academic Press.

Adler, P.A., & Adler, P. (1988). Intense loyalty in organizations: A case study of college athletics. *Administrative Science Quarterly, 33*, 401–417.

Adorno, T.W., Frenkel-Brunswik, E., Levinson, D.J., & Sanford, R.N. (1950). *The authoritarian personality.* New York: Harper.

Albanese, R., & Van Fleet, D.D. (1985). Rational behavior in groups: The free-riding tendency. *Academy of Management Review, 10*, 244–255.

Alderfer, C.P. (1972). *Existence, relatedness, and growth.* New York: Free Press.

Allen, M.P., Panian, S.K., & Lotz, R.E. (1979). Managerial succession and organizational performance: A recalcitrant problem revisited. *Administrative Science Quarterly, 24*, 167–180.

Allport, G.W. (1965). *Pattern and growth in personality.* New York: Holt, Rinehart & Winston.

Altman, I. (1968). Choicepoints in the classification of scientific knowledge. In B.P. Indik & F.K. Berrien (Eds.), *People, groups and organizations* (pp. 47–69). New York: Columbia University Press.

Altman, I. (1975). *The environment and social behavior.* Monterey, CA: Brooks/Cole.

Amabile, T.M. (1979). Effects of external evaluations on artistic creativity. *Journal of Personality and Social Psychology, 37*, 221–233.

Anastasi, A. (1988). *Psychological testing* (6th ed.). New York: Macmillan.

Anderson, C.A., & Anderson, D.C. (1984). Ambient temperature and violent crime: Tests of the linear and curvilinear hypothesis. *Journal of Personality and Social Psychology, 46*, 91–97.

Anderson, C.A., & DeNeve, K.M. (1992). Temperature, aggression, and the negative affect escape model. *Psychological Bulletin, 111*, 347–351.

Anderson, D.F. (1979). Sport spectatorship: Appropriation of an identity or appraisal of self. *Review of Sport & Leisure, 4*, 115–127.

Anderson, N.H. (1968). Likableness ratings of 555 personality-trait words. *Journal of Personality and Social Psychology, 9*, 272–279.

Archer, D., & Gartner, R. (1984). *Violence and crime in cross-national perspective.* New Haven, CT: Yale University Press.

Ardrey, R. (1966). *The territorial imperative.* New York: Atheneum.

Arms, R.L., Russell, G.W., & Sandilands, M.L. (1979). Effects of viewing aggressive sports on the hostility of spectators. *Social Psychology Quarterly, 42*, 275–279.

Atkins, A., Hilton, I., Neigher, W., & Bahr, A. (1972, September). *Anger, fight, fantasy, and catharsis.* Paper presented at the meeting of the American Psychological Association, Honolulu, HI.

Atkinson, J.W. (Ed.). (1958). *Motives in fantasy, action, and society.* Princeton, NJ: Van Nostrand.

Atkinson, J.W., & Feather, N.T. (1966). *A theory of achievement motivation.* New York: Wiley.

Aveni, A.F. (1977). The not-so-lonely crowd: Friendship groups in collective behavior. *Sociometry, 40*, 96–99.

Averill, L.A. (1950). The impact of a changing culture upon pubescent ideals. *School and Society, 72*, 49–53.

Babbit, T., Rowland, G.L., & Franken, R.E. (1990). Sensation seeking and participation in aerobic exercise classes. *Personality and Individual Differences, 11*, 181–183.

Bach, G., & Goldberg, H. (1983). *Creative aggression: The art of assertion*. Garden City, NY: Doubleday.

Back, A., & Kim, D. (1984). The future course of the Eastern martial arts. *Quest, 36*, 7–14.

Bales, R.F. (1953). The equilibrium problem in small groups. In T. Parsons, R.F. Bales & E.A. Shils (Eds.), *Working papers in the theory of action* (pp. 111–161). Glencoe, IL: Free Press.

Bales, R.F., & Slater, P.E. (1955). Role differentiation in small decision-making groups. In T. Parsons & R.F. Bales (Eds.), *Family, socialization and interaction process* (pp. 259–306). Glencoe, IL: Free Press.

Balswick, J., & Ingoldsby, B. (1982). Heroes and heroines among American adolescents. *Sex Roles, 8*, 243–249.

Bandura, A. (1969). Social-learning theory of identificatory processes. In D.A. Goslin (Ed.), *Handbook of socialization theory and research* (pp. 213–262). Chicago: Rand McNally.

Bandura, A. (1973). *Aggression: A social learning analysis*. Englewood Cliffs, NJ: Prentice Hall.

Bandura, A. (1977). Self-efficacy: Toward a unifying theory of behavioral change. *Psychological Review, 84*, 191–215.

Bandura, A. (1982). The self and mechanisms of agency. In J. Suls (Ed.), *Psychological perspectives on the self* (Vol. 1). Hillsdale, NJ: Erlbaum.

Bandura, A. (1983). Psychological mechanisms of aggression. In R.G. Geen & E.I. Donnerstein (Eds.), *Aggression: Theoretical and empirical reviews* (Vol. 1, pp. 1–40). New York: Academic Press.

Bandura, A. (1986). *Social foundations of thought and action*. Englewood Cliffs, NJ: Prentice-Hall.

Bandura, A., Underwood, B., & Fromson, M.E. (1975). Disinhibition of aggression through diffusion of responsibility and dehumanization of victims. *Journal of Research in Personality, 9*, 253–269.

Bar fight pictures to avoid race riots. (1910, July 6). *The New York Times*, p. 3.

Barling, J., & Abel, M. (1983). Self-efficacy beliefs and tennis performance. *Cognitive Therapy and Research, 7*, 265–272.

Barnes, J. (1983). *Sports and the law in Canada*. Toronto: Butterworths.

Barnett, S.A. (1988). *Biology and freedom*. New York: Cambridge University Press.

Barney, R.K. (1985). The hailed, the haloed, and the hallowed: Sport heroes and their qualities—An analysis and hypothetical model for their commemoration. In N. Muller & J. Ruhl (Eds.), *Sport history* (pp. 88–103). Niederhausen, Germany: Schors-Verlag.

Barnsley, R.H., & Thompson, A.H. (1988). Birthdate and success in minor hockey: The key to the NHL. *Canadian Journal of Behavioural Science, 20*, 167–176.

Barnsley, R.H., Thompson, A.H., & Barnsley, P.E. (1985). Hockey success and birthdate: The relative age effect. *Canadian Association for Health, Physical Education, and Recreation, 51*, 23–28.

Barnsley, R.H., Thompson, A.H., & Legault, P. (in press). Family planning: Football style. The relative age effect in football. *International Review for the Sociology of Sport*.

Baron, J.N., & Reiss, P.C. (1985). Same time, next year: Aggregate analyses of the mass media and violent behavior. *American Sociological Review, 50*, 347–363.

Baron, R.A. (1977). *Human aggression.* New York: Plenum.

Baron, R.A. (1983). *Behavior in organizations: Understanding and managing the human side of work.* Boston: Allyn and Bacon.

Baron, R.A. (1987). Effects of negative air ions on interpersonal attraction: Evidence for intensification. *Journal of Personality and Social Psychology, 52,* 547–553.

Baron, R.A., & Bell, P.A. (1976). Aggression and heat: The influence of ambient temperature, negative affect, and a cooling drink on physical aggression. *Journal of Personality and Social Psychology, 33,* 245–255.

Baron, R.A., & Ransberger, V.M. (1978). Ambient temperature and the occurrence of collective violence: The "long hot summer" revisited. *Journal of Personality and Social Psychology, 36,* 351–360.

Baron, R.A., Russell, G.W., & Arms, R.L. (1985). Negative ions and behavior: Impact on mood, memory, and aggression among Type A and Type B persons. *Journal of Personality and Social Psychology, 48,* 746–754.

Baron, R.S., Moore, D., & Sanders, G.S. (1978). Distraction as a source of drive in social facilitation research. *Journal of Personality and Social Psychology, 36,* 816–824.

Bass, B.M. (1962). *The Orientation Inventory.* Palo Alto, CA: Consulting Psychologists Press.

Baumeister, R.F. (1984). Choking under pressure: Self-consciousness and paradoxical effects of incentives on skillful performance. *Journal of Personality and Social Psychology, 46,* 610–620.

Baumeister, R.F. (1985, April). The championship choke. *Psychology Today,* pp. 48–52.

Baumeister, R.F., Hutton, D.G., & Cairns, K.J. (1990). Negative effects of praise on skilled performance. *Basic and Applied Social Psychology, 11,* 131–148.

Baumeister, R.F., & Steinhilber, A. (1984). Paradoxical effects of supportive audiences on performance under pressure: The home field disadvantage in sports championships. *Journal of Personality and Social Psychology, 47,* 85–93.

Beckhouse, L., Tanur, J., Weiler, J., & Weinstein, E. (1975). And some men have leadership thrust upon them. *Journal of Personality and Social Psychology, 31,* 557–566.

Beer, J., & Beer, J. (1989). Relationship of eye color to professional baseball players' batting statistics given on bubblegum cards. *Perceptual and Motor Skills, 69,* 632–634.

Bell, P.A. (1992). In defense of the negative affect escape model of heat and aggression. *Psychological Bulletin, 111,* 342–346.

Bell, P.A., & Yee, L.A. (1989). Skill level and audience effects on performance of a karate drill. *The Journal of Social Psychology, 129,* 191–200.

Benagh, J. (1978). Fan violence a growing threat. *The Sporting News.*

Bennett, J.C. (1988, fall). No room for fighting. *School Safety,* 28–29.

Bennett, J.C. (1991). The irrationality of the catharsis theory of aggression as justification for educators' support of interscholastic football. *Perceptual and Motor Skills, 72,* 415–418.

Bennett, R.M., Buss, A.H., & Carpenter, J.A. (1969). Alcohol and human physical aggression. *Quarterly Journal of Studies on Alcohol, 30,* 870–877.

Berczeller, E. (1967). The "aesthetic feelings" and Aristotle's *catharsis* theory. *Journal of Psychology, 65,* 261–267.

Berkowitz, L. (1962). *Aggression: A social psychological analysis.* New York: McGraw-Hill.

Berkowitz, L. (1965). Some aspects of observed aggression. *Journal of Personality and Social Psychology, 2,* 359–369.

Berkowitz, L. (Ed.). (1969). *Roots of aggression.* New York: Atherton.

Berkowitz, L. (1970). Experimental investigations of hostility catharsis. *Journal of Consulting and Clinical Psychology, 35*, 1–7.

Berkowitz, L. (1973). Sports, competition, and aggression. *Physical Educator, 30*, 59–61.

Berkowitz, L. (1974). Some determinants of impulsive aggression: Role of mediated associations with reinforcements for aggression. *Psychological Review, 81*, 165–176.

Berkowitz, L. (1981, June). How guns control us. *Psychology Today*, pp. 11–12.

Berkowitz, L. (1988). Frustrations, appraisals, and aversively stimulated aggression. *Aggressive Behavior, 14*, 3–11.

Berkowitz, L. (1989). Frustration-aggression hypothesis: Examination and reformulation. *Psychological Bulletin, 106*, 59–73.

Berkowitz, L., & Alioto, J.T. (1973). The meaning of an observed event as a determinant of its aggressive consequences. *Journal of Personality and Social Psychology, 28*, 206–217.

Berkowitz, L., & Geen, R.G. (1966). Film violence and the cue properties of available targets. *Journal of Personality and Social Psychology, 3*, 525–530.

Berkowitz, L., & LePage, A. (1967). Weapons as aggression-eliciting stimuli. *Journal of Personality and Social Psychology, 7*, 202–207.

Berlyne, D.E. (1960). *Conflict, arousal and curiosity*. New York: McGraw-Hill.

Bernard, J. (1968). The eudaemonists. In S.Z. Klausner (Ed.), *Why men take chances* (pp. 6–47). Garden City, NY: Anchor.

Berscheid, E., & Walster, E.H. (1969). *Interpersonal attraction*. Reading, MA: Addison-Wesley.

Biaggio, M.K. (1987). A survey of psychologists' perspectives on catharsis. *Journal of Psychology, 121*, 243–248.

Bibby, R.W. (1991). *Project Can 90* (Release #5). Lethbridge, Alberta: University of Lethbridge, Department of Sociology.

Bindra, D. (1959). *Motivation*. New York: Ronald Press.

Bird, A.M. (1977). Development of a model for predicting team performance. *Research Quarterly, 48*, 24–32.

Bird, A.M., & Brame, J.M. (1978). Self versus team attributions: A test of the "I'm OK, but the team's so-so" phenomenon. *Research Quarterly, 49*, 260–268.

Bittker, T.E. (1970). The choice of collective violence in intergroup conflict. In D.N. Daniels, M.F. Gilula & F.M. Ochberg (Eds.), *Violence and the struggle for existence* (pp. 165–192). Boston, MA: Little, Brown.

Björkqvist, K. (1985). Desensitization to film violence in aggressive and nonaggressive boys. In K. Björkqvist (Ed.), *Violent films, anxiety and aggression* (pp. 45–50). Helsinki, Finland: Societas Scientiarum Fennica.

Blumenfeld, W.S. (1985). Ability of *Sports Illustrated* to predict 10 college football conference standings. *Perceptual and Motor Skills, 61*, 1004.

Bond, C.F., Jr., & Titus, L.J. (1983). Social facilitation: A meta-analysis of 241 studies. *Psychological Bulletin, 94*, 265–292.

Boorstin, D. (1968). From hero to celebrity: A human pseudo-event. In H. Lubin (Ed.), *Heroes and anti-heroes* (pp. 325–340). San Francisco: Chandler.

Borden, R.J., & Taylor, S.P. (1973). The social instigation and control of physical aggression. *Journal of Applied Social Psychology, 3*, 354–361.

Borden, R.J., & Taylor, S.P. (1976). Pennies for pain: A note on instrumental aggression toward a pacifist by vanquished, victorious, and evenly-matched opponents. *Victimology, 1*, 154–157.

Boyanowsky, E.O., & Griffiths, C.T. (1982). Weapons and eye contact as instigators or inhibitors of aggressive arousal in police-citizen interaction. *Journal of Applied Social Psychology, 12*, 398–407.

Branscombe, N.R., & Wann, D.L. (1992a). Physiological arousal and reactions to out-group members during competitions that implicate an important social identity. *Aggressive Behavior, 18*, 85–93.

Branscombe, N.R., & Wann, D.L. (1992b). Role of identification with a group, arousal, categorization processes, and self-esteem in sport spectator aggression. *Human Relations, 45*, 1013–1033.

Branscombe, N.R., Wann, D.L., & Noel, J.G. (1992). *Loyal and disloyal group members: Ingroup extremity when an important social identity is threatened.* Manuscript submitted for publication.

Bratton, R., Clark, L., Dyer, S., Harding, C., & Roberts, G. (1978, November). *Attitudes of fans toward violence in professional wrestling.* Paper presented at the meeting of the Canadian Society for Psychomotor Learning and Sport Psychology Congress, Toronto, Canada.

Bredemeier, B.J. (1975). The assessment of reactive and instrumental athletic aggression. In D.M. Landers (Ed.), *Psychology of sport and motor behavior* (pp. 71–83). State College, PA: Pennsylvania State University.

Bredemeier, B.J., Weiss, M.R., Shields, D.L., & Cooper, B.A.B. (1986). The relationship of sport involvement with children's moral reasoning and aggression tendencies. *Journal of Sport Psychology, 8*, 304–318.

Brickner, M.A., Harkins, S.G., & Ostrom, T.M. (1986). Effects of personal involvement: Thought-provoking implications for social loafing. *Journal of Personality and Social Psychology, 51*, 763–769.

Brill, A.A. (1929). The way of the fan. *North American Review, 226*, 400–434.

Brissett, M., & Nowicki, S., Jr. (1973). Internal versus external control of reinforcement and reaction to frustration. *Journal of Personality and Social Psychology, 25*, 35–44.

Brown, M.C. (1982). Administrative succession and organizational performance: The succession effect. *Administrative Science Quarterly, 27*, 1–16.

Burger, J.M. (1985). Temporal effects on attributions for academic performances and reflected-glory basking. *Social Psychology Quarterly, 48*, 330–336.

Burnham, J.R. (1968). *Effects of experimenter's expectancies on children's ability to learn to swim.* Unpublished master's thesis, Purdue University, West Lafayette, IN.

Buros, O.K. (Ed.). (1978). *The eighth mental measurements yearbook.* Lincoln, NE: Buros Institute of Mental Measurements.

Burton, R.V. (1963). Generality of honesty revisited. *Psychological Review, 70*, 481–499.

Bushman, B.J., & Cooper, H.M. (1990). Effects of alcohol on human aggression: An integrative research review. *Psychological Bulletin, 107*, 341–354.

Buss, A.H. (1961). *The psychology of aggression.* New York: Wiley.

Buss, A.H., Booker, A., & Buss, E. (1972). Firing a weapon and aggression. *Journal of Personality and Social Psychology, 22*, 296–302.

Buss, A.H., & Durkee, A. (1957). An inventory for assessing different kinds of hostility. *Journal of Consulting Psychology, 21*, 343–349.

Buss, A.H., & Finn, S.E. (1987). Classification of personality traits. *Journal of Personality and Social Psychology, 52*, 432–444.

Buss, A.H., & Perry, M. (1992). The aggression questionnaire. *Journal of Personality and Social Psychology, 63*, 452–459.

Butt, D.S. (1976). *Psychology of sport: The behavior, motivation, personality, and performance of athletes.* New York: Van Nostrand Reinhold.

Butt, D.S. (1979). Short scales for the measurement of sport motivation. *International Journal of Sports Psychology, 10*, 203–216.

Butt, D.S. (1987). *Psychology of sport: The behavior, motivation, personality, and performance of athletes* (2nd ed.). New York: Van Nostrand Reinhold.

Butt, D.S. (1990). The sexual response as exercise: A brief review and theoretical proposal. *Sports Medicine, 9*, 330–343.

Buys, C.J. (1978). Humans would do better without groups. *Personality and Social Psychology Bulletin, 4*, 123–125.

Calder, B.J., & Staw, B.M. (1975). Self-perception of intrinsic and extrinsic motivation. *Journal of Personality and Social Psychology, 31*, 599–605.

Campbell, D.P. (1967). The vocational interests of beautiful women. *Personnel and Guidance Journal*, June, 968–972.

Campbell, D.T., & Stanley, J.C. (1966). *Experimental and quasi-experimental designs for research*. Chicago: Rand McNally.

Carlyle, T. (1840). *On heroes and hero worship*. London: Oxford University Press.

Carron, A.V. (1982). Cohesiveness in sport groups: Interpretations and considerations. *Journal of Sport Psychology, 4*, 123–128.

Carron, A.V., Widmeyer, W.N., & Brawley, L.R. (1985). The development of an instrument to assess cohesion in sport teams: The Group Environment Questionnaire. *Journal of Sport Psychology, 7*, 244–266.

Carron, A.V., Widmeyer, W.N., & Brawley, L.R. (1988). Group cohesion and individual adherence to physical activity. *Journal of Sport & Exercise Psychology, 10*, 127–138.

Carver, C.S., Coleman, A.E., & Glass, D.C. (1976). The coronary-prone behavior pattern and the suppression of fatigue on a treadmill test. *Journal of Personality and Social Psychology, 33*, 460–466.

Carver, C.S., DeGregorio, E., & Gillis, R. (1981). Challenge and Type-A behavior among intercollegiate football players. *Journal of Sport Psychology, 3*, 140–148.

Carver, C.S., & Glass, D.C. (1978). Coronary-prone behavior pattern and interpersonal aggression. *Journal of Personality and Social Psychology, 36*, 361–366.

Castine, S.C., & Roberts, G.C. (1974). Modeling in the socialization process of the black athlete. *International Review of Sport Sociology, 9*, 59–74.

Cattell, R.B., Eber, H.W., & Tatsuoka, M.M. (1970). *Handbook for the sixteen personality factor questionnaire (16 PF)*. Champaign, IL: Institute for Personality and Ability Testing.

Cavanaugh, B.S., & Silva, J.M., III (1980). Spectator perceptions of fan misbehavior: An attitudinal inquiry. In C.H. Nadeau, W.R. Halliwell, K.M. Newell, & G.C. Roberts (Eds.), *Psychology of motor behavior and sport, 1979* (pp. 189–198). Champaign, IL: Human Kinetics.

Ceci, S.J., & Liker, J.K. (1986). A day at the races: A study of IQ, expertise, and cognitive complexity. *Journal of Experimental Psychology: General, 115*, 255–266.

Celozzi, M.J. (1977). *The stimulating versus cathartic effects of viewing televised violence in ice hockey and the relationship of subsequent levels of aggression and hostility*. Unpublished doctoral dissertation, University of Southern Mississippi.

Cervantes, L.F. (1965). *The dropout: Causes and cures*. Ann Arbor, MI: University of Michigan Press.

Chakravarty, S.N. (1983, October 10). Character is destiny. *Forbes*, pp. 114–123.

Charry, J.M., & Hawkinshire, F.B.W. (1981). Effects of atmospheric electricity on some substrates of disordered social behavior. *Journal of Personality and Social Psychology, 41*, 185–197.

Chelladurai, P. (1984). Discrepancy between preferences and perceptions of leadership behavior and satisfaction of athletes in varying sports. *Journal of Sport Psychology, 6*, 27–41.

Chelladurai, P. (in press). Leadership in sports: A review. *International Journal of Sports Psychology*.

Chelladurai, P., & Carron, A.V. (1983). Athletic maturity and preferred leadership. *Journal of Sport Psychology, 5*, 371–380.

Chelladurai, P., & Saleh, S.D. (1978). Preferred leadership in sports. *Canadian Journal of Applied Sport Sciences, 3*, 85–92.

Chelladurai, P., & Saleh, S.D. (1980). Dimensions of leader-behavior in sports: Development of a leadership scale. *Journal of Sport Psychology, 2*, 34–45.

Chemers, M.M. (1970). The relationship between birth order and leadership style. *The Journal of Social Psychology, 80*, 243–244.

Chichester, F. (1967). *"Gypsy Moth" circles the world*. London: Hodder and Stoughton.

Christie, R., & Geis, F. (1970). *Studies in Machiavellianism*. New York: Academic Press.

Cialdini, R.B. (1985). *Influence: Science and practice*. Glenview, IL: Scott, Foresman.

Cialdini, R.B., Borden, R.J., Thorne, A., Walker, M., Freeman, S., & Sloan, L. (1976). Basking in reflected glory: Three (football) field studies. *Journal of Personality and Social Psychology, 34*, 366–375.

Coates, C.J., Leong, D.J. (1988). A psychosocial approach to family violence: Application of conceptual systems theory. In G.W. Russell (Ed.), *Violence in intimate relationships* (pp. 177–201). Great Neck, NY: PMA Publishing.

Conger, J.A., & Kanungo, R.N. (1987). Toward a behavioral theory of charismatic leadership in organizational settings. *Academy of Management Review, 12*, 637–647.

Cook, T.D., & Campbell, D.T. (1979). *Quasi-experimentation: Design and analysis issues for field settings*. Chicago: Rand McNally.

Cooper, D., Livingood, A.B., & Kurz, R.B. (1981). Children's choice of sports heroes and heroines: The role of child-hero similarity. *Psychological Documents, 11*, 85. [Ms. No. 2376]

Cooper, R., & Payne, R. (1967). *Personality orientations and performance in football teams: Leaders' and subordinates' orientations related to team success*. (Rep. No. 1). Birmingham, England: University of Aston, Dept. of Industrial Administration.

Cottrell, N.B. (1972). Social facilitation. In C.G. McClintock (Ed.), *Experimental social psychology* (pp. 185–236). New York: Holt, Rinehart & Winston.

Courneya, K.S. (1990). Importance of game location and scoring first in college baseball. *Perceptual and Motor Skills, 71*, 624–626.

Courneya, K.S., & Carron, A.V. (1991). Effects of travel and length of home stand/road trip on the home advantage. *Journal of Sport and Exercise Psychology, 13*, 42–49.

Courneya, K.S., & Carron, A.V. (1992). The home advantage in sport competition: A literature review. *Journal of Sport and Exercise Psychology, 14*, 13–27.

Crews, D.J., Shirreffs, J.H., Thomas, G., Krahenbuhl, G.S., & Helfrich, H.M. (1986). Psychological and physiological attributes associated with performance of selected players of the Ladies Professional Golf Association tour. *Perceptual and Motor Skills, 63*, 235–238.

Criswell, J.H. (1961). The sociometric study of leadership. In L. Petrullo & B.M. Bass (Eds.), *Leadership and interpersonal behaviors* (pp. 10–29). New York: Holt, Rinehart and Winston.

Curtis, B., Smith, R.E., & Smoll, F.L. (1979). Scrutinizing the skipper: A study of leadership behaviors in the dugout. *Journal of Applied Psychology, 64*, 391–400.

Daley, R. (1963). *The cruel sport*. New York: Bonanza.

Darrah, E.M. (1898, May). A study of children's ideals. *Popular Science Monthly, 53*, 88–98.

Darrow, C., & Lowinger, P. (1968). The Detroit uprising: A psychological study. In J. Masserman (Ed.), *The dynamics of dissent. Science and Psychoanalysis*, Vol. 13. New York: Grune & Stratton.

274   References

Darwin, C. (1965). *The expression of the emotions in man and animals*. Chicago: University of Chicago Press. (Original work published 1872).

Davids, K., & Nutter, A. (1988). The cohesion-performance relationship of English national league volleyball teams. *Journal of Human Movement Studies, 15*, 205–213,

Davis H., IV. (1990). Cognitive style and nonsport imagery in elite ice hockey performance. *Perceptual and Motor Skills, 71*, 795–801.

Deci, E.L. (1975). *Intrinsic motivation*. New York: Plenum.

Deci, E.L., Betley, G., Kahle, J., Abrams, L., & Porac, J. (1981). When trying to win: Competition and intrinsic motivation. *Personality and Social Psychology Bulletin, 7*, 79–83.

Deci, E.L., & Ryan, R.M. (1985). *Intrinsic motivation and self-determination in human behavior*. New York: Plenum.

Deford, F. (1976, May 3). Religion in sport. *Sports Illustrated*, pp. 42–44, 57–60.

Deford, F. (1969, June 9). What price heroes? *Sports Illustrated*, pp. 33–40.

De Freitas, B., & Schwartz, G. (1979). Effects of caffeine in chronic psychiatric patients. *American Journal of Psychiatry, 136*, 1337–1338.

DeGree, C.E., & Snyder, C.R. (1985). Adler's psychology (of use) today: Personal history of traumatic life events as a self-handicapping strategy. *Journal of Personality and Social Psychology, 48*, 1512–1519.

Dervin, D. (1985). A psychoanalysis of sports. *Psychoanalytic Review, 72*, 277–299.

Deutsch, M., & Krauss, R.M. (1960). The effect of threat upon interpersonal bargaining. *Journal of Abnormal and Social Psychology, 61*, 181–189.

DeZonia, R.H. (1958). *The relationship between psychological distance and effective task performance*. Unpublished doctoral dissertation, University of Illinois, Urbana.

Diab, L.N. (1970). A study of intragroup and intergroup relations among experimentally produced small groups. *Genetic Psychology Monographs, 82*, 49–82.

Didillon, H., & Vandewiele, M. (1985). Individuals whom the youth in Central Africa would like to resemble. *Perceptual and Motor Skills, 61*, 442.

Dollard, J., Doob, L., Miller, N., Mowrer, O.H., & Sears, R.R. (1939). *Frustration and aggression*. New Haven, CT: Yale University Press.

Donner, L. (1990). Television and violence. In L.J. Hertzberg, G.F. Ostrum, & J.R. Field (Eds.), *Violent behavior* (Vol. 1; pp. 151–166). Great Neck, NY: PMA Publishing.

Donnerstein, E., & Wilson, D.W. (1976). Effects of noise and perceived control on ongoing and subsequent aggressive behavior. *Journal of Personality and Social Psychology, 34*, 774–781.

Doob, A.M., & Wood, L. (1972). Catharsis and aggression: Effects of annoyance and retaliation on aggressive behavior. *Journal of Personality and Social Psychology, 22*, 156–162.

Duchon, D., & Jago, A.G. (1981). Equity and the performance of major league baseball players: An extension of Lord and Hohenfeld. *Journal of Applied Psychology, 66*, 728–732.

Dunand, M.A. (1986). Violence et panique dans le stade de football de Bruxelles en 1985: Approche psychosociale des evenements. *Cahiers de Psychologie Cognitive, 6*, 235–266.

Dunand, M.A., Berkowitz, L., & Leyens, J.P. (1984). Audience effects when viewing aggressive movies. *British Journal of Social Psychology, 23*, 69–76.

Dutton, D.G. (1988). *The domestic assault of women*. Boston: Allyn and Bacon.

Eastwood, J.M. (1974). The effects of viewing a film of professional hockey on aggression. *Medicine and Science in Sports, 6*, 158–163.

Ebbesen, E.B., Duncan, B., & Konecni, V.J. (1975). Effects of content of verbal aggression on future verbal aggression: A field experiment. *Journal of Experimental Social Psychology, 11*, 192–204.

Eberspächer, H. (1982). *Sportpsychologie*. Hamburg, Germany: Rowohlt.

Edwards, A.L. (1954). *Personal Preference Schedule: Manual*. New York: The Psychological Corporation.

Edwards, J. (1979). The home field advantage. In J.H. Goldstein (Ed.), *Sports, games, and play* (pp. 409–438). Hillsdale, NJ: Erlbaum.

Eibl-Eibesfeldt, I. (1979). *The biology of peace and war*. New York: Viking.

Eitzen, D.S., & Yetman, N.R. (1972). Managerial change, longevity and organizational effectiveness. *Administrative Science Quarterly, 17*, 110–116.

Epstein, S., & Fenz, W.D. (1965). Steepness of approach and avoidance gradients in humans as a function of experience: Theory and experiment. *Journal of Experimental Psychology, 70*, 1–12.

Evans, C.R., & Dion, K.L. (1991). Group cohesion and performance: A meta-analysis. *Small Group Research, 22*, 175–186.

Evans, R.I. (1974). A conversation with Konrad Lorenz about aggression, homosexuality, pornography, and the need for a new ethic. *Psychology Today, 8*, 82–93.

Everett, A. (1988). The role of personality in violent relationships. In G.W. Russell (Ed.), *Violence in intimate relationships* (pp. 135–148). Great Neck, NY: PMA Publishing.

Exner, J.E., Jr. (1986). *The Rorschach: A comprehensive system, Volume 1. Basic foundations* (2nd ed.). New York: Wiley.

Eysenck, H.J., Nias, D.K.B., & Cox, D.N. (1982). Sport and personality. *Advances in Behaviour Research and Therapy, 4*, 1–56.

Fabianic, D. (1984). Managerial succession, organizational effectiveness and franchise relocation in professional baseball. *Journal of Sport Behavior, 7*, 3–12.

Fasteau, M.F. (1975). *The male machine*. New York: Dell.

Feather, N.T., & Simon, J.G. (1971). Causal attributions for success and failure in relation to expectations of success based upon selective or manipulative control. *Journal of Personality, 39*, 527–541.

Feltz, D.L. (1982). Path analysis of the causal elements in Bandura's theory of self-efficacy and an anxiety-based model of avoidance behavior. *Journal of Personality and Social Psychology, 42*, 764–781.

Fenigstein, A. (1979). Does aggression cause a preference for viewing media violence? *Journal of Personality and Social Psychology, 37*, 2307–2317.

Ferguson, T.J., Rule, B.G., & Lindsay, R.C.L. (1982). The effects of caffeine and provocation on aggression. *Journal of Research in Personality, 16*, 60–71.

Ferrari, J.R. (1991). Self-handicapping by procrastinators: Protecting self-esteem, social esteem, or both? *Journal of Research in Personality, 25*, 245–261.

Festinger, L., Schachter, S., & Back, K. (1950). *Social pressures in informal groups*. New York: Harper.

Fiedler, F.E. (1967). *A theory of leadership effectiveness*. New York: McGraw-Hill.

Fiedler, F.E. (1970). Leadership experience and leader performance: Another hypothesis shot to hell. *Organizational Behavior and Human Performance, 5*, 1–14.

Fiedler, F.E. (1971). Validation and extension of the contingency model of leadership effectiveness: A review of empirical findings. *Psychological Bulletin, 76*, 128–148.

Fiedler, F.E. (1978). The contingency model and the dynamics of the leadership process. In L. Berkowitz (Ed.), *Advances in experimental social psychology* (Vol. 11, pp. 59–112). New York: Academic Press.

Fiedler, F.E., & Chemers, M.M. (1984). *Improving leadership effectiveness: The leader match concept* (2nd ed.). New York: Wiley.

Fiedler, F.E., & Garcia, J.E. (1987). *New approaches to effective leadership.* New York: Wiley.

Fiedler, F.E., McGuire, M.A., & Richardson, M. (1989). The role of intelligence and experience in successful group performance. *Journal of Applied Sport Psychology, 1,* 132–149.

Fiedler, F.E., Potter, E.H., & McGuire, M.A. (1988). *Stress and effective leadership decisions* (Tech. Rep. No. 88–3). Seattle: University of Washington.

Fitzsimmons, P.A., Landers, D.M., Thomas, J.R., & van der Mars, H. (1991). Does self-efficacy predict performance in experienced weightlifters? *Research Quarterly for Exercise and Sport, 62,* 424–431.

Fleming, I., Baum, A., & Weiss, L. (1987). Social density and perceived control as mediators of crowding stress in a high-density neighborhood. *Journal of Personality and Social Psychology, 52,* 899–906.

Foreman, P. (1953). Panic theory. *Sociology and Social Research, 37,* 295–304.

Forgas, J.P., Brennan, G., Howe, S., Kane, J.F., & Sweet, S. (1980). Audience effects on squash players' performance. *The Journal of Social Psychology, 111,* 41–47.

Forward, J.R., & Williams, J.R. (1970). Internal-external control and black militancy. *Journal of Social Issues, 26,* 75–92.

Foundation for Child Development (1977). *National survey of children.* 345 East 46 Street, New York.

Frank, M.G., & Gilovich, T. (1988). The dark side of self-and social perception: Black uniforms and aggression in professional sports. *Journal of Personality and Social Psychology, 54,* 74–85.

Fredrickson, J.W., Hambrick, D.C., & Baumrin, S. (1988). A model of CEO dismissal. *Academy of Management Review, 13,* 255–270.

Freedman, J.L. (1984). Effect of television violence on aggressiveness. *Psychological Bulletin, 96,* 227–246.

Freedman, J.L. Levy, A.S., Buchanan, R.W., & Price, J. (1972). Crowding and human aggressiveness. *Journal of Experimental Social Psychology, 8,* 528–548.

Freischlag, J., & Hardin, D. (1975). The effects of social class and school achievement on the composition of sport crowds. *Sport Sociology Bulletin, 4,* 36–46.

French, E.G. (1956). Motivation as a variable in work-partner selection. *Journal of Abnormal and Social Psychology, 53,* 96–99.

French, E.G. (1958). Development of a measure of complex motivation. In J.W. Atkinson (Ed.), *Motives in fantasy, action, and society* (pp. 242–248). New York: Van Nostrand.

Gabrenya, W.K., Wang, Y., & Latané, B. (1985). Social loafing on an optimizing task. *Journal of Cross-Cultural Psychology, 16,* 223–242.

Gaebelein, J., & Taylor, S.P. (1971). The effects of competition and attack on physical aggression. *Psychonomic Science, 24,* 65–67.

Gamson, W.A., & Scotch, N.A. (1964). Scapegoating in baseball. *American Journal of Sociology, 60,* 69–72.

Gantner, A.B., & Taylor, S.P. (1988). Human physical aggression as a function of diazepam. *Personality and Social Psychology Bulletin, 14,* 479–484.

Gantner, A.B., & Taylor, S.P. (1992). Human physical aggression as a function of alcohol and threat of harm. *Aggressive Behavior, 18,* 29–36.

Gayton, W.F., Matthews, G.R., & Burchstead, G.N. (1986). An investigation of the validity of the Physical Self-efficacy Scale in predicting marathon performance. *Perceptual and Motor Skills, 63,* 752–754.

Gayton, W.F., Matthews, G.R., & Nickless, C.J. (1987). The home field disadvantage in sports championships: Does it exist in hockey? *Journal of Sport Psychology, 9,* 183–185.

Geen, R.G. (1976). The study of aggression. In R.G. Geen & E.C. O'Neal (Eds.), *Perspectives on aggression* (pp. 1–9). New York: Academic Press.

Geen, R.G. (1980). The effects of being observed on performance. In P.B. Paulus (Ed.), *Psychology of group influence* (pp. 61–97). Hillsdale, NJ: Erlbaum.

Geen, R.G. (1983). Aggression and television violence. In R.G. Geen & E.I. Donnerstein (Eds.), *Aggression: Theoretical and empirical reviews* (Vol. 2, pp. 103–125). New York: Academic Press.

Geen, R.G. (1990). *Human aggression.* Pacific Grove, CA: Brooks/Cole.

Geen, R.G., & Gange, J.J. (1977). Drive theory of social facilitation: Twelve years of theory and research. *Psychological Bulletin, 84,* 1267–1288.

Geen, R.G., & McCown, E.J. (1984). Effects of noise and attack on aggression and physiological arousal. *Motivation and Emotion, 8,* 231–241.

Geen, R.G., & Quanty, M.B. (1977). The catharsis of aggression: An evaluation of a hypothesis. In L. Berkowitz (Ed.), *Advances in experimental social psychology* (Vol. 10, pp. 1–37). New York: Academic Press.

Geen, R.G., Stonner, D., & Shope, G.L. (1975). The facilitation of aggression by aggression: Evidence against the catharsis hypothesis. *Journal of Personality and Social Psychology, 31,* 721–726.

Gerth, H., & Mills, C.W. (1953). *Character and social structure.* New York: Harcourt, Brace.

Gibb, C.A. (1969). Leadership. In G. Lindzey & E. Aronson (Eds.), *The handbook of social psychology* (Vol. 4, pp. 205–282). Reading, MA: Addison-Wesley.

Gill, D.L. (1986). *Psychological dynamics of sport.* Champaign, IL: Human Kinetics.

Gilovich, T., Vallone, R., & Tversky, A. (1985). The hot hand in basketball: On the misperception of random sequences. *Cognitive Psychology, 17,* 295–314.

Glass, D.C. (1977). *Behavior patterns, stress, and coronary disease.* Hillsdale, NJ: Erlbaum.

Godden, D.R., & Baddeley, A.D. (1975). Context-dependent memory in two natural environments: On land and underwater. *British Journal of Psychology, 66,* 325–331.

Goldstein, A.P., & Keller, H. (1987). *Aggressive behavior: Assessment and intervention.* New York: Pergamon.

Goldstein, J.H. (1979). Outcomes in professional team sports: Chance, skill, and situational factors. In J.H. Goldstein (Ed.), *Sports, games and play: Social and psychological viewpoints* (pp. 401–408). Hillsdale, NJ: Erlbaum.

Goldstein, J.H. (Ed.). (1983). *Sports violence.* New York: Springer-Verlag.

Goldstein, J.H. (1985). Athletic performance and spectator behavior: The humanistic concerns of sports psychology. In W.L. Umphlett (Ed.), *American sport culture: The humanistic dimensions* (pp. 159–179). Lewisburg, PA: Bucknell University Press.

Goldstein, J.H., & Arms, R.L. (1971). Effects of observing athletic contests on hostility. *Sociometry, 34,* 83–90.

Goldstein, J.H., Davis, R.W., & Herman, D. (1975). Escalation of aggression: Experimental studies. *Journal of Personality and Social Psychology, 31,* 162–170.

Goldstein, J.H., Davis, R.W., Kernis, M., & Cohn, E.S. (1981). Retarding the escalation of aggression. *Social Behavior and Personality, 9,* 65–70.

Goodhart, P., & Chataway, C. (1968). *War without weapons.* London: W.H. Allen.

Goodman, P. (1964). Letter to the editor. *Scientific American, 210,* 8.

Goranson, R.E. (1970). Media violence and aggressive behavior: A review of experimental research. In L. Berkowitz (Ed.), *Advances in experimental social psychology* (Vol. 5, pp. 1–31). New York: Academic Press.

Goranson, R.E. (1978). *Sports violence and the catharsis hypothesis*. Paper presented at the meeting of the Canadian Society for Psychomotor Learning and Sport Psychology, Toronto, Canada.

Goranson, R.E. (1982). *The impact of televised hockey violence* (Report No. 1). The LaMarsh Research Programme, Toronto: York University.

Gould, S.J. (1991). *Bully for Brontosaurus*. New York: W.W. Norton.

Graen, G., Alvares, K., Orris, J.B., & Martella, S.A. (1970). Contingency model of leadership effectiveness: Antecedent and evidential results. *Psychological Bulletin, 74,* 285–296.

Greenberg, J. (1986). Differential intolerance for inequity from organizational individual agents. *Journal of Applied Social Psychology, 16,* 191–196.

Greenstein, F.I. (1964). New light on changing American values: A forgotten body of survey data. *Social Forces, 42,* 441–450.

Greenwell, J., & Dengerink, H.A. (1973). The role of perceived versus actual attack in human physical aggression. *Journal of Personality and Social Psychology, 26,* 66–71.

Greer, D.L. (1983). Spectator booing and the home advantage: A study of social influence in the basketball arena. *Social Psychology Quarterly, 46,* 252–261.

Griffith, C.R. (1922). A comment upon the psychology of the audience. *Psychological Monographs, 30,* 36–47.

Grove, J.R., Hanrahan, S.J., & McInman, A. (1991). Success/failure bias in attributions across involvement categories in sport. *Personality and Social Psychology Bulletin, 17,* 93–97.

Grudge over lost game ends in murder, suicide. (1990, April 23) *The Lethbridge Herald,* p. A8.

Grusky, O. (1963a). Managerial succession and organizational effectiveness. *American Journal of Sociology, 69,* 21–31.

Grusky, O. (1963b). The effects of formal structure on managerial recruitment: A study of baseball organization. *Sociometry, 26,* 345–353.

Guerin, B. (1986). Mere presence effects in humans: A review. *Journal of Experimental Social Psychology, 22,* 38–77.

Guttmann, A. (1981). Sports spectators from antiquity to the Renaissance. *Journal of Sport History, 8,* 5–27.

Guttmann, A. (1983). Roman sports violence. In J.H. Goldstein (Ed.), *Sports violence* (pp. 7–19). New York: Springer-Verlag.

Guttmann, A. (1986). *Sports spectators*. New York: Columbia University Press.

Hall, J.F. (1971). *Verbal learning and retention*. New York: J.B. Lippincott.

Halpern, D.F., & Coren, S. (1988). Do right-handers live longer? *Nature, 333,* 213.

Hamblin, R.L. (1958). Leadership and crises. *Sociometry, 21,* 322–335.

Hammerschlag, C.A., & Astrachan, B.M. (1971). The Kennedy Airport snow-in: An inquiry into intergroup phenomena. *Psychiatry, 34,* 301–308.

Harder, J.W. (1991). Equity theory versus expectancy theory: The case of major league baseball free agents. *Journal of Applied Psychology, 76,* 458–464.

Hardy, C.J., & Latané, B. (1988). Social loafing in cheerleaders: Effects of team membership and competition. *Journal of Sport & Exercise Psychology, 10,* 109–114.

Harkins, S.G., & Jackson, J.M. (1985). The role of evaluation in eliminating social loafing. *Personality and Social Psychology Bulletin, 11,* 457–465.

Harkins, S.G., & Petty, R.E. (1982). Effects of task difficulty and task uniqueness on social loafing. *Journal of Personality and Social Psychology, 43,* 1214–1229.

Harkins, S.G., & Szymanski, K. (1989). Social loafing and group evaluation. *Journal of Personality and Social Psychology, 56*, 934–941.

Harrell, W.A. (1981). Verbal aggressiveness in spectators at professional hockey games: The effects of tolerance of violence and amount of exposure to hockey. *Human Relations, 34*, 643–655.

Harries, K.D., & Stadler, S.J. (1988). Heat and violence: New findings from Dallas field data, 1980–1981. *Journal of Applied Social Psychology, 18*, 129–138.

Harris, H.A. (1972). *Sport in Greece and Rome*. London: Thames and Hudson.

Harris, J.C. (1986). Athletic exemplars in context: General exemplar selection patterns in relation to sex, race and age. *Quest, 38*, 95–115.

Harris, M.B. (1974). Mediators between frustration and aggression in a field experiment. *Journal of Experimental Social Psychology, 10*, 561–571.

Hartshorne, H., & May, M.A. (1928). *Studies in the nature of character*. (Vol. 1: Studies in deceit). New York: Macmillan.

Hastorf, A.H., & Cantril, H. (1954). They saw a game: A case study. *Journal of Abnormal and Social Psychology, 49*, 129–134.

Hathaway, S.R., & McKinley, J.C. (1989). *Minnesota Multiphasic Personality Inventory-2*. Minneapolis, MN: University of Minnesota Press.

Haupt, H.A., & Rovere, G.D. (1984). Anabolic steroids: A review of the literature. *The American Journal of Sports Medicine, 12*, 469–484.

Heaton, A.W., & Sigall, H. (1989). The "championship choke" revisited: The role of fear of acquiring a negative identity. *Journal of Applied Social Psychology, 19*, 1019–1033.

Heaton, A.W., & Sigall, H. (1991). Self-consciousness, self-presentation, and performance under pressure: Who chokes, and when? *Journal of Applied Social Psychology, 21*, 175–188.

Heider, F. (1958). *The psychology of interpersonal relations*. New York: Wiley.

Helmreich, R.L., Beane, W., Lucker, G.W., & Spence, J.T. (1978). Achievement motivation and scientific attainment. *Personality and Social Psychology Bulletin, 4*, 222–226.

Helmreich, R.L., & Spence, J.T. (1978). The Work and Family Orientation Questionnaire: An objective instrument to assess components of achievement motivation and attitudes toward family and career. *JSAS Catalog of Selected Documents in Psychology, 8*, 35. (Ms. No. 1677).

Helmreich, R.L., Spence, J.T., Beane, W.E., Lucker, G.W., & Matthews, K.A. (1980). Making it in academic psychology: Demographic and personality correlates of attainment. *Journal of Personality and Social Psychology, 39*, 896–908.

Herrmann, H.U. (1977). *Die fussballfans*. Schorndorf, Germany: Karl Hofmann.

Hicks, L.E. (1970). Some properties of ipsative, normative, and forced-choice normative measures. *Psychological Bulletin, 74*, 167–184.

Hirt, E.R., & Kimble, C.E. (1981, May). *The home-field advantage in sports: Differences and correlates*. Paper presented at the meeting of the Midwestern Psychological Association, Detroit, MI.

Hirt, E.R., Zillmann, D., Erickson, G.A., & Kennedy, C. (in press). The costs and benefits of allegiance: Changes in fans' self-ascribed competencies after team victory versus defeat. *Journal of Personality and Social Psychology*.

Hofling, C.K., Brotzman, E., Dalrymple, S., Graves, N., & Pierce, C.M. (1966). An experimental study in nurse-physician relationships. *Journal of Nervous and Mental Diseases, 143*, 171–180.

Hokanson, J.E. (1970). Psychophysiological evaluation of the catharsis hypothesis. In E.I. Megargee & J.E. Hokanson (Eds.), *The dynamics of aggression* (pp. 74–86). New York: Harper & Row.

Hollander, E.P. (1964). *Leaders, groups, and influence.* New York: Oxford University Press.

Hollander, E.P., & Julian, J.W. (1970). Studies in leader legitimacy, influence, and innovation. In L. Berkowitz (Ed.), *Advances in experimental social psychology* (Vol. 5, pp. 33–69). New York: Academic Press.

Hollander, E.P., & Offerman, L.R. (1990). Power and leadership in organizations: Relationships in transition. *Journal of Applied Psychology, 45,* 179–189.

Holt, R.R. (1970). On the interpersonal and intrapersonal consequences of expressing or not expressing anger. *Journal of Consulting and Clinical Psychology, 35,* 8–12.

Hornberger, R.H. (1959). The differential reduction of aggressive responses as a function of interpolated activities. *American Psychologist, 14,* 354.

Houston, B.K., & Snyder, C.R. (Eds.). (1988). *Type A behavior pattern: Research, theory, and interventions.* New York: Wiley.

Houston, M.E. (1979). Nutrition and ice hockey performance. *Canadian Journal of Applied Sport Sciences, 4,* 98–99.

Huddleston, S., Doody, S.G., & Ruder, M.K. (1985). The effect of prior knowledge on the social loafing phenomenon on performance in a group. *International Journal of Sport Psychology, 16,* 176–182.

Husman, B.F. (1955). Aggression in boxers and wrestlers as measured by projective techniques. *Research Quarterly, 26,* 421–425.

Hyman, H.H. (1975). Reference individuals and reference idols. In L.A. Coser (Ed.), *The idea of social structure* (pp. 265–282). New York: Harcourt Brace Jovanovich.

Iso-Ahola, S.E. (1980). Attributional determinants of decisions to attend football games. *Scandanavian Journal of Sports Sciences, 2,* 39–46.

Jackson, J.M. (1986). In defense of social impact theory: Comment on Mullen. *Journal of Personality and Social Psychology, 50,* 511–513.

Jeavons, C.M., & Taylor, S.P. (1985). The control of alcohol-related aggression: Redirecting the inebriate's attention to socially approved conduct. *Aggressive Behavior, 11,* 93–101.

Jenkins, C.D., Zyzanski, S.J., & Rosenman, R.H. (1979). *Jenkins Activity Survey.* New York: Psychological Corporation.

Jerome, J.K. (1900). *Three men on the bummel.* Bristol, England: Arrowsmith.

Johnsgard, K., Ogilvie, B.C., & Merritt, K. (1975). The stress seekers: A psychological study of sports parachutists, racing drivers, and football players. *Journal of Sports Medicine, 15,* 158–169.

Johnson, D.W., Maruyama, G., Johnson, R., Nelson, D., & Skon, L. (1981). Effects of cooperative, competitive, and individualistic goal structures on achievement: A meta-analysis. *Psychological Bulletin, 89,* 47–62.

Johnson, N.R. (1987a). Panic and the breakdown of social order: Popular myth, social theory, empirical evidence. *Sociological Focus, 20,* 171–183.

Johnson, N.R. (1987b). Panic at "The Who Concert Stampede": An empirical assessment. *Social Problems, 34,* 362–373.

Johnson, S.D., Gibson, L., & Linden, R. (1978). Alcohol and rape in Winnipeg, 1966–1975. *Journal of Studies on Alcohol, 39,* 1887–1894.

Johnson, W.R., & Hutton, D.C. (1955). Effects of a combative sport upon personality dynamics as measured by a projective test. *Research Quarterly, 26,* 49–53.

Jones, E.E., & Berglas, S. (1978). Control of attributions about the self through self-hand-icapping strategies: The appeal of alcohol and the role of underachievement. *Personality and Social Psychology Bulletin, 4*, 200–206.

Jones, K.V. (1985). The thrill of victory: Blood-pressure variability and the Type A behavior pattern. *Journal of Behavioral Medicine, 8*, 277–285.

Josephson, W.L. (1987). Television violence and children's aggression: Testing the priming, social script, and disinhibition predictions, *Journal of Personality and Social Psychology, 53*, 882–890.

Katz, D., & Schanck, R.L. (1938). *Social psychology*. New York: Wiley.

Keefer, R., Goldstein, J.H., & Kasiarz, D. (1983). Olympic games participation and warfare. In J.H. Goldstein (Ed.), *Sports violence* (pp. 183–193). New York: Springer-Verlag.

Kellermann, A.L., & Reay, D.T. (1986). An analysis of firearm-related deaths in the home. *New England Journal of Medicine, 314*, 1557–1560.

Kelley, H.H. (1972). Attribution in social interaction. In E.E. Jones et al. (Eds.), *Attribution: Perceiving the causes of behavior*. Morristown, NJ: General Learning Press.

Kelly, B.R., & McCarthy, J.F. (1979). Personality dimensions of aggression: Its relationship to time and place of action in ice hockey. *Human Relations, 32*, 219–225.

Kerr, J.H., & Svebak, S. (1989). Motivational aspects of preference for, and participation in, 'risk' and 'safe' sports. *Personality and Individual Differences, 10*, 797–800.

Kerr, N.L. (1983). Motivation losses in small groups: A social dilemma analysis. *Journal of Personality and Social Psychology, 45*, 819–828.

Kerr, N.L., & Bruun, S.E. (1983). Dispensability of member effort and group motivation losses: Free-rider effects. *Journal of Personality and Social Psychology, 44*, 78–94.

Kerr, N.L., & Yukelson, D. (1977, April). *Audience size and social facilitation*. Paper presented at the meeting of the Western Psychological Association, Seattle, WA.

Kerr, S., & Jermier, J.M. (1978). Substitutes for leadership: Their meaning and measurement. *Organizational Behavior and Human Performance, 22*, 375–403.

Kidd, A.H., & Walton, N.Y. (1966). Dart throwing as a method of reducing extrapunitive aggression. *Psychological Reports, 19*, 88–90.

Kingsmore, J.M. (1970). The effect of a professional wrestling and a professional basketball contest upon the aggressive tendencies of spectators. In G.S. Kenyon (Ed.), *Contemporary psychology of sport* (pp. 311–315). Chicago: Athletic Institute.

Kirshenbaum, J. (1989, February 27). An American disgrace. *Sports Illustrated*, pp. 16–19.

Klapp, O.E. (1962). *Heroes, villains and fools*. Englewood Cliffs, NJ: Prentice-Hall.

Klapp, O.E. (1969). *Collective search for identity*. New York: Holt, Rinehart & Winston.

Klausner, S.Z. (1968). The intermingling of pain and pleasure: The stress-seeking personality in its social context. In S.Z. Klausner (Ed.), *Why men take chances* (pp. 137–168). Garden City, NY: Anchor.

Kleck, G., & Mcelrath, K. (1991). The effects of weaponry on human violence. *Social Forces, 69*, 669–692.

Klein, A.L. (1976). Changes in leadership appraisal as a function of the stress of a simulated panic situation, *Journal of Personality and Social Psychology, 34*, 1143–1154.

Knight, G.P., & Dubro, A.F. (1984). Cooperative, competitive, and individualistic social values: An individualized regression and clustering approach. *Journal of Personality and Social Psychology, 46*, 98–105.

Knott, P.D., Lasater, L., & Schuman, R. (1974). Aggression-guilt and conditionability for aggressiveness. *Journal of Personality, 42,* 332–344.

Konar-Goldband, E., Rice, R.W., & Monkarsh, W. (1979). Time-phased interrelationships of group atmosphere, group performance, and leader style. *Journal of Applied Psychology, 64,* 401–409.

Konecni, V.J. (1975). Annoyance, type and duration of postannoyance activity, and aggression: The "cathartic effect." *Journal of Experimental Psychology: General, 104,* 76–102.

Konecni, V.J. (1984). Methodological issues in human aggression research. In R.M. Kaplan, V.J. Konecni & R.W. Novaco (Eds.), *Aggression in children and youth* (pp. 1–43). The Hague: Martinus Nijhoff.

Konecni, V.J., & Doob, A.M. (1972). Catharsis through displacement of aggression. *Journal of Personality and Social Psychology, 23,* 379–387.

Koocher, G.P. (1971). Swimming, competence, and personality change, *Journal of Personality and Social Psychology, 18,* 275–278.

Kravitz, D.A., & Martin, B. (1986). Ringelmann rediscovered: The original article. *Journal of Personality and Social Psychology, 50,* 936–941.

Kuhlmann, W. (1975). Violence in professional sports. *Wisconsin Law Review, 3,* 771–790.

Kushell, E., & Newton, R. (1986). Gender, leadership style, and subordinate satisfaction: An experiment. *Sex Roles, 14,* 203–209.

Laird, D.A. (1923). Changes in motor control under the influence of razzing. *Journal of Experimental Psychology, 6,* 236–246.

Lang, K., & Lang, G.E. (1961). *Collective dynamics.* New York: Thomas Y. Crowell.

Lange, A.R., Goeckner, D.J., Adesso, V.J., & Marlatt, G.A. (1975). Effects of alcohol on aggression in male social drinkers. *Journal of Abnormal Psychology, 84,* 508–518.

Latané, B. (1981). The psychology of social impact. *American Psychologist, 36,* 343–356.

Latané, B., & Harkins, S.G. (1976). Cross-modality matches suggest anticipated stage fright a multiplicative power function of audience size and status. *Perception and Psychophysics, 20,* 482–488.

Latané, B., Harkins, S.G., & Williams, K. (1980). *Many hands make light the work: Social loafing as a social disease.* Unpublished manuscript, The Ohio State University.

Latané, B., & Nida, S. (1980). Social impact theory and group influence: A social engineering perspective. In P.B. Paulus (Ed.), *Psychology of group influence* (pp. 3–34). Hillsdale, NJ: Erlbaum.

Latané, B., Williams, K., & Harkins, S.G. (1979). Many hands make light the work: The causes and consequences of social loafing. *Journal of Personality and Social Psychology, 37,* 823–832.

Lau, R.R., & Russell, D. (1980). Attributions in the sports pages. *Journal of Personality and Social Psychology, 39,* 29–38.

Lay, C.H. (1986). At last, my research article on procrastination. *Journal of Research in Personality, 20,* 474–495.

Lay, C.H., & Burns, P. (1991). Intentions and behavior in studying for an examination: The role of trait procrastination and its interaction with optimism. *Journal of Social Behavior and Personality, 6,* 605–617.

Lee, M.J. (1985). Self-esteem and social identity in basketball fans: A closer look at basking in reflected glory. *Journal of Sport Behavior, 8,* 210–223.

Lee, M.J., Coburn, T., & Partridge, R. (1983). The influence of team structure in determining leadership function in Association Football. *Journal of Sport Behavior, 6,* 59–66.

Lefkowitz, M.M., Walder, L.O., Eron, L.D., & Huesmann, L.R. (1973). Preference for televised contact sports as related to sex differences in aggression. *Developmental Psychology, 9*, 417–420.

Lehman, B.H. (1928). *Carlyle's theory of the hero.* Durham, NC: Duke University Press.

Lehman, D.R., & Reifman, A. (1987). Spectator influence on basketball officiating. *Journal of Social Psychology, 127,* 673–675.

Lenk, H. (1977). *Team dynamics.* Champaign, IL: Stipes.

Lennon, J.X., & Hatfield, F.C. (1980). The effects of crowding and observation of athletic events on spectator tendency toward aggressive behavior. *Journal of Sport Behavior, 3,* 61–67.

Leuck, M.R., Krahenbuhl, G.S., & Odenkirk, J.E. (1979). Assessment of spectator aggression at intercollegiate basketball contests. *Review of Sport and Leisure, 4,* 40–52.

LeUnes, A.D., Hayward, S., & Daiss, S. (1988). Annotated bibliography on the Profile of Mood States in sport, 1975–1988. *Journal of Sport Behavior, 11,* 213–240.

LeUnes, A.D., & Nation, J.R. (1982). Saturday's heroes: A psychological portrait of college football players. *Journal of Sport Behavior, 5,* 139–149.

LeUnes, A.D., & Nation, J.R. (1989). *Sport psychology: An introduction.* Chicago: Nelson-Hall.

Levenson, M.R. (1990). Risk taking and personality. *Journal of Personality and Social Psychology, 58,* 1073–1080.

Levin, H.S., Eisenberg, H.M., & Benton, A.L. (1989). *Mild head injury.* New York: Oxford University Press.

Lewis, G. (1983). *Real men like violence.* Kenthurst, Australia: Kangaroo Press.

Lewis, G., & Redmond, G. (1974). *Sport heritage: A guide to halls of fame, special collections and museums in the United States and Canada.* New York: Barnes.

Lewis, J.M. (1989). A value-added analysis of the Heysel stadium soccer riot. *Current Psychology: Research and Reviews, 8,* 15–29.

Lewis, J.M., & Veneman, J.M. (1987). Crisis resolution: The Bradford fire and English society. *Sociological Focus, 20,* 155–168.

Lirgg, C.D., & Feltz, D.L. (1991). Teacher versus peer models revisited: Effects on motor performance and self-efficacy. *Research Quarterly for Exercise and Sport, 62,* 217–224.

Listiak, A. (1974). Legitimate deviance and social class: Bar behaviour during Grey Cup week. *Sociological Focus, 7,* 13–44.

Loew, C.A. (1967). Acquisition of a hostile attitude and its relationship to aggressive behavior. *Journal of Personality and Social Psychology, 5,* 335–341.

London, P. (1970). The rescuers: Motivational hypotheses about Christians who saved Jews from the Nazis (pp. 241–250). In J. Macaulay & L. Berkowitz (Eds.), *Altruism and helping behavior: Social psychological studies of some antecedents and consequences.* New York: Academic Press.

Lord, R.G., DeVader, C.L., & Alliger, G.M. (1986). A meta-analysis of the relation between personality traits and leadership perceptions: An application of validity generalization procedures. *Journal of Applied Psychology, 71,* 402–410.

Lord, R.G., & Hohenfeld, J.A. (1979). Longitudinal field assessment of equity effects on the performance of major league baseball players. *Journal of Applied Psychology, 64,* 19–26.

Lorenz, K. (1966). *On aggression.* New York: Harcourt, Brace & World.

Lott, A.J., & Lott, B.E. (1965). Group cohesiveness as interpersonal attraction: A review of relationships with antecedent and consequent variables. *Psychological Bulletin, 64*, 259–309.

Loy, J.W., Jr., Curtis, J.E., & Hillen, J.M. (1987). Effects of formal structure on managerial recruitment: Comparisons of Japanese and North American professional baseball clubs. *Sociology of Sport Journal, 4*, 1–16.

Loy, J.W., Jr., Curtis, J.E., & Sage, J.N. (1978). Relative centrality of playing position and leadership recruitment in team sports. *Exercise and Sport Sciences Reviews, 6*, 257–284.

Loy, J.W., Jr., McPherson, B.D., & Kenyon, G. (1978). *Sport and social systems*. Reading, MA: Addison-Wesley.

Loy, J.W., Jr., & Sage, J.N. (1970). The effects of formal structure on organizational leadership: An investigation of interscholastic baseball. In G.S. Kenyon (Ed.), *Contemporary psychology of sport* (pp. 363–373). Chicago: The Athletic Institute.

MacDonald, J.M. (1961). *The murderer and his victim*. Springfield, IL: C.C. Thomas.

Maddi, S.R. (1968). *Personality theories: A comparative analysis*. Homewood, IL: Dorsey.

Mandell, R.D. (1976). The invention of the sports record. *Stadion, 2*, 250–264.

Mann, L. (1969). Queue culture: The waiting line as a social system. *American Journal of Sociology, 75*, 340–354.

Mann, L. (1974). On being a sore loser: How fans react to their team's failure. *Australian Journal of Psychology, 26*, 37–47.

Mann, L. (1979). Sports crowds viewed from the perspective of collective behavior. In J.H. Goldstein (Ed.), *Sports, games, and play* (pp. 337–368). Hillsdale, NJ: Erlbaum.

Mann, L. (1989). Sports crowds and the collective behavior perspective. In J.H. Goldstein (Ed.), *Sports, games, and play* (2nd ed., pp. 299–331). Hillsdale, NJ: Erlbaum.

Mann, L., & Pearce, P. (1978). Social psychology of the sports spectator. In D.J. Glencross (Ed.), *Psychology and sport* (pp. 173–201). New York: McGraw-Hill.

Mark, M.M., Mutrie, N., Brooks, D.R., & Harris, D.V. (1984). Causal attributions of winners and losers in individual competitive sports: Toward a reformulation of the self-serving bias. *Journal of Sport Psychology, 6*, 184–196.

Markovsky, B., & Berger, S.M. (1983). Crowd noise and mimicry. *Personality and Social Psychology Bulletin, 9*, 90–96.

Marsh, P. (1978). *Aggro: The illusion of violence*. London: J.M. Dent.

Marsh, P. (1982). Social order on the British soccer terraces. *International Social Science Journal, 34*, 247–256.

Marshall, J.E., & Heslin, R. (1975). Boys and girls together: Sexual composition and the effect of density and group size on cohesiveness. *Journal of Personality and Social Psychology, 31*, 952–961.

Marshall, R. (1927). Precipitation and presidents. *The Nation, 124*, 315–316.

Martens, R. (1976). The paradigmatic crises in American sport personology. In A. Fisher (Ed.), *Psychology of sport: Issues and insights* (pp. 415–431). Palo Alto, CA: Mayfield.

Mashiach, A. (1980). A study to determine the factors which influence American spectators to go to see the summer Olympics in Montreal, 1976. *Journal of Sport Behavior, 3*, 17–28.

Maslow, A.H. (1968). *Toward a psychology of being* (2nd ed.). New York: Van Nostrand.

Massengale, J., & Farrington, S. (1977). The influence of playing position centrality on the careers of college football coaches. *Review of Sport and Leisure, 2*, 107–115,

Matthews, K.A., Helmreich, R.L., Beane, W.E., & Lucker, G.W. (1980). Pattern A, achievement striving, and scientific merit: Does pattern A help or hinder? *Journal of Personality and Social Psychology, 39*, 962–967.

McAuley, E., & Gill, D. (1983). Reliability and validity of the Physical Self-efficacy Scale in a competitive sport setting. *Journal of Sport Psychology, 5*, 410–418.

McAuley, E., & Gross, J.B. (1983). Perceptions of causality in sport: An application of the Causal Dimension Scale. *Journal of Sport Psychology, 5*, 72–76.

McClelland, D.C. (1953). *The achievement motive.* New York: Appleton Century Crofts.

McClelland, D.C. (1958). Risk-taking in children with high and low need for achievement. In J.W. Atkinson (Ed.), *Motives in fantasy, action, and society.* Princeton, NJ: Van Nostrand.

McClelland, D.C. (1987). *Human motivation.* New York: Cambridge University Press.

McClelland, D.C., Atkinson, J.W., Clark, R.A., & Lowell, E.L. (1953). *The achievement motive.* New York: Appleton-Century-Crofts.

McCutcheon, L.E. (1984). The home advantage in high school athletics. *Journal of Sport Behavior, 7*, 135–138.

McDougall, W. (1908). *An introduction to social psychology.* London: Methuen.

McElroy, M.A., & Kirkendall, D.R. (1980). Significant others and professionalized sport attitudes. *Research Quarterly for Exercise and Sport, 51*, 645–653.

McEvoy, A., & Erickson, E.L. (1981). Heroes and villains: A conceptual strategy for assessing their influence. *Sociological Focus, 14*, 111–122.

McGowan, J., & Gormly, J. (1976). Validation of personality traits: A multicriteria approach. *Journal of Personality and Social Psychology, 34*, 791–795.

McNair, D.M., Lorr, M., & Droppleman, L.F. (1971). *Manual for the Profile of Mood States.* San Diego, CA: Educational & Industrial Testing Service.

Mehlman, R.C., & Snyder, C.R. (1985). Excuse theory: A test of the self-protective role of attributions. *Journal of Personality and Social Psychology, 49*, 994–1001.

Mehrabian, A. (1968). Male and female scales of the tendency to achieve. *Educational and Psychological Measurement, 28*, 493–502.

Mehrabian, A. (1976). *Public places, and private spaces: Psychology of work, play and living environments.* New York: Fitzhenry & Whiteside.

Milgram, S. (1974). *Obedience to authority.* New York: Cambridge University Press.

Milgram, S., & Toch, H. (1969). Collective behavior: Crowds and social movements. In G. Lindzey & E. Aronson (Eds.), *The handbook of social psychology* (Vol. 4, pp. 507–610). Reading, MA: Addison-Wesley.

Miller, A.G., & Thomas, R. (1972). Cooperation and competition among Blackfoot Indian and urban Canadian children. *Child Development, 43*, 1104–1110.

Miller, D.T., & Ross, M. (1975). Self-serving biases in the attribution of causality: Fact of fiction? *Psychological Bulletin, 82*, 213–225.

Miller, N.E. (1941). The frustration-aggression hypothesis. *Psychological Review, 48*, 337–342.

Miller, T.Q., Heath, L., Molcan, J.R., & Dugoni, B.L. (1991). Imitative violence in the real world: A reanalysis of homicide rates following championship prize fights. *Aggressive Behavior, 17*, 121–134.

The Miller Lite report on American attitudes toward sports (1983). Milwaukee: Miller Brewing Company.

Millon, T. (1969). *Modern psychopathology.* Philadelphia, PA: W.B. Saunders.

Mintz, A. (1951). Non-adaptive group behavior. *Journal of Abnormal and Social Psychology, 46*, 150–159.

Mischel, W. (1961). Delay of gratification, need for achievement, and acquiescence in another culture. *Journal of Abnormal and Social Psychology, 62,* 543–552.

Mischel, W. (1977). On the future of personality measurement. *American Psychologist, 32,* 246–254.

Mischel, W. (1986). *Introduction to personality* (4th ed.). New York: Holt, Rinehart and Winston.

Mitchell, R.E. (1971). Some social implications of higher density housing. *American Sociological Review, 36,* 18–29.

Mizruchi, M.S. (1991). Urgency, motivation, and group performance: The effect of prior success on current success among professional basketball teams. *Social Psychology Quarterly, 54,* 181–189.

Moorhouse, H.F. (1984). Professional football and working class culture: English theories and Scottish evidence. *Sociological Review, 32,* 285–315.

Moreno, J.L. (1953). *Who shall survive?* Beacon, NY: Beacon.

Morgan, W.P. (1980). The trait psychology controversy. *Research Quarterly for Exercise and Sport, 51,* 50–76.

Morrison, D.G., & Wheat, R.D. (1986). Pulling the goalie revisited. *Interfaces, 16,* 28–34.

Mosher, D.L. (1991). Macho men, machismo, and sexuality. In J. Bancroft (Ed.), *Annual Review of Sex Research, 2,* 199–247.

Mosher, D.L. (in press). *Scripting the macho man: Theory, research, and measurement of hypermasculinity.* New York: Guilford.

Mosher, D.L., & Anderson, R.D. (1986). Macho personality, sexual aggression, and reactions to guided imagery of realistic rape. *Journal of Research in Personality, 20,* 77–94.

Mosher, D.L., & Sirkin, M. (1984). Measuring a macho personality constellation. *Journal of Research in Personality, 18,* 150–163.

Mosher, D.L., & Tomkins, S.S. (1988). Scripting the macho man: Hypermasculine socialization and enculturation. *Journal of Sex Research, 25,* 60–84.

Mossholder, K.W. (1980). Effects of externally mediated goal setting on intrinsic motivation: A laboratory experiment. *Journal of Applied Psychology, 65,* 202–210.

Moyer, K.E. (1987). *Violence and aggression: A physiological perspective.* New York: Paragon House.

Mudrack, P.E. (1989a). Defining group cohesiveness: A legacy of confusion? *Small Group Behavior, 20,* 37–49.

Mudrack, P.E. (1989b). Group cohesiveness and productivity: A closer look. *Human Relations, 42,* 771–785.

Mugno, D.A., & Feltz, D.L. (1985). The social learning of aggression in youth football in the United States. *Canadian Journal of Applied Sport Sciences, 10,* 26–35.

Mullen, B. (1985). Strength and immediacy of sources: A meta-analytic evaluation of the forgotten elements of social impact theory. *Journal of Personality and Social Psychology, 49,* 1458–1466.

Mullen, B. (1986). Effects of strength and immediacy in group contexts: Reply to Jackson. *Journal of Personality and Social Psychology, 50,* 514–516.

Murray, H.A., et al. (1938). *Explorations in personality.* New York: Oxford University Press.

Murray, J., & Feshbach, S. (1978). Let's not throw the baby out with the bathwater: The catharsis hypothesis revisited. *Journal of Personality, 46,* 462–473.

Musante, L., MacDougall, J.M., & Dembroski, T.M. (1984). The Type A behavior pattern and attributions for success and failure. *Personality and Social Psychology Bulletin, 10*, 544–553.

Myers, A.E. (1962). Team competition, success, and the adjustment of group members. *Journal of Abnormal and Social Psychology, 65*, 325–332.

Narancic, V.G. (1972). The psychology of swearing among sportsmen. *Journal of Sports Medicine, 12*, 207–210.

Nash, J.E., & Lerner, E. (1981). Learning from the pros: Violence in youth hockey. *Youth & Society, 13*, 229–244.

Nation, J.R., & LeUnes, A. (1983a). A personality profile of the black athlete in college football. *Psychology, 20*, 1–3.

Nation, J.R., & LeUnes, A. (1983b). Personality characteristics of intercollegiate football players as determined by position, classification, and redshirt status. *Journal of Sport Behavior, 6*, 92–102.

Nepalese look for survivors of stampede at soccer game. (1988, March 14). *New York Times*.

Nichols, M.P., & Zax, M. (1977). *Catharsis in psychotherapy*. New York: Gardner.

Nighswander, J.K., & Mayer, G.R. (1969). Catharsis: A means of reducing elementary school students' aggressive behaviors? *Personnel and Guidance Journal, 47*, 461–466.

Noble, G. (1975). *Children in front of the small screen*. Beverly Hills, CA: Sage.

Noll, R.G. (1974). Attendance and price setting. In R.G. Noll (Ed.), *Government and the sports business* (pp. 115–157). Washington, DC: The Brookings Institution.

Nosanchuk, T.A. (1981). The way of the warrior: The effects of traditional martial arts training on aggressiveness. *Human Relations, 34*, 435–444.

Nosanchuk, T.A., & MacNeil, M.L.C. (1989). Examination of the effects of traditional and modern martial arts training on aggressiveness. *Aggressive Behavior, 15*, 153–159.

Novaco, R.W. (1975). *Anger control: The development and evaluation of an experimental treatment*. Lexington, MA: Heath.

Novaco, R.W. (1986). Anger as a clinical and social problem. In R.J. Blanchard & D.C. Blanchard (Eds.), *Advances in the study of aggression* (Vol. 2, pp. 1–67). New York: Academic Press.

Nowicki, S., Jr. (1982). Competition-cooperation as a mediator of locus of control and achievement. *Journal of Research in Personality, 16*, 157–164.

Nowlis, V. (1965). Research with the Mood Adjective Check List. In S.S. Tompkins & C. Izard (Eds.), *Affect, cognition, and personality* (pp. 352–389). New York: Springer.

Oberndorf, C.P. (1951). Psychopathology of work. *Bulletin of the Menninger Clinic, 15*, 77–84.

Ogilvie, B.C. (1974, October). The sweet psycho jolt of danger. *Psychology Today*, pp. 92–94.

Ogilvie, B.C., & Pool, C.C. (1974). Aerobatic pilots: Why do they fly that way? *The Physician and Sportsmedicine, 2*, 63–65.

O'Leary, M.R., & Dengerink, H.A. (1973). Aggression as a function of the intensity and pattern of attack. *Journal of Experimental Research in Personality, 7*, 61–70.

O'Leary, V.E. (1974). Some attitudinal barriers to occupational aspirations in women. *Psychological Bulletin, 81*, 809–826.

Olweus, D. (1978). *Aggression in the schools: Bullies and whipping boys*. Washington, DC: Hemisphere.

Olweus, D. (1979). Stability of aggressive reaction patterns in males: A review. *Psychological Bulletin, 86*, 852–875.

175 at football game injured fleeing fumes. (1986, September 21). *New York Times*, I, p. 24:6.

Orlick, T. (1978). *Winning through cooperation*. Washington, DC: Acropolis.

Ostrow, A.C. (1974). The aggressive tendencies of male intercollegiate tennis team players as measured by selected psychological tests. *New Zealand Journal of Health, Physical Education, and Recreation, 6*, 19–21.

Ostrow, A.C. (1976). Goal-setting behavior and need achievement in relation to competitive motor activity. *Research Quarterly, 47*, 174–183.

Ostrow, A.C. (Ed.). (1990). *Directory of psychological tests in the sport and exercise sciences*. Morgantown, WV: Fitness Information Technology.

Page, M.M., & Scheidt, R.J. (1971). The elusive weapons effect: Demand awareness, evaluation apprehension and slightly sophisticated subjects. *Journal of Personality and Social Psychology, 20*, 591–596.

Page, R.A., & Moss, M.K. (1976). Environmental influences on aggression: The effects of darkness and proximity of victim. *Journal of Applied Social Psychology, 6*, 126–133.

Patterson, A.H. (1974). Hostility catharsis: A naturalistic quasi-experiment. *Personality and Social Psychology Bulletin, 1*, 195–197.

Paulhus, D., Molin, J., & Schuchts, R. (1979). Control profiles of football players, tennis players, and nonathletes. *Journal of Social Psychology, 108*, 199–205.

Paulus, P.B. (Ed.). (1989). *Psychology of group influence* (2nd ed.). Hillsdale, NJ: Erlbaum.

Paulus, P.B., Judd, B.B., & Bernstein, I.H. (1976, April). *Social facilitation and sports*. Paper presented at the meeting of the North American Society for Psychology of Sport and Physical Activity, Austin, TX.

Paulus, P.B., Shannon, J.C., Wilson, D.L., & Boone, T.D. (1972). The effect of spectator presence on gymnastic performance in a field situation. *Psychonomic Science, 29*, 88–90.

Penman, K.A., Hastad, D.N., & Cords, W.L. (1974). Success of the authoritarian coach. *Journal of Social Psychology, 92*, 155–156.

Pennebaker, J.A., & Lightner, J.M. (1980). Competition of internal and external information in an exercise setting. *Journal of Personality and Social Psychology, 39*, 165–174.

Peper, D. (1980). *Aggression und katharsis im sport: Motivationstheoretischer beitrag zur funktion von motorischer aktivitat und zielerreichung*. Unpublished doctoral dissertation, University of Saarbrucken, Germany.

Perrow, C. (1984). *Normal accidents: Living with high-risk technologies*. New York: Basic Books.

Pervin, L.A. (1970). *Personality: Theory, assessment, and research*. New York: Wiley.

Peters, L.H., Hartke, D.D., & Pohlmann, J.T. (1985). Fiedler's contingency theory of leadership: An application of the meta-analysis procedures of Schmidt and Hunter. *Psychological Bulletin, 97*, 274–285.

Peterson, C. (1980). Attribution in the sports pages: An archival investigation of the covariation hypothesis. *Social Psychology Quarterly, 43*, 136–141.

Petrie, B.M. (1975). Sport and politics. In D.W. Ball & J.W. Loy (Eds.), *Sport and social order* (pp. 189–237). Reading, MA: Addison-Wesley.

Pfeffer, J., & Davis-Blake, A. (1986). Administrative succession and organizational performance: How administrator experience mediates the succession effect. *Academy of Management Journal, 29*, 72–83.

Phillips, C.L. (1985). Sport group-behavior and officials' perceptions. *International Journal of Sports Psychology, 16*, 1–11.

Phillips, D.P. (1983). The impact of mass media violence on U.S. homicides. *American Sociological Review, 48*, 560–568.

Phillips, D.P. (1986). Natural experiments on the effects of mass media violence on fatal aggression: Strength and weaknesses of a new approach. In L. Berkowitz (Ed.), *Advances in experimental social psychology* (Vol. 19, pp. 207–250), New York: Academic Press.

Pihl, R.O., Smith, M., & Farrell, B. (1984). Alcohol and aggression in men: A comparison of brewed and distilled beverages. *Journal of Studies on Alcohol, 45*, 278–282.

Pilkington, C.J., Richardson, D.R., & Utley, M.E. (1988). Is conflict stimulating?: Sensation seekers' responses to interpersonal conflict. *Personality and Social Psychology Bulletin, 14*, 596–603.

Pilz, G.A. (1989). Social factors influencing sport and violence: On the "problem" of football fans in West Germany. *Concilium-International Review of Theology, 5*, 32–43.

Pittsburgh victory fete erupts into riot: Many hurt, arrested. (1971, October 18). *The New York Times*, p. 50.

Podborski turns back on ski sponsors. (1984, February 24). *The Lethbridge Herald*.

Pollard, R. (1986). Home advantage in soccer: A retrospective analysis. *Journal of Sports Sciences, 4*, 237–248.

Pope, H.G., Jr., & Katz, D.L. (1988). Affective and psychotic symptoms associated with anabolic steroid use. *American Journal of Psychiatry, 145*, 487–490.

Pope, H.G., Jr., & Katz, D.L. (1990). Homicide and near-homicide by anabolic steroid users. *Journal of Clinical Psychiatry, 51*, 28–31.

Price, V.A. (1982). *Type A behavior pattern*. New York: Academic Press.

Price, V.A. (1988). Research and clinical issues in treating Type A behavior. In B.K. Houston & C.R. Snyder (Eds.), *Type A behavior pattern: Research, theory, and intervention* (pp. 275–311). New York: Wiley.

Pritchard, R.D., Campbell, K.M., & Campbell, D.J. (1977). Effects of extrinsic financial rewards on intrinsic motivation. *Journal of Applied Psychology, 62*, 9–15.

Pritchard, R.D., Dunnette, M.D., & Jorgenson, D.O. (1972). Effects of perceptions of equity and inequity on worker performance and satisfaction. *Journal of Applied Psychology, 56*, 75–94.

Proctor, R.C., & Eckerd, W.M. (1976). *"Toot-toot"* or spectator sports: Psychological and therapeutic implications. *American Journal of Sports Medicine, 4*, 78–83.

Pyszczynski, T., & Greenberg, J. (1987). Toward an integration of cognitive and motivational perspectives on social inference: A biased hypothesis-testing model. In L. Berkowitz (Ed.), *Advances in experimental social psychology* (Vol. 20, pp. 297–340). New York: Academic Press.

Quanty, M.B. (1976). Aggression catharsis: Experimental investigations and implications. In R.G. Geen & E.C. O'Neal (Eds.), *Perspectives on aggression* (pp. 99–132). New York: Academic Press.

Rabbie, J.M. (1989). Football violence in the Heizel Stadium: A management crisis (Review of *Het Heizel drama: Rampzalig organiseren en kritieke beslissingen*). *Current Psychology: Research & Reviews, 8*, 50–56.

Rainbow man at the game for the Lord. (1987, January 24). *The Edmonton Journal*. p. E5.

Ransford, H.E. (1968). Isolation, powerlessness, and violence: A study of attitudes and participation in the Watts riot. *American Journal of Sociology, 73*, 581–591.

Rees, C.R. (1983). Instrumental and expressive leadership in team sports: A test of leadership role differentiation theory. *Journal of Sport Behavior, 6*, 17–27.

Rees, C.R., & Segal, M.W. (1984). Role differentiation in groups: The relationship between instrumental and expressive leadership. *Small Group Behavior, 15*, 109–123.

Reifman, A.S., Larrick, R.P., & Fein, S. (1991). Temper and temperature on the diamond: The heat-aggression relationship in major league baseball. *Personality and Social Psychology Bulletin, 17,* 580–585.

Rhodewalt, F., Saltzman, A.T., & Wittmer, J. (1984). Self-handicapping among competitive athletes: The role of practice in self-esteem protection. *Basic and Applied Social Psychology, 5,* 197–209.

Rhodewalt, F., & Strube, M.J. (1985). A self-attribution-reactance model of recovery from injury in Type A individuals. *Journal of Applied Social Psychology, 15,* 330–344.

Richmond, B.O., & Weiner, G.P. (1973). Cooperation and competition among young children as a function of ethnic grouping, grade, sex, and reward condition. *Journal of Educational Psychology, 64,* 329–334.

Riess, M., & Taylor, J. (1984). Ego-involvement and attributions for success and failure in a field setting. *Personality and Social Psychology Bulletin, 10,* 536–543.

Roberts, G.C. (1974). Effect of achievement motivation and social environment on risk taking. *The Research Quarterly, 45,* 42–55.

Robinson, D.W. (1985). Stress seeking: Selected behavioral characteristics of elite rock climbers. *Journal of Sport Psychology, 7,* 400–404.

Robinson, J.P., Shaver, P.R., & Wrightsman, L.S. (Eds.). (1991). *Measures of personality and social psychological attitudes.* New York: Academic Press.

Rosecrance, J. (1986). You can't tell the players without a scorecard: A typology of horse players. *Deviant Behavior, 7,* 77–97.

Rosen, B.C., & D'Andrade, R.G. (1959). The psychosocial origin of achievement motivation. *Sociometry, 22,* 185–218.

Rosenberg, M. (1973). Which significant others? *American Behavioral Scientist, 16,* 829–860.

Rosenthal, R. (1969). Interpersonal expectation. In R. Rosenthal & R.L. Rosnow (Eds.), *Artifact in behavioral research* (pp. 181–277). New York: Academic Press.

Rosenthal, R., & Jacobson, L. (1968). *Pygmalion in the classroom: Teacher expectation and pupils' intellectual development.* New York: Holt, Rinehart & Winston.

Rosenthal, R., & Rosnow, R.L. (1984). *Essentials of behavioral research.* New York: McGraw-Hill.

Rosnow, R.L. (1965). Bias in evaluating the presidential debates: A "splinter" effect. *Journal of Social Psychology, 67,* 211–219.

Rosnow, R.L., & Robinson, E.J. (Eds.). (1967). *Experiments in persuasion.* New York: Academic Press.

Rotter, J.B. (1966). Generalized expectancies for internal versus external control of reinforcement. *Psychological Monographs, 80* (Whole No. 609).

Rotton, J., & Frey, J. (1985). Air pollution, weather, and violent crimes: Concomitant time-series analysis of archival data. *Journal of Personality and Social Psychology, 49,* 1207–1220.

Rotton J., Frey, J., Barry, T., Milligan, M., & Fitzpatrick, M. (1979). The air pollution experience and physical aggression. *Journal of Applied Social Psychology, 9,* 397–412.

Rotton, J., & Kelly, I.W. (1985). Much ado about the full moon: A meta-analysis of the lunar-lunacy research. *Psychological Bulletin, 97,* 286–306.

Rowland, G.L., Franken, R.E., & Harrison, K. (1986). Sensation seeking and participation in sporting activities. *Journal of Sport Psychology, 8,* 212–220.

Rule, B.G., & Nesdale, A.R. (1976). Emotional arousal and aggressive behavior. *Psychological Bulletin, 83,* 851–863.

Runfola, R.T. (1974, October 27). He is a hockey player, 17, black and convicted of manslaughter. *The New York Times*, p. S2.

Russell, G.W. (1974). Machiavellianism, locus of control, aggression, performance and precautionary behaviour in ice hockey. *Human Relations, 27*, 825–837.

Russell, G.W. (1979). Hero selection by Canadian ice hockey players: Skill or aggression? *Canadian Journal of Applied Sport Sciences, 4*, 309–313.

Russell, G.W. (1981a). A comparison of hostility measures. *The Journal of Social Psychology, 113*, 45–55.

Russell, G.W. (1981b). Aggression in sport. In P.F. Brain & D. Benton (Eds.), *A multidisciplinary approach to aggression research* (pp. 431–446). North Holland: Elsevier.

Russell, G.W. (1981c). Spectator moods at an aggressive sports event. *Journal of Sport Psychology, 3*, 217–227.

Russell, G.W. (1983a). Crowd size and density in relation to athletic aggression and performance. *Social Behavior and Personality, 11*, 9–15.

Russell, G.W. (1983b). Psychological issues in sports aggression. In J.H. Goldstein (Ed.), *Sports violence* (pp. 157–181). New York: Springer-Verlag.

Russell, G.W. (1986). Does sports violence increase box office receipts? *International Journal of Sports Psychology, 17*, 173–183.

Russell, G.W. (1991). Athletes as targets of aggression. In R. Baenninger (Ed.), *Targets of violence and aggression* (pp. 211–252). North Holland: Elsevier.

Russell, G.W. (1992a). Battling Amazons: Responses to female fighters. In K. Björkqvist & P. Niemelä (Eds), *Of mice and women: Aspects of female aggression* (pp. 251–260). Orlando, FL: Academic Press.

Russell, G.W. (1992b, September). Personalities in the crowd: Those who would escalate a riot. Paper presented at the meeting of the International Society for Research on Aggression, Siena, Italy.

Russell, G.W. (in press). *Response of the macho male to viewing a combatant sport. Journal of Social Behavior and Personality.*

Russell, G.W., & deGraaf, J. (1985). Lunar cycles and human aggression: A replication. *Social Behavior and Personality, 13*, 143–146.

Russell, G.W., Di Lullo, S.L., & Di Lullo, D. (1989). Effects of viewing competitive and violent versions of a sport. *Current Psychology: Research and Reviews, 7*, 313–321.

Russell, G.W., & Drewry, B.R. (1976). Crowd size and competitive aspects of aggression in ice hockey: An archival study. *Human Relations, 29*, 723–735.

Russell, G.W., & Dua, M. (1983). Lunar influences on human aggression. *Social Behavior and Personality, 11*, 41–44.

Russell, G.W., Horn, V.E., & Huddle, M.J. (1988). Male responses to female aggression. *Social Behavior and Personality, 16*, 47–53.

Russell, G.W., Huddle, M.J., & Corson, M.C. (1988). At close quarters: Personal space requirements of men in intimate heterosexual dyads. In G.W. Russell (Ed.), *Violence in intimate relationships* (pp. 253–267). Great Neck, NY: PMA Publishing.

Russell, G.W., & McClusky, M.G. (1985, May) *The exemplars of adolescents: Their influence and quality.* Paper presented at the meeting of the Banff Annual Seminar in Cognitive Science, Banff, Alberta, Canada.

Russell, G.W., & Pigat, L. (1991). Effects of modeled censure/support of media violence and need for approval on aggression. *Current Psychology: Research and Reviews, 10*, 121–128.

Russell, G.W., & Russell, A.M. (1984). Sports penalties: An alternative means of assessing aggression. *Social Behavior and Personality, 12*, 69–74.

Ryan, E.D. (1970). The cathartic effect of vigorous motor activity on aggressive behavior. *Research Quarterly, 41*, 542–551.

Ryan, E.D., & Lakie, W.L. (1965). Competitive and noncompetitive performance in relation to achievement motive and manifest anxiety. *Journal of Personality and Social Psychology, 1*, 342–345.

Sandiford, K.A.P. (1982). English cricket crowds during the Victorian age. *Journal of Sport History, 9*, 5–22.

Scanlon, T., & Passer, M. (1980). Self-serving biases in the competitive sport setting: An attributional dilemma. *Journal of Sport Psychology, 2*, 124–136.

Schedlowski, M., & Tewes, U. (1992). Physiological arousal and perception of bodily state during parachute jumping. *Psychophysiology, 29*, 95–103.

Scheer, J.K., & Ansorge, C.J. (1979). Influence due to expectations of judges: A function of internal-external locus of control. *Journal of Sport Psychology, 1*, 53–58.

Scheff, T.J., & Bushnell, D.D. (1984). A theory of catharsis. *Journal of Research in Personality, 18*, 238–264.

Schmitt, B.H., Gilovich, T., Goore, N., & Joseph, L. (1986). Mere presence and social facilitation: One more time. *Journal of Experimental Social Psychology, 22*, 242–248.

Schmitt, R.L., & Leonard W.L., II. (1986). Immortalizing the self through sport. *The American Journal of Sociology, 91*, 1088–1111.

Schollaert, P.T., & Smith, D.H. (1987). Team racial composition and sports attendance. *Sociological Quarterly, 28*, 71–87.

Schroder, H.M., Driver, M.J., & Streufert, S. (1967). *Human information processing.* New York: Holt, Rinehart & Winston.

Schuh, A.J. (1986). Performance measures of game activity and team effectiveness in competitive youth soccer. *Bulletin of the Psychonomic Society, 24*, 381–384.

Schultz, D.P. (Ed.). (1964a). *Panic behavior.* New York: Random House.

Schultz, D.P. (1964b). Panic in organized collectivities. *Journal of Social Psychology, 63*, 353–359.

Schultz, D.P. (1964c). Theories of panic: A review. *Journal of Social Psychology, 66*, 31–40.

Schwartz, B., & Barsky, S.F. (1977). The home advantage. *Social Forces, 55*, 641–661.

Schweitzer, K., Zillmann, D., Weaver, J.B., & Luttrell, E.S. (1992). Perception of threatening events in the emotional aftermath of a televised college football game. *Journal of Broadcasting & Electronic Media, 36*, 75–82.

Shaw, M.E. (1976). *Group dynamics: The psychology of small group behavior* (2nd ed.). New York: McGraw-Hill.

Shaw, M.E., & Wright, J.M. (1967). *Scales for the measurement of attitudes.* New York: McGraw-Hill.

Sheldon, W.H. (1940). *The varieties of human physique.* New York: Harper.

Sherif, M., & Sherif, C.W. (1969). *Social psychology.* New York: Harper & Row.

Showalter, S.W. (1985). Sports polls: Predictive or promotional? *Journalism Quarterly, 62*, 100–104.

Silva, J.M., III. (1979). Behavioral and situational factors affecting concentration and skill performance. *Journal of Sport Psychology, 1*, 221–227.

Silva, J.M., III. & Andrew, J.A. (1987). An analysis of game location and basketball performance in the Atlantic Coast Conference. *International Journal of Sports Psychology, 18*, 188–204.

Sipes, R.G. (1973). War, sports and aggression: An empirical test of two rival theories. *American Anthropologist, 75*, 64–86.

Six at City College crushed to death (1991, December 29). *New York Times*, p. 1.

Skogan, W.G. (1979). Crime in contemporary America. In H.D. Graham & T.R. Gurr (Eds.), *Violence in America: Historical and comparative perspectives* (pp. 375–391). Beverly Hills, CA: Sage.

Sloan, L.R. (1979). The function and impact of sports for fans: A review of theory and contemporary research. In J.H. Goldstein (Ed.), *Sports, games, and play* (pp. 219–262). Hillsdale, NJ: Erlbaum.

Smith, G.J. (1973). The sport hero: An endangered species. *Quest, 19*, 59–70.

Smith, G.J. (1976). An examination of the phenomenon of sports hero worship. *Canadian Journal of Applied Sport Sciences, 1*, 259–270.

Smith, G.J., Patterson, B., Williams, T., & Hogg, J. (1981). A profile of the deeply committed male sports fan. *Arena Review, 5*, 26–44.

Smith, H.P., & Rosen, E.W. (1958). Some psychological correlates of worldmindedness and authoritarianism. *Journal of Personality, 26*, 170–183.

Smith, M.D. (1974). Significant others' influence on the assaultive behavior of young hockey players. *International Review of Sport Sociology, 3–4/9*, 45–58.

Smith, M.D. (1978). From professional to youth hockey violence: The role of the mass media. In M.A.B. Gammon (Ed.), *Violence in Canada* (pp. 269–281). Agincourt, Ontario: Methuen.

Smith, M.D. (1979). Social determinants of violence in hockey: A review. *Canadian Journal of Applied Sport Sciences, 4*, 76–82.

Smith, M.D. (1983). *Violence and sport.* Toronto: Butterworths.

Smith, R.J. (1978). *The psychopath in society.* New York: Academic Press.

Smith, Tom. W. (1986). The polls: The most admired man and woman. *Public Opinion Quarterly, 50*, 573–583.

Smith, T.W., Snyder, C.R., & Handelsman, M.M. (1982). On the self-serving function of an academic wooden leg: Test anxiety as a self-handicapping strategy. *Journal of Personality and Social Psychology, 42*, 314–321.

Snyder, C.R., Higgins, R.L., & Stucky, R.J. (1983). *Excuses: Masquerades in search of grace.* New York: Wiley/Interscience.

Snyder, C.R., Lassegard, M.A., & Ford, C.E. (1986). Distancing after group success and failure: Basking in reflected glory and cutting off reflected failure. *Journal of Personality and Social Psychology, 51*, 382–388.

Snyder, E.E. (1991). Sociology of nostalgia: Sport halls of fame and museums in America. *Sociology of Sport Journal, 8*, 228–238.

Snyder, E.E., & Spreitzer, E. (1979). Structural strains in the coaching role and alignment actions. *Review of Sport and Leisure, 4*, 97–109.

Spence, J.T., Pred, R.S., & Helmreich, R.L. (1989). Achievement strivings, scholastic aptitude, and academic performance: A follow-up to "Impatience versus achievement strivings in the Type A pattern." *Journal of Applied Psychology, 74*, 176–178.

Stallings, W.M., & Gillmore, G.M. (1972). Estimating the interjudge reliability of the Ali–Frazier fight. *Journal of Applied Psychology, 56*, 435–436.

Stebbins, R.A. (1987). *Canadian football: The view from the helmet.* London, Canada: Centre for Social and Humanistic Studies, University of Western Ontario.

Stein, A.A. (1976). Conflict and cohesion: A review of the literature. *Journal of Conflict Resolution, 20*, 143–172.

Stogdill, R.M. (1972). Group productivity, drive, and cohesiveness. *Organizational Behavior and Human Performance, 8*, 26–43.

Stogdill, R.M. (1974). *Handbook of leadership.* New York: Free Press.

Storr, A. (1968). *Human aggression.* New York: Anthaneum.

Straub, R.O., Grunberg, N.E., Street, S.W., & Singer, J.E. (1990). Dominance: Another facet of Type A. *Journal of Applied Social Psychology, 20*, 1051–1062.

Straub, W.F. (1982). Sensation seeking among high and low-risk male athletes. *Journal of Sport Psychology, 4*, 246–253.

Strong, E.K. (1951). *Manual for Vocational Interest Blank for men*. Palo Alto, CA: Stanford University Press.

Strube, M.J., & Garcia, J.E. (1981). A meta-analytical investigation of Fiedler's contingency model of leadership effectiveness. *Psychological Bulletin, 90*, 307–321.

Strube, M.J., Miles, M.E., & Finch, W.H. (1981). The social facilitation of a simple task: Field tests of alternative explanations. *Personality and Social Psychology Bulletin, 7*, 701–707.

Suedfeld, P., Corteen, R.S., & McCormick, C. (1986). The role of integrative complexity in military leadership: Robert E. Lee and his opponents. *Journal of Applied Social Psychology, 16*, 498–507.

Suls, J., & Wills, T.A. (Eds.). (1991). *Social comparison: Contemporary theory and research*. Hillsdale, NJ: Erlbaum.

Sumner, J., & Mobley, M. (1981). Are cricket umpires biased? *New Scientist, 91*, 29–31.

Tarnok, M.P. (1984). *Spectator violence: Its influence on the marketing strategies of professional sports enterprises*. Unpublished honors thesis. New York University.

Taylor, I. (1987). Putting the boot into a working-class sport: British soccer after Bradford and Brussels. *Sociology of Sport Journal, 4*, 171–191.

Taylor, J. (1987). Predicting athletic performance with self-confidence and somatic and cognitive anxiety as a function of motor and physiological requirements in six sports. *Journal of Personality, 55*, 1–15.

Taylor, S.L., O'Neal, E.C., Langley, T., Houston Butcher, A. (1991). Anger arousal, deindividuation, and aggression. *Aggressive Behavior, 17*, 193–206.

Taylor, S.P., & Gammon, C.B. (1976). Aggressive behavior of intoxicated subjects: The effect of third-party intervention. *Journal of Studies on Alcohol, 37*, 917–930.

Taylor, S.P., Gammon, C.B., & Capasso, D.R. (1976). Aggression as a function of the interaction of alcohol and threat. *Journal of Personality and Social Psychology, 34*, 938–941.

Taylor, S.P., & Leonard, K.E. (1983). Alcohol and human physical aggression. In R.G. Geen & E.I. Donnerstein (Eds.), *Aggression: Theoretical and empirical reviews* (Vol. 2, pp. 77–101). New York: Academic Press.

Taylor, S.P., & Pisano, R. (1971). Physical aggression as a function of frustration and physical attack. *Journal of Social Psychology, 84*, 261–267.

Taylor, S.P., Vardaris, R.M., Rawtich, A.B., Gammon, C.B., Cranston, J.W., & Lubetkin, A.I. (1976). The effects of alcohol and delta-9–tetrahydrocannabinol on human physical aggression. *Aggressive Behavior, 2*, 153–161.

Tesler, B.S., & Alker, H.A. (1983). Football games: Victory, defeat, and spectators' power preferences. *Journal of Research in Personality, 17*, 72–80.

't Hart, P., & Pijnenburg, B. (1988). *Het Heizel drama: Rampzalig organiseren en kritieke beslissingen*. Brussels, Belgium: H.D. Samsom.

Thibaut, J.W., & Kelley, H.H. (1959). *The social psychology of groups*. New York: Wiley.

Thirer, J. (1978). The effect of observing filmed violence on the aggressive attitudes of female athletes and non-athletes. *Journal of Sport Behavior, 1*, 28–36.

Thomas, M.H., Horton, R.W., Lippincott, E.C., & Drabman, R.S. (1977). Desensitization to portrayals of real-life aggression as a function of exposure to television violence. *Journal of Personality and Social Psychology, 35*, 450–458.

Thomas, R.M. (1986, June 4). 7 of 10 say they are fans. *The New York Times,* p. 43.

Thompson, A.H., Barnsley, R.H., & Stebelsky, G. (1991). "Born to play ball": The relative age effect and major league baseball. *Sociology of Sport Journal, 8,* 146–151.

Tice, D.M., Buder, J., & Baumeister, R.F. (1985). Development of self-consciousness: At what age does audience pressure disrupt performance? *Adolescence, 20,* 301–305.

Tinbergen, N. (1968). On war and peace in animals and man. *Science, 160,* 1411–1418.

Toch, H. (1984). *Violent men.* Cambridge, MA: Schenkman.

Toukomaa, P. (1969). *Value development among Finnish schoolboys.* Tampere, Finland: Research Institute of the University of Tampere.

Trice, H.M., & Beyer, J.M. (1984). Studying organizational cultures through rites and ceremonials. *Academy of Management Review, 9,* 653–669.

Triplett, N. (1898). The dynamogenic factors in pacemaking and competition. *American Journal of Psychology, 9,* 507–533.

Trope, Y. (1980). Self-assessment, self-enhancement, and task preference. *Journal of Personality and Social Psychology, 16,* 116–129.

Trulson, M.E. (1986). Martial arts training: A novel "cure" for juvenile delinquency. *Human Relations, 39,* 1131–1140.

Turnbull, D., & Brown, M. (1977). Attitudes towards homosexuality and male and female reactions to homosexual and heterosexual slides. *Canadian Journal of Behavioural Science, 9,* 68–80.

Turner, C.W., Simons, L.S., Berkowitz, L., & Frodi, A. (1977). The stimulating and inhibiting effects of weapons on aggressive behavior. *Aggressive Behavior, 3,* 355–378.

Turner, E.T. (1970). The effects of viewing college football, basketball and wrestling on the elicited aggressive responses of male spectators. *Medicine and Science in Sports, 2,* 100–105.

Turner, R.H., & Killian, L.M. (1972). *Collective behavior* (2nd ed.). Englewood Cliffs, NJ: Prentice Hall.

Ungar, S., & Sev'er, A. (1989). "Say it ain't so, Ben": Attributions for a fallen hero. *Social Psychology Quarterly, 52,* 207–212.

Vallerand, R.J. (1983). Effect of differential amounts of positive verbal feedback on the intrinsic motivation of male hockey players. *Journal of Sport Psychology, 5,* 100–107.

Vallerand, R.J., & Reid, G. (1984). On the causal effects of perceived competence on intrinsic motivation: A test of cognitive evaluation theory. *Journal of Sport Psychology, 6,* 94–102.

Vamplew, W. (1980). Sports crowd disorder in Britain, 1870–1914: Causes and controls. *Journal of Sport History, 7,* 5–20.

Vamplew, W. (1983). Unsporting behavior: The control of football and horse-racing crowds in England, 1875–1914. In J.H. Goldstein (Ed.), *Sports violence* (pp. 21–31). New York: Springer-Verlag.

Vander Velden, L. (1986). Heroes and bad winners: Cultural differences. In L. Vander Velden & J.H. Humphrey (Eds.), *Psychology and sociology of sport: Current selected research* (Vol. 1, pp. 205–220). New York: AMS Press.

Varca, P. (1980). An analysis of home and away game performance of male college basketball teams. *Journal of Sport Psychology, 2,* 245–257.

Vecchio, R.P. (1990). Theoretical and empirical examination of cognitive resource theory. *Journal of Applied Psychology, 75,* 141–147.

Vokey, J.R., & Russell, G.W. (1992). On penalties in sport as measures of aggression. *Social Behavior and Personality, 20,* 219–226.

Wade, N. (1972). Anabolic steroids: Doctors denounce them, but athletes aren't listening. *Science, 176*, 1399–1403.

Wahba, M.A., & Birdwell, L.G. (1976). Maslow reconsidered: A review of research on the need hierarchy theory. *Organizational Behavior and Human Performance, 15*, 212–240.

Wallace, M.D., & Suedfeld, P. (1988). Leadership performance in crisis: The longevity-complexity link. *International Studies Quarterly, 32*, 439–451.

Walters, R.H. (1966). Implications of laboratory studies of aggression for the control and regulation of violence. *The Annals of the American Academy of Political and Social Science, 364*, 60–72.

Wann, D.L., & Branscombe, N.R. (1990a). Die-hard and fair-weather fans: Effects of identification on BIRGing and CORFing tendencies. *Journal of Sport and Social Issues, 14*, 103–117.

Wann, D.L., & Branscombe, N.R. (1990b). Person perception when aggressive or nonaggressive sports are primed. *Aggressive Behavior, 16*, 27–32.

Watkins, D. (1986). Attributions in the New Zealand sports pages. *Journal of Social Psychology, 126*, 817–819.

Webb, E.J., Campbell, D.T., Schwartz, R.D., Sechrest, L., & Grove, J.B. (1981). *Nonreactive measures in the social sciences* (2nd ed.). Boston, MA: Houghton Mifflin.

Weidner, G., & Matthews, K.A. (1978). Reported physical symptoms elicited by unpredictable events and the Type A coronary-prone behavior pattern. *Journal of Personality and Social Psychology, 36*, 1213–1220.

Weinberg, R.S. (1986). Relationship between self-efficacy and cognitive strategies in enhancing endurance performance. *International Journal of Sports Psychology, 17*, 280–293.

Weinberg, R.S., Gould, D., & Jackson, A. (1979). Expectations and performance: An empirical test of Bandura's self-efficacy theory. *Journal of Sport Psychology, 1*, 320–331.

Weinberg, R.S., & Jackson, A. (1990). Building self-efficacy in tennis players: A coach's perspective. *Journal of Applied Sport Psychology, 2*, 164–174.

Weinberg, R.S., Smith, J., Jackson, A., & Gould, D. (1984). Effect of association, dissociation and positive self-talk strategies on endurance performance. *Canadian Journal of Applied Sport Sciences, 9*, 25–32.

Weiner, B. (1979). A theory of motivation for some classroom experiences. *Journal of Educational Psychology, 71*, 3–25.

Weiner, B., Frieze, I., Kukla, L.R., Rest, S., & Rosenbaum, R.M. (1971). Perceiving the causes of success and failure. In E.E. Jones et al. (Eds.) *Attribution: Perceiving the causes of behavior*. Morristown, NJ: General Learning Press.

Weiss, M.R., & Freidrichs, W.D. (1986). The influence of leader behaviors, coach attributes, and institutional variables on performance and satisfaction of collegiate basketball teams. *Journal of Sport Psychology, 8*, 332–346.

White, G., Katz, J., & Scarborough, K.E. (in press). The impact of professional football games on battering. *Violence and Victims*.

Widmeyer, W.N., Brawley, L.R., & Carron, A.V. (1990). The effects of group size in sport. *Journal of Sport & Exercise Psychology, 12*, 177–190.

Wilkins, J.L., Scharff, W.H., & Schlottmann, R.S. (1974). Personality type, reports of violence, and aggressive behavior. *Journal of Personality and Social Psychology, 30*, 243–247.

Williams, J.M., Dunning, E.G., & Murphy, P.J. (1984). *Hooligans abroad: The behaviour and control of English fans in continental Europe*. London: Routledge & Kegan Paul.

Williams, J.M., & Widmeyer, W.N. (1991). The cohesion-performance outcome relationship in a coacting sport. *Journal of Sport & Exercise Psychology, 13*, 364–371.

Williams, K.D., Harkins, S.G., & Latané, B. (1981). Identifiability as a deterrent to social loafing: Two cheering experiments. *Journal of Personality and Social Psychology, 40*, 303–311.

Williams, K.D., Nida, S.A., Baca, L.D., & Latané, B. (1989). Social loafing and swimming: Effects of identifiability on individual and relay performance of intercollegiate swimmers. *Basic and Applied Social Psychology, 10*, 73–81.

Winkler, J.D., & Taylor, S.E. (1979). Preference, expectations, and attributional bias: Two field studies. *Journal of Applied Social Psychology, 9*, 183–197.

Winter, D.G. (1973). *The power motive.* New York: Free Press.

Winterbottom, M.R. (1958). The relation of need for achievement to learning experiences in independence and mastery. In J.W. Atkinson (Ed.), *Motives in fantasy, action, and society* (pp. 453–478). New York: Van Nostrand.

Wolfenstein, M., & Kliman, G. (Eds.). (1965). *Children and the death of a president.* New York: Doubleday.

Worchel, S., Andreoli, V.A., & Folger, R. (1977) Intergroup cooperation and intergroup attraction: The effect of previous interaction and outcome of combined effort. *Journal of Experimental Social Psychology, 13*, 131–140.

Worchel, S., Hardy, T.W., & Hurley, R. (1976). The effects of commercial interruption of violent and nonviolent films on viewers' subsequent aggression. *Journal of Experimental Social Psychology, 12*, 220–232.

Wright, E.F., Jackson, W., Christie, S.D., McGuire, G.R., & Wright, R.D. (1991). The home-course disadvantage in golf championships: Further evidence for the undermining effect of supportive audiences on performance under pressure. *Journal of Sport Behavior, 14*, 51–60.

Wurtele, S.K. (1986). Self-efficacy and athletic performance: A review. *Journal of Social and Clinical Psychology, 4*, 290–301.

Yarmey, A.D. (1990). *Understanding police and police work.* New York: New York University Press.

Young, K. (1946). *Handbook of social psychology.* London: Kegan Paul, Trench, Trubner & Co.

Young, Kevin. (1986). "The killing field": Themes in mass media responses to the Heysel Stadium riot. *International Review for Sociology of Sport, 21*, 253–265.

Young, Kevin. (1988). Performance, control, and public image of behavior in a deviant subculture: The case of rugby. *Deviant Behavior, 9*, 275–293.

Zaccaro, S.J., Peterson, C., & Walker, S. (1987). Self-serving attributions for individual and group performance. *Social Psychology Quarterly, 50*, 257–263.

Zajonc, R.B. (1965). Social facilitation. *Science, 149*, 269–274.

Zajonc, R.B. (1968). Attitudinal effects of mere exposure. *Journal of Personality and Social Psychology Monographs Supplement, 9*, 1–27.

Zajonc, R.B. (1980). Compresence. In E.B. Paulus (Ed.), *Psychology of group influence* (pp. 35–60). Hillsdale, NJ: Erlbaum.

Zani, B., & Kirchler, E. (1991). When violence overshadows the spirit of sporting competition: Italian football fans and their clubs. *Journal of Community & Applied Social Psychology, 1*, 5–21.

Zeigler, E.F. (1987). Babe Ruth or Lou Gehrig: A United States dilemma. *The Physical Educator, 44*, 325–329.

Zillmann, D. (1979). *Hostility and aggression.* Hillsdale, NJ: Erlbaum.

Zillmann, D., & Bryant, J. (1974). Effects of residual excitation on the emotional response to provocation and delayed aggressive behavior. *Journal of Personality and Social Psychology, 30*, 782–791.

Zillmann, D., Johnson, R.C., & Day, K.D. (1974). Provoked and unprovoked aggressiveness in athletes. *Journal of Research in Personality, 8*, 139–152.

Zimbardo, P.G., & Leippe, M.R. (1991). *The psychology of attitude change and social influence.* New York: McGraw-Hill.

Zimring, F.E. (1985). Violence and firearms policy. In L.A. Curtis (Ed.), *American violence and public policy* (pp. 133–152). New Haven, CT: Yale University Press.

Zuckerman, M. (1979). *Sensation seeking: Beyond the optimal level of arousal.* Hillsdale, NJ: Erlbaum.

Zuckerman, M. (1983). Sensation seeking and sports. *Personality and Individual Differences, 4*, 285–293.

Author Index

Subject Index

Sports Index